12

Cognitive Behavioral Therapy for Chronic Illness and Disability

Renée R. Taylor

Cognitive Behavioral Therapy for Chronic Illness and Disability

With 94 Figures

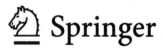 Springer

Renée R. Taylor
Department of Occupational Therapy (MC 811)
University of Illinois
1919 West Taylor Street
Chicago, IL 60612
USA
rtaylor@uic.edu

Library of Congress Control Number: 2005923751

ISBN-10: 0-387-25309-2   e-ISBN 0-387-25310-6
ISBN-13: 978-0387-25309-1

Printed on acid-free paper.

Printed in the United States of America.   (SPI/SBA)

9 8 7 6 5 4 3 2 1

springeronline.com

This book is dedicated to my mother and to the memory of my father. Thank you for your love and support.

Preface

The linkage between chronic illness, impairment, psychological adjustment, and health-related behavior is a topic of significant and wide-ranging concern worldwide. This book was developed to offer empirically based practical guidance to providers of psychotherapy and rehabilitation services for people with chronic illnesses and impairments. It should also be of use to researchers involved in conducting, evaluating, and thinking critically about the efficacy of cognitive-behavioral approaches to the management and treatment of these chronic conditions.

Three important developments have influenced the writing of this book. First, the book reflects my experience as a clinical psychologist evaluating and treating individuals with chronic illness and impairment in practice. Second, it was shaped by my research into the nature and consequences of these conditions and the therapeutic services designed to address them. Finally, the book is the result of personal experience living with, caring for, and witnessing the lives of close family members with chronic illnesses and impairments.

The conditions covered in this book will be grouped in terms of four cross-cutting symptom categories: fatigue, pain, sleep dysfunction, and gastrointestinal difficulties. Because these symptom categories may be shared by individuals with chronic illnesses or impairments, the term "chronic conditions" will be used in this book to incorporate individuals with chronic illnesses or impairments. These four categories were selected because they represent broad symptom groupings that are commonly observed and experienced across a number of the most prevalent chronic conditions facing the international population. Fatigue, pain, sleep dysfunction, and/or gastrointestinal difficulties occur with all of the following conditions or as a result of treatments for these conditions: heart disease, cancer, diabetes, stroke, HIV/AIDS, all forms of arthritis, lower back pain, thyroid disease, multiple sclerosis, lupus, and Crohn's Disease (among countless others). Additionally, these cross-cutting symptoms also represent some of the most commonly observed problems in individuals with physical impairments and difficult-to-treat syndromes such as chronic fatigue syndrome, fibromyalgia and other chronic pain disorders, multiple chemical sensitivities, and irritable bowel syndrome.

In an effort to illustrate applications of therapeutic strategies in the most straightforward way possible, the same four cases, each describing an individual with a condition that involves one of the four cross-cutting symptoms, will be presented and utilized throughout the book. These case examples illustrate how approaches to cognitive behavioral therapy can vary depending upon variations in the symptomatology of chronic conditions. Both long- and short-term approaches to therapy are presented to illustrate the extent to which timing and setting demands can affect treatment goals and methods used.

It should be noted that the term "disability" is used in the title because in contemporary usage it continues to be the term that most professionals would understand as referring to individuals that have some type of enduring limitation of functional capacity. This book does not aim, specifically, to address the numerous social and environmental issues experienced by individuals with chronic illnesses and impairments (e.g., disability oppression and discrimination, stigmatization, limited access, the phenomenology of disability, and disability identity). It is widely acknowledged that these issues, in addition to numerous other key aspects of disability experience, have a significant influence upon an individual's beliefs about his or her own illness or impairment. Although some of these issues are covered in the book and incorporated into recommended therapy procedures, full and adequate treatment of the social and environmental issues that accompany chronic illness and disability is admittedly beyond the scope of this book. For full treatment of these issues, readers are referred to the works of renowned authors such as James Charlton (1998), Michael Oliver (1990), and Simi Linton (1998). In order to be consistent with the argument that disability is created when a person with impairment confronts environmental barriers, the term "impairment" will be used throughout to refer to limitations of functional capacity.

This book draws most heavily upon the contemporary work of Aaron Beck (1996) and Judith Beck's (1995) cognitive therapy. Major theoretical ideas and techniques from cognitive therapy are applied as a framework for understanding and treating individuals with a wide range of chronic illnesses and impairments. Beckian cognitive therapy was chosen as the central framework because Beck's cognitive theory of psychopathology and cognitive therapy strategies have been subjected to a high level of critical thought and empirical examination (Beck 1996; Clark, Beck, and Alford 1999; Dobson and Dozois 2001; Ingram, Miranda, and Segal 1998). Moreover, there is substantial evidence to suggest that cognitive therapy is the most well-researched and successful approach to therapy for a growing number of conditions, including a number of chronic illnesses (Dobson and Dozois 2001; White 2001; Winterowd and Beck, and Gruener 2003). Although the book draws most heavily upon Beckian cognitive therapy, many other approaches and techniques covered in this book have been drawn from the broader domain of cognitive behavioral therapy (e.g., Greenberger and Padesky 1995; Nicassio and Smith 1995; Turk, Michenbaum, and Genest 1983). To reflect the incorporation of these more broadly derived methods, the more comprehensive term "cognitive behavioral therapy" will be used.

The development of this book was also influenced by existing theoretical and empirical knowledge from three additional domains, which will be labeled "areas of related knowledge" for purposes of definition and clarity. I chose to include areas of related knowledge because cognitive therapy has been described as an integrative psychosocial treatment and a flexible and continually evolving approach to psychotherapy (Beck 1991; Beutler, Harwood, and Caldwell 2001). Beck (1991) has explained that the main operant of cognitive therapy, cognitive change, is a variable that has been found to cut across all therapies that have reported effective outcomes. Accordingly, Beckian cognitive therapists are permitted to select interventions from a variety of theoretical orientations, provided that they are appropriately applied in any given case (Beutler et al. 2001).

Specifically, the three areas of related knowledge that will be incorporated in this book include self psychology (Gardner 1991; Kohut 1971), positive psychology (Seligman and Csikszentmihalyi 2000), and the model of human occupation (Kielhofner 2002). I selected these three bodies of knowledge with the specific aim of using theoretical knowledge and strategies offered in these areas to supplement or highlight three specific aspects of the therapeutic process that are controversial, underdeveloped or underemphasized within the current cognitive behavioral therapy literature—and particularly within the literature that covers the application of cognitive behavioral therapy to chronic illness and impairment. Broadly speaking, these include empathy, hope, and volition. These specific areas of related knowledge are included as modest, supplemental resources, with the understanding that Beckian cognitive therapy is the central orientation guiding the theoretical framework and treatment strategies described in this book. These areas of related knowledge are only intended to supplement existing theoretical and empirical knowledge of the application of cognitive behavioral therapy approaches to specific chronic conditions; they are not presented as a means of suggesting a new model or orientation to psychotherapy.

Finally, the ideas presented in this volume should be viewed as early in their development. As such they will require further clinical and empirical evaluation and ongoing dialogue about their application. It is hoped that this book and its organization around cross-cutting symptom areas might lead to the further refinement and focus in outcomes studies of the use of cognitive behavioral therapy for chronic illness and impairment.

Chicago, Illinois, USA   **Renée R. Taylor**

Acknowledgments

A number of people have contributed to the thinking, contents, and development of this book. First I would like to thank the psychotherapy clients and research participants that I have had the privilege of knowing, working with, and learning from. Their unwitting contributions to my knowledge of chronic illness and impairment have formed the basis for this book. I would also like to thank Dr. David Greenberg for introducing me to cognitive behavioral therapy and for educating me about its practice in health care and rehabilitation settings. I would like to thank Dr. Gary Kielhofner for introducing me to the model of human occupation and to its application in mental health settings, and I would like to thank Dr. Betty Contorer for introducing me to the theory and practice of self psychology. In addition, I am very grateful to a small group of clinical supervisors and mentors who, in particular, have influenced my general development as a practitioner: Drs. Catherine Pines, Sheila Ribordy, Richard Volden, Sarah Kallick, Larry Craven, and James O'Keefe. In addition, I would like to extend special thanks Michelle Query and Jennifer Utz for serving as my graduate assistants and helping with numerous organizational and editorial tasks. I would also like to thank Megan Agner for her support in conducting literature searches and entering references for this manuscript. Finally, special thanks go to Sharon Panulla, Executive Editor, Joseph, Zito, Assistant Editor, Michael Koy, Senior Production Editor, Julia S. Brainin, Copyeditor, and the rest of the production staff at Springer for their unwavering consistency, support, and care in editing and producing this manuscript.

Contents

Section One

Theoretical Foundations and General Practice Guidelines

Introduction

This first section of the book reviews the theoretical foundations of cognitive behavioral therapy and specifies general guidelines for practicing cognitive behavioral therapy with individuals with chronic conditions. Chapter 1 introduces four cases that will serve as a basis for application of key concepts presented throughout the book. Chapter 2 provides an overview of cognitive behavioral therapy and highlights its relevance to persons with chronic conditions. Chapter 3 covers issues facing professionals involved in the treatment of individuals with chronic conditions, discusses the linkage between cognition, stress and chronic illness, and provides a rationale for the application of cognitive behavioral therapy to individuals with chronic conditions. Chapters 4 through 9 describe specific cognitive behavioral approaches as they are applied to people with chronic conditions. Chapter 10 discusses the complexities of cognitive behavioral therapy for clients with chronic conditions and the necessity of adjusting traditional approaches to accommodate these unique issues.

1

Introduction: The Four Case Examples

This book addresses the application of cognitive behavioral therapy to persons with chronic illness and/or impairment. Rather than emphasizing diagnostic categories, it focuses on cross-cutting symptom categories of fatigue, pain, sleep dysfunction, and gastrointestinal problems. Individually or in combination, these symptom categories most frequently characterize chronic conditions. While each of these categories of symptoms requires some special considerations, the book will illustrate how the major therapeutic strategies of cognitive behavioral therapy can be applied across them.

In this chapter, four case examples are introduced, each presenting with one of the four major symptom categories. The first case example focuses on fatigue as the primary symptom and describes the experiences of Nina, a 35-year-old woman with chronic fatigue syndrome. The second focuses on pain as the primary symptom and describes the experience of Paulette, a 42-year-old woman with rheumatoid arthritis. The third case example highlights the role of sleep disorder in chronic illness and describes Curtis, a 60-year-old man with advanced prostate cancer. The fourth case example focuses on gastrointestinal difficulties as the primary symptom and describes Alex, a 23 year-old man with Crohn's Disease. These case examples are composite representations of actual cases seen by the author. Significant sociodemographic details, diagnostic information, aspects of the medical history, and background information have been altered so that it is impossible to trace any of the case examples to the individuals that were actually treated.

These case examples reappear throughout the book and serve as bases for illustrating the application of key concepts of cognitive behavioral therapy. They each vary in terms of the degree to which Axis I and II psychiatric overlay is also present to illustrate nuances involving therapy pacing, differing approaches to the integration of related knowledge, and to reveal the real-world complexities that can arise when conducting cognitive behavioral therapy with individuals with chronic illness.

The choice to present some of the case examples as having psychiatric overlay was made in an effort to best reflect variation in the types of clients with chronic conditions that would most likely be referred for psychotherapy. Though the author's belief is that all individuals experiencing the focal symptoms of this book have the potential to benefit from cognitive behavioral therapy approaches to symptom management, individuals with a greater degree of overlapping psycho-pathology are more likely to be seen in clinical psychotherapy practice than those without. Importantly, the choice to present some clients with psychiatric overlay is not intended to stigmatize individuals with chronic conditions or to suggest that most individuals with chronic conditions will also exhibit clinically significant psychopathology.

Nina: A Woman with Severe Fatigue

Nina is a 35-year-old married woman of mixed European-American origin. She has a bachelor's degree and is the mother of a 10-year-old daughter. Before the onset of her illness and subsequent impairment, Nina worked as a salesperson for a small, family-owned packaging company. She specialized in the design and sale of packaging for athletic products. Her job involved being on the road and in and out of her car, calling on as many as five clients within a 70-mile radius of her home on a daily basis. Nina's job also required her to fly out of town to various major cities within the U.S. at least once a month. In addition to her job, Nina also liked to participate in sports; she had always been an avid athlete along with her husband, a physical therapist. Together they had always enjoyed participating in a number of activities together, including skiing, sailing, horseback riding, and snowmobiling.

Diagnosis and Health History

With the exception of a series of severe infectious illnesses during childhood (e.g., chicken pox, mumps, whooping cough, and multiple episodes of influenza) and a concussion she sustained while snowmobiling at the age of 30, Nina considers herself to have been in excellent health for most of her life. Two years ago, Nina became ill with mononucleosis and was hospitalized for four days because of a sustained high fever and inflammation within her throat that was so severe it obstructed her breathing.

After she returned home from the hospital, Nina's fatigue and other infectious symptoms continued. Although there were brief periods of time (e.g., five to seven days) when she felt strong enough to function, these periods would typically be followed by fatigue and symptoms that were almost as severe as her initial episode of mononucleosis. Her recurrent episodes of debilitating fatigue were accompanied by recurrent sore throats, chronically swollen lymph nodes, pain in multiple joints and muscles, severe difficulties with short-term memory and concentration, unrefreshing sleep, and dizziness/fainting episodes that occurred when sitting upright or standing still for longer than a few minutes at a time.

Nina describes her fatigue as an "all-encompassing feeling of mental and physical exhaustion." Of her physical fatigue she notes, "I am exhausted and yet my heart is beating and my body feels like an electric current is running through it."

Nina describes the mental fatigue as "feeling and acting spacey – in a dangerous way that scares my husband sometimes." She also complains of losing her ability to concentrate, becoming unusually forgetful, and occasionally becoming disoriented and confused. She reports that these symptoms concern her most when she is driving and suddenly realizes she does not know where she is. Despite her fatigue, she can't sleep or even rest very well.

In addition to her myriad symptoms, Nina, a strikingly beautiful and athletic woman prior to her illness, lost a significant amount of weight. In addition, she developed a pale and ashen complexion and complained that her hair had become dry and brittle. Her limited energy made it difficult for her to maintain all the personal care activities she had previously done to "look her best." One of her friends commented that she appeared to have aged a decade in less than a year.

When Nina's symptoms had persisted for six months, she began what for the next year was a series of visits to various physicians specializing in infectious diseases, rheumatology, endocrinology, neurology and cardiology. Nina found most of these visits to be highly discouraging and unhelpful. Because blood testing and radiology results revealed no apparent cause for her symptoms, Nina was often referred back to her general practitioner with no diagnosis or treatment recommendations. When she was provided with an explanation for her symptoms, she was diagnosed as having somaticized depression or anxiety and referred to a psychiatrist. Following several consultations, one physician specializing in infectious diseases referred her to a general practitioner who specialized in post-infectious fatigue syndromes.

Six months ago, Nina was diagnosed with chronic fatigue syndrome by this physician. Following the diagnosis, he prescribed a series of different antidepressant medications, antianxiety medications, analgesics, and stimulants. With the exception of the analgesics, all of the medications failed to provide any significant or lasting relief for her symptoms. Moreover, some of them produced side effects that Nina was unable to tolerate. Nina's physician also recommended that she cut back on more stressful work-related activities, begin a graded exercise program, and consider a career change. Nina has consistently rejected those recommendations, maintaining that she has already cut back on her activities enough. Because she felt her physician did not understand her and was not competent enough to treat her, Nina was considering changing physicians. However, given her prior history of negative interactions with health care providers, she was reluctant to seek additional referrals and did not know to whom she should turn.

Recent Psychosocial History

Following a four-month leave of absence from her job due to her illness, Nina returned to work, only to discover that her boss had requested that his son take over all of her sales accounts during her long absence. She was told she would have to start from scratch to develop new accounts. This meant tracking new products and cold-calling potential clients to offer them alternatives to their current packaging choices. Because Nina had always believed that sales was a very visual and image-oriented profession and she believed she once benefited from her attractive physical appearance, she had significant concerns about how she would ever be able to regain the sales volume she once had.

In the face of these concerns and despite the unfair and discriminatory behavior of her company, Nina began to set appointments and to call on new clients in an effort to develop relationships and reestablish a customer base. However, her productivity and capacity to make these calls had declined significantly. Compared to her previous rate of calling on up to five customers per day, Nina now considers herself lucky to be able to call on two customers per week.

In addition to her job-related concerns, Nina also reported that her family relationships had changed. Though her husband remains supportive, he has also stopped his involvement in sports and has gained a significant amount of weight. In Nina's opinion, he always appears exhausted, depressed and emotionally withdrawn.

Nina's 10-year-old daughter now does dishes, helps clean the house, and even helps her mother with basic dressing tasks during times when Nina's husband is not available. In addition, she has decreased her contact with friends and her involvement in after-school sports and extracurricular activities. Although Nina's daughter appears to have coped with the all the changes by assisting her mother and assuming more responsibility within the family, she has become highly anxious and more pressured about her schoolwork. Nina reports feeling very guilty and responsible for the changes in her family that she perceives to have come about as a result of her illness.

Background Information

Nina reported that she grew up in a supportive family but that she often felt pressured to perform well both academically and as an athlete. Nina has one brother, aged 30. Nina's parents remained married until they both died in a major car accident when Nina was 23 years old. In addition to her husband, Nina's aunt and uncle became a major source of social support following her parents' death. With the exception of a brief episode of simple bereavement following her parents' death, Nina denied any prior symptoms of psychiatric problems or emotional distress.

Reason for Referral

For six months, Nina's physician had been recommending that she see a psychologist for psychotherapy. The physician recommended psychotherapy for three reasons:

- Nina had not responded well to any of the prescribed medications or treatments he has recommended. The physician believed that psychological variables may have been interfering with Nina's ability to follow a recommended treatment regime.

- Nina reported increased stress and conflict related to her relationship with her husband and daughter and she was concerned about their well-being.
- As time passed, Nina appeared increasingly demoralized and anxious about her symptoms and about her level of impairment in completing usual daily activities. She was tearful at almost every appointment and would often call her physician between appointments, sobbing on the phone and pleading with him to find some other way to help her. She was no longer able to participate in athletic activities, which had been very important to her. She was feeling overwhelmed by her work and finding it increasingly difficult to maintain an optimistic outlook on life.

Each time the physician suggested that Nina seek counseling, she rejected his referral for psychotherapy, insisting that her symptoms are "in her body and not in her head." Though Nina had repeatedly rejected the physician's recommendations for therapy, ultimately she was willing to see a psychotherapist that specialized in the treatment of individuals with fatigue. The turning point came when her physician indicated that he knew of a therapist that specialized in treating individuals with chronic illnesses that involved fatigue. He informed Nina that this therapist was very collaborative in her approach and that the work would mainly involve identifying strategies for managing her disabling fatigue.

Paulette: A Woman with Severe Pain

Paulette is a 42-year-old woman of unknown ethnicity. She has a master's degree in special education and works part-time as a special education teacher at a local grammar school. She lives with her second husband and her two adolescent sons from a previous marriage.

Diagnosis and Health History

Paulette reported a history of good health prior to her diagnosis of rheumatoid arthritis (RA). Paulette recalls that she was first diagnosed with RA at the age of 24, following the birth of her first child. Routine blood testing revealed an elevated sedimentation rate. This led her obstetrician to run additional blood tests, which revealed a positive anti-CCP, a positive rheumatoid factor, and an elevated level of C-reactive protein. She was diagnosed with rheumatoid arthritis and referred to a rheumatologist.

At that time, Paulette was experiencing periodic pain flare-ups that involved soreness, stiffness, and aching, particularly in the joints of her fingers and wrists. This was accompanied by soft tissue swelling and redness in the fingers of both hands and wrists. However, she was able to maintain the basic functions of her job well enough with the use of various non-steroidal anti-inflammatory drugs (NSAIDs). The rheumatologist prescribed a second medication designed to slow the progression of the disease and prevent joint destruction and deformity (a disease-modifying anti-rheumatic drug, or DMARD). After trying several DMARDs, Paulette decided to stop taking them. She reported that she did not see any immediate results and that they caused her to have a number of uncomfortable side effects, including rashes and severe gastrointestinal symptoms. In addition to discontinuing her DMARD therapy, Paulette did not return to see this rheumatologist because she did not find her to be very supportive or helpful. Instead she chose to obtain prescribed NSAIDs from her obstetrician.

Since her 20s and in the absence of careful management, Paulette's condition has progressed. Paulette now experiences stiffness, limited joint mobility and range of motion, and pain flare-ups that are more frequent, more pervasive, and more severe. Because the flare-ups are so severe, the pain does not respond even to high dosages of the various non-steroidal anti-inflammatory medications that she has been using to treat her symptoms. As a result, Paulette now sees a rheumatologist regularly for corticosteroid injections. She has developed obvious malformation in the joints of her hands and feet, and she is showing some evidence of muscle atrophy. During flare-ups, Paulette also experiences pervasive fatigue, sleep difficulties, and occasional fevers. She has quit her volunteer activities and is beginning to wonder whether she can continue working, even on a part-time basis.

Paulette is now considering trying anti-rheumatic medications again because the rheumatologist informed her that her pain, joint degeneration, and mobility limitations would only get worse if she did not take one of these drugs. However, she has not yet accepted any prescriptions for this class of medications because she is fearful of their side effects. Depending on the specific DMARD, side effects can include rash, diarrhea, liver and bone marrow damage, kidney damage, and visual problems. However, because of concerns about other long-term side effects of repeated corticosteroid injections, her rheumatologist is threatening to discontinue the injections if Paulette does not decide to take the prescribed anti-rheumatic medication.

The rheumatologist has also recommended that Paulette consult a physical therapist and an occupational therapist to work on improving her joint range of motion, to obtain hand splints to wear to improve joint alignment, and to begin a graded aqua-therapy exercise program to increase overall physical functioning, decrease pain, and increase mobility. However, because Paulette's health insurance is very limited and does not cover rehabilitation services, Paulette has not pursued these recommendations.

Recent Psychosocial History

In addition to her job as a special education teacher, Paulette had also enjoyed volunteering once a week at the local nursing home, going to casinos, doing artwork, clothes shopping, attending her youngest son's musical concerts, and watching her eldest son participate on various sports teams. However, in the past two years she has slowly given up many of the activities she once enjoyed. Paulette acknowledged that she has struggled with periods of feeling sad, apathetic, and hopeless for most of her life. Paulette describes herself as a "chronic worrier" and has felt very anxious and agitated at times, particularly during her first marriage. Until now, her mood and symptoms of RA had never interfered to the extent that they affected her ability to work and function in her roles as wife and mother.

When she is not working, Paulette currently spends most of her time in her home and only participates in activities that she feels are obligatory. She reports that her pain and stiffness prevent her from getting out to parties and social gatherings like she used to. She reports feeling depressed, physically unattractive, lonely, and sad.

Background Information

Paulette has an extensive history of interpersonal difficulties and losses, dating back to early childhood. As an infant, Paulette was severely burned on her legs by the boyfriend of her biological mother. Because her biological mother was unable to provide adequate care and protection for her infant, Paulette was placed into protective custody within a foster home. Her biological mother was 15 years old at the time of the incident. After two and a half years, her biological mother stopped visiting Paulette and relinquished all parenting rights. Paulette was placed for adoption at the age of three.

Paulette was adopted into a family of four boys, who were all biological offspring of her adoptive parents. Her father was the principal of a local high school and her mother taught kindergarten. She described her brothers as "more or less okay – they provided me with a lot of advice and stuck up for me at school." She described her adoptive father as loving and supportive of her. In addition, Paulette had a particularly close relationship with her paternal grandmother. She described her adoptive mother as "hot and cold and sometimes verbally abusive toward us, depending on her mood."

Paulette and her ex-husband had a long history of marital conflict, with two isolated episodes of domestic violence during which Paulette's ex-husband struck her on the side of the face with his hand early in their marriage. After a period of separations and reunifications, Paulette was divorced from her husband when she was 30 years old. She raised her two boys mostly on her own until she married her current husband at the age of 38.

Paulette's current husband, a 43-year-old master carpenter, enjoys hunting and playing cards with friends. Paulette loves her current husband and describes him as "much more supportive than [her] first husband." However, she is concerned that her current husband may have a drinking problem. She is also concerned that he may be losing interest in her. On numerous occasions she has witnessed him become inappropriately angry with her or with one of her two sons, particularly when he is drinking. Paulette reported that these problems began soon after they were married but have gotten worse as her illness has progressed.

Paulette has had a number of previous experiences with various forms of counseling and psychotherapy, but she has never received cognitive behavioral therapy. Paulette received crisis counseling within the emergency room both times after her ex-husband hit her. Her first experience with a longer-term counseling relationship was domestic violence counseling that she received at a local shelter during her first marriage. She also received court-mandated divorce mediation sessions with her ex-husband in order to plan for their anticipated divorce. She reported that she found the mediation sessions helpful in "keeping the divorce proceedings civil" but "otherwise useless."

Following her divorce, Paulette developed symptoms of anxiety and depression and sought psychotherapy from a psychodynamically oriented psychotherapist. In describing this episode of treatment, she reported that the "only helpful aspect of that two-year journey into hell was the first session or two." That therapeutic relationship ended poorly and without resolution. Paulette reported that she left feeling like she had wasted her time and money on someone that ultimately "looked down on [her]" and "made [her] think negatively about [her] mother." From that point on, Paulette had been reluctant to seek further psychotherapy.

Reason for Referral: Severe Pain

Paulette referred herself for psychotherapy when faced with the dilemma of her rheumatologist threatening to discontinue her corticosteroid injections. She had read about the benefits of cognitive behavioral therapy for managing pain in a magazine article that was published by a self-help organization for individuals with arthritis. She obtained a referral for a cognitive behavioral therapist in her area from this organization. Her rheumatologist supported her decision to seek cognitive behavioral therapy and provided Paulette with a list of goals to take to therapy. However, Paulette's primary goal was to find relief from her pain.

Curtis: A Man with Secondary Insomnia

Curtis is a 60-year-old married man that identifies as African-American. He has been married for 25 years and has one daughter, aged 20. He has an Associate's Degree in business and has worked in retail for most of his life. He currently works as a furniture salesman.

Diagnosis and Health History

With the exception of mild hypertension and some orthopedic problems resulting from old injuries, Curtis had no prior history of any major physical illness and he had no history of sleep difficulties. Approximately one month ago, Curtis was diagnosed with prostate cancer by a urologist. At first Curtis had thought that the cancer would be entirely curable through surgical removal of the prostate. However, following surgery that originally aimed to remove the prostate, Curtis was informed that his cancer was inoperable and would likely metastasize within the next six months to one year. Following this news, Cutis developed difficulty getting to sleep, multiple awakenings during sleep, and frequent nightmares. He began napping during the day and was caught three times sleeping on the job when business was slow.

Recent Psychosocial History

Curtis had no history of mental illness and had never been seen in psychotherapy. He had been coping well with his diagnosis of prostate cancer until he learned that his cancer was inoperable. At that point he developed insomnia, nightmares, anxiety attacks and reactive symptoms of depression. Curtis responded positively to a prescribed anti-depressant medication, and with ongoing support from his wife, daughter, and extended family, all of his emotional symptoms subsided within approximately three months.

Background Information

Curtis had a successful 25-year marriage to his wife, a strong relationship with their daughter, and an extended kinship network of family and friends that he described as "close." Curtis described his relationship with his wife as "a very loving and close partnership." He had a history of ongoing and relatively stable employment in various kinds of retail sales positions and described himself as a "sociable," "peaceful," and "well-liked" person. Curtis was the eldest of two children. He and his younger sister were raised by both parents in an urban neighborhood. His father worked as a mechanic and his mother worked as a cashier. He described his father as "hardworking, with a good sense of humor" and his mother as "strong," "self-confident," and "a good mother."

Reason for Referral: Secondary Insomnia

Although Curtis's emotional symptoms responded well to the antidepressant, his insomnia only seemed to be getting worse. After three months Curtis was referred to a sleep specialist for a sleep study. Following the sleep study he was diagnosed with secondary insomnia. The formal DSM-IV diagnosis was "dyssomnia not otherwise specified." This diagnosis was given because the sleep specialist had difficulty determining whether the sleep disorder was solely the result of his depression, a direct result of a physiological process involved in his cancer, or a side effect from a cancer medication or treatment. A change in antidepressant medication was recommended, and Curtis was prescribed Nefazodone, a serotonin-2 receptor antagonist with sedating and sleep-inducing properties. Although this helped attenuate some of his difficulties initiating sleep, the effects were mild in comparison to the magnitude of his insomnia. His urologist referred him to a cognitive behavioral therapist to learn more about the management of his sleep disorder and to learn sleep hygiene techniques. At this point Curtis decided to accept this recommendation.

Alex: A Man with Gastrointestinal Dysfunction

Alex is a 23-year-old man of mixed European-American origin. He has a Bachelor's degree in psychology and is currently enrolled as a graduate student in social work program. Alex has never been married and has no children.

Diagnosis and Health History

During late adolescence, Alex periodically experienced episodes of severe gastrointestinal upset that were occasionally accompanied by what felt like a mild fever. These episodes involved symptoms of severe, persistent diarrhea and abdominal pain. At first, he attributed these episodes to having recurrent bouts of a "stomach flu." He did not seek medical attention because they tended to "come and go on their own." Alex explained that his family had always minimized health concerns, and that people did not go to the doctor unless something was "really wrong." Alex described himself as physically strong and very healthy during childhood, and, with the exception of minor colds and episodes of influenza, this had been his only recurrent health problem.

As Alex entered young adulthood, he noticed that these episodes and their symptoms appeared to be getting worse and more frequent with time. At the age of 21, Alex had a similar episode, but this time it involved profuse vomiting, rectal bleeding, severe fatigue and weakness, and stomach pain, which he described as unbearable. Alex went to the emergency room and underwent surgery for a bowel obstruction. At that time, Alex was diagnosed with Crohn's Disease.

In the two years following his diagnosis, Alex had no major relapses. He followed all treatment recommendations, and his adherence to his prescribed medications was excellent. He graduated from college with honors and entered graduate school. However, during his graduate school training, his symptoms reemerged and, at the age of 23, he experienced another relapse.

Recent Psychosocial History

In addition to graduate school, Alex also enjoyed watching movies, working on computers, going out with friends, and dating. Alex had no history of psychiatric problems and had never received counseling or psychotherapy. Until his recent relapse, Alex had been coping very well with having Crohn's disease.

Given that he had worked so hard to maintain healthy GI functioning and given that it occurred approximately two weeks before final exams, Alex had much more difficulty adjusting to this relapse than he did to his initial diagnosis two years prior. He was shocked and angered by the relapse, and had some significant concerns about the potential effects of his worsening health on his academic performance. His physician explained that it is not unusual for second obstructions to occur following a surgery because scar tissue develops and the disease simply relocates itself to the next available part of the bowel.

This explanation only made Alex feel demoralized and less hopeful about his future. Alex had once read that some individuals with Crohn's disease that progresses into the large intestine are forced to have their entire large intestine removed and have to wear a colostomy bag. Alex worried about this possibility and was also concerned that he would not be able to fulfill his dreams, which included graduating from social work school, finding a partner that would accept him, and possibly starting a family. Because his intestine was not yet completely obstructed and his symptoms and pain were not as severe as they had been, Alex had some time to buy before the date of his surgery.

Background Information

Alex is the only child of working-class parents. His father had a high-school education and worked full-time in a meat packing company. His mother also had a high-school education and worked part-time as a waitress. Alex grew up in a small rural community. Alex's uncle, who took over the family farm after the early death of Alex's grandfather, lived in a neighboring town. While Alex was growing up, he and his parents often helped his uncle on the farm, particularly during harvest time. Alex's parents had always valued education, and they encouraged him to attend college. Alex described his father as "strict," his mother as "a worrier," and his uncle as "a workaholic." He also mentioned that "otherwise they're pretty normal."

Alex had a history of average to above-average performance in school, was skilled at fixing computers, and was an avid reader. In addition, Alex enjoyed being with people, was very comfortable in social situations, and had a large network consisting of close friends, friends from graduate school, neighbors, and other acquaintances. He decided that he wanted to become a medical social worker following his diagnosis with Crohn's disease.

Reason for Referral: Gastrointestinal Problems

Alex's graduate school advisor recommended that he seek psychotherapy for two reasons:

- She was aware of Alex's recent health difficulties
- It was becoming clear to her that Alex was struggling to maintain his grades and was becoming increasingly preoccupied about his overall performance within the training program

Although Alex was receptive to his advisor's recommendation, he requested that she refer him to someone skilled in short-term therapy. He reported that he did not wish to enter a long-term therapy relationship at this time because he was concerned that he would not have enough time to address his concerns before finals week and before his surgery. Due to the nature of his request, his advisor referred him to a therapist specializing in cognitive behavioral therapy.

Conclusion

This chapter introduced four individuals who will be featured as case examples throughout this book. Information about each client's health and psychosocial history was presented, and the reason for referral for cognitive behavioral therapy was provided. Additional information about each case (including psychiatric diagnosis, cognitive behavioral therapy assessment findings, and information about the course and outcomes of therapy) will be presented later in the book. Throughout this first section the cases will be used to illustrate various aspects of the cognitive behavioral therapy process. In Section Two the cases will be used to illustrate use of related knowledge. The cases will be concluded with outcomes in Section Three.

2

Overview of Cognitive Behavioral Therapy

When an individual is initially diagnosed with a chronic illness or acquires a new impairment, a number of very realistic concerns and fears may rapidly come to mind. These include worry about physical pain (Will I be able to endure this pain?) overall quality of life (Will I ever be able to eat what I like again? How will this affect my sex life?), and mortality (Am I going to die?). There may be apprehensiveness about the perceptions and opinions of others (What will people think when they see I am wearing a wig?) and desirability to others (Who would want to marry me now?). There may be economic concern (How will I pay for all the medical expenses?) and questions about how the condition will this affect his or her involvement in daily activities, roles, and responsibilities (Will I be able to keep my job? What kind of a parent will I be?). An individual may also wonder how the condition will affect close friends, partners, or family members and worry about who will take care of dependent children or elders.

These are only a few of the many potential concerns that a person with a chronic condition might have. Cognitive behavioral therapy is an approach that can be used by psychotherapists and other medical and rehabilitation professionals to address such concerns. It can facilitate improved quality of life and adaptation for individuals with chronic conditions.

What is Cognitive-Behavioral Therapy?

A variety of approaches to therapy are generally considered to fall within the broader domain of cognitive behavioral therapy (Dobson and Dozios, 2001). These approaches share three assumptions:

- Cognition affects behavior
- Cognition can be monitored and altered
- Behavior change is mediated by cognitive change

Cognitive behavioral therapy always involves cognitive mediation of behavior as the fundamental core of treatment.

According to Dobson, (2001), cognitive behavioral therapies can be grouped under three broad categories:

- Coping skills methods
- Problem-solving methods
- Cognitive restructuring methods

These categories reflect differences in the degree of emphasis on cognitive versus behavioral change (Dobson and Dozios, 2001). A more comprehensive analysis of the nuanced differences between many approaches to cognitive behavioral therapy can be found in Dobson, (2001). This book reflects some degree of integration of all three of these approaches to cognitive behavioral therapy.

It is generally accepted that the different categories of therapy are best suited for different kinds of presenting problems (Dobson and Dozios, 2001). For example, the coping skills therapies are best applied to clients that are reacting to problems or situations occurring outside of themselves. These approaches focus on changing cognitions that serve to exacerbate the consequences of a negative event and on improving cognitive and behavioral approaches to coping with that event. Cognitive restructuring methods are best applied to problems emerging from within the psyche and thus require a more comprehensive and multilevel approach to cognitive change.

The theory and procedures of cognitive therapy (Beck, 1995; Beck, 1996) will be emphasized most centrally in this book. This approach emphasizes the way in which systematic errors in thinking and unrealistic cognitive appraisals of events can lead to negative emotions and maladaptive behaviors. Because this book also draws upon knowledge produced within the broader area of cognitive behavioral therapy, cognitive behavioral therapy will be the term that is used. Though at first glance cognitive behavioral approaches may be classified more narrowly as relying primarily on cognitive restructuring methods, recent applications to individuals with chronic conditions consider the necessity of working with realistic cognitions that occur as clients face adverse life circumstances (Moorey, 1996).

Cognitive behavioral therapy is a structured form of therapy guided by the cognitive model. The cognitive model proposes that dysfunctional thinking and unrealistic cognitive appraisals of certain life events can negatively influence feelings and behavior and that this process is reciprocal, generative of further cognitive impairment, and common to all psychological problems (Beck, 1985, 1991, 1995, 1999). Because this model will be emphasized and elaborated throughout the book, this chapter will limit itself to an overview of only the core concepts.

Core Concepts

As shown in Figure 1, the core of Beck's (1991, 1995, 1999) cognitive model incorporates a hierarchy involving three levels of cognition:

- Core beliefs
- Intermediate beliefs
- Automatic thoughts and images

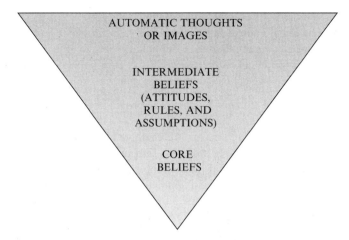

FIGURE 1. A Hierarchy of Three Levels of Cognition

Core beliefs are the most entrenched and inner level of beliefs. The core beliefs of well-adjusted individuals allow them to interpret, appraise, and respond to life events in realistic and adaptive ways. When dysfunctional, core beliefs represent distortions of reality and tend to be global, rigid, and overgeneralized (e.g., "I am a burden to others.") (Beck, 1995).

Intermediate beliefs are defined as often unarticulated attitudes, rules, expectations, or assumptions (conditional statements). The following are examples of intermediate beliefs:

- "Sick people are a burden."
- "No one wants to hear about another person's medical problems."
- "People get sick because they don't take care of themselves."
- "If I fail to follow any of my physician's recommendations, I'll be punished with a relapse."
- "I will be an example of the worst prognosis of this disease."
- "If I ignore my symptoms I won't be such a burden to others."

Importantly, intermediate beliefs influence an individual's view of a situation, and ultimately, his or her thinking, feelings, and behavior.

Automatic thoughts are defined as the most superficial level of cognition. The following are examples of a negative automatic thought:

- "I won't be able to get up today."
- "Those people were offended by my appearance."
- "That pain means I'm getting worse."
- "I can tell they will be relieved when I'm gone."

As the examples show, automatic thoughts are the actual sayings or images that go through one's mind in a given situation.

These three aspects of cognition are organized in terms of a hierarchy such that core beliefs drive intermediate beliefs and both ultimately manifest themselves in terms of automatic thoughts. Core beliefs serve to organize and process incoming information (Beck, 1991, 1996). Both core beliefs and intermediate beliefs arise as a result of people's attempts to interpret and make sense of their life experiences and environment. The way in which they approach this interpretation depends largely on the approaches to thinking they learned earlier in their development (Beck, 1995).

The Goal of Cognitive Behavioral Therapy

The goal of cognitive behavioral therapy is to teach a client to replace distorted thinking and unrealistic cognitive appraisals with more realistic and adaptive appraisals. The initial stages of therapy involve educating clients about the relationships between situational triggers, automatic thoughts, and emotional, behavioral, and physiological reactions according to the cognitive model (Beck, 1995).

The initial stages of therapy also involve creating homework assignments, behavioral experiments and learning experiences that teach clients to identify, monitor, and evaluate the validity of automatic thoughts. This generally leads to a degree of symptom relief. The later stages of therapy involve identifying and modifying the intermediate and core beliefs that underlie the automatic thoughts, cut across situations, and predispose individuals to engage in dysfunctional thinking. The final stages of therapy focus on relapse prevention and on empowering the client to function as his or her own therapist. Judith Beck (1995) has outlined 10 general principles that define the cognitive behavioral approach. These are summarized in Table 1. These principles and the corresponding specific techniques of cognitive behavioral therapy as they apply more uniquely to individuals with chronic conditions will be elaborated in subsequent chapters.

Why Cognitive Behavioral Therapy?

There are three general reasons why cognitive behavioral therapy is particularly useful for individuals with chronic conditions. These are that cognitive behavioral therapy

- Is useful for treating psychological symptoms that can accompany a chronic condition or become exacerbated as a result of stressors associated with the chronic experience of illness or impairment,
- Readily addresses the practical problems and unique challenges that clients with chronic conditions face, and
- Has substantial empirical support for its efficacy.

Each of these reasons is discussed below.

TABLE 1. Beck's general principles of cognitive behavioral therapy.

- Therapists construct an ongoing case conceptualization based on the cognitive model and make revisions to that conceptualization as more information becomes available.
- Therapists make multiple efforts to ensure a strong therapeutic relationship. This includes ongoing solicitation of feedback from the client about the relationship.
- Therapists expect collaboration and active participation on the part of the client.
- The therapeutic relationship is characterized by collaborative empiricism and guided discovery.
- Therapists emphasize structured approaches to goal setting based upon the enumeration of specific problems.
- In the initial stages of therapy, therapists emphasize problems occurring in present time.
- Therapists educate clients about their conditions and about the cognitive model in order to promote self-treatment and prevent relapses.
- Therapists and clients set goals regarding the overall length of treatment so that clients will bear in mind that treatment is generally time-limited.
- Therapists ensure that sessions are structured and that they include a specific agenda.
- Clients learn to identify, evaluate, and respond to dysfunctional cognitions through Socratic questioning.
- Therapists are permitted to utilize techniques from other orientations

Solving Practical Problems and Psychological Symptoms

In addition to treating undiagnosed psychiatric disorders or isolated symptoms of anxiety or depression, cognitive behavioral therapy can serve a number of other important functions for clients with chronic conditions (White 2001). Cognitive behavioral therapy can address a number of practical issues faced by a client and his or her health care professionals. These include, but are not limited to, the ten uses presented in Table 2.

TABLE 2. Ten reasons to use cognitive behavioral therapy for clients with chronic conditions.

- Facilitate compliance with medical treatments
- Provide emotional support and stability to a newly diagnosed client in crisis
- Prevent or reduce behaviors that have negative consequences for a client's health (eating disorders, overactivity or underactivity, smoking, substance abuse)
- Increase clients' access to social, economic, and physical resources
- Empower clients to take responsibility for their own health care and decrease reliance on medical providers and family members for care
- Facilitate a sense of perceived control over symptoms and teach clients to become their own therapist
- Provide clients with health-related education and a framework within which to make decisions about treatment options
- Improve health status and immune functioning through stress management
- Address nonspecific symptoms of chronic conditions that are often difficult to manage and treat with medication or other medical treatments alone
- Reduce a client's overall health expenditures due to anxiety-related somatic symptoms or misinterpretation of minor symptoms as serious problems, overutilization of medication, and excessive doctor-shopping

Addressing Unique Challenges of Psychotherapy with Clients with Chronic Conditions and Impairments

The practice of psychotherapy with individuals with chronic conditions presents unique challenges that are not always encountered in general psychotherapy practice with individuals without chronic conditions (Guthrie, 1996). The inevitable stressors and losses associated with chronic illness are invariably linked to a heightened intensity and wider range of psychological symptoms and emotional reactions to everyday stressors. Clients with chronic illness may also be more likely to present in states of crisis and can present existential issues that involve suicide or other issues associated with death and dying.

In many cases, clinicians are presented with ambiguity regarding issues involving differential diagnosis and the origin of symptoms. For example, anxiety and depressive disorders are sometimes difficult to identify in individuals with chronic conditions given the significant amount of overlap between physical symptoms that may be common to both disorders. Symptoms such as low self-worth, depressed or anxious mood, hopelessness, suicidal ideation, and adhedonia can serve as key discriminators between psychological and physical conditions. Identifying cognitive errors, such as catastrophic thinking about a nonterminal chronic condition that does not warrant this kind of thinking, can also serve as an important discriminator.

Another challenge involves difficulties differentiating between somatic presentations of psychological symptoms and the actual physical disorder itself. Still other challenges may involve alterations in the way clients are referred for therapy, changes to the length of sessions, and new settings in which psychotherapy takes place. There may also need to be adjustments to the pace of psychotherapy based upon client stress levels and reactions to the change process.

One of the most significant of these challenges involves achieving an accurate understanding of the client's physical, emotional, and cognitive experience of chronic illness and the ongoing synergies between them. Cognitive assessments and other more informal approaches to ongoing evaluation, such as Socratic questioning, serve an integral aspect of cognitive behavioral therapy. The heavy reliance on ongoing assessment in cognitive behavioral approaches is ideal for clients with chronic conditions because assessments offer a direct and highly structured means of ongoing monitoring of cognitions, affective experience, physical symptoms, and behaviors. This not only facilitates clients' awareness of the cognitive model, or conceptualization of their problem, but it also leads to self-monitoring and self-management of symptoms.

Empirical Support

Other reasons for using cognitive behavioral therapy to treat individuals with chronic conditions include the fact that it has the most empirical support, and is arguably the psychotherapy of choice, for many chronic illnesses, including HIV/AIDS, cancer, rheumatoid arthritis and other chronic pain disorders, insomnia, gastrointestinal disorders, and chronic fatigue syndrome (White, 2001). A growing number of research studies point to positive outcomes of cognitive behavioral approaches that involve reductions in symptom severity and improvements in self-efficacy, physical functioning, and quality of life (e.g., Antoni et al., 2001; Haddock et al., 2003; Lorig, Manzonson, and Holman, 1993)

Why Include Related Knowledge along with Cognitive Behavioral Therapy?

Although the primary focus of this text is on the use of cognitive behavioral theory and approaches, it will include the use of other "related" knowledge and approaches. An increasing number of studies have shown that cognitive behavioral therapy is in an ideal position to be the therapy of choice to treat individuals with a wide range of chronic conditions. However, like all approaches, cognitive behavioral approaches in general do have limitations (Beck, 1996). These limitations may be more pronounced when considering chronic conditions that often involve complex symptom pictures that include both physical and psychological components.

One of the main strengths of the cognitive behavioral approach is that it allows for the incorporation of techniques from other orientations. Related knowledge and therapeutic strategies offered by other orientations can serve to strengthen, supplement, and add to existing cognitive behavioral techniques in the treatment of individuals with chronic conditions. In this book, three areas of related knowledge will be highlighted as offering certain perspectives and therapeutic strategies not emphasized in traditional approaches to cognitive behavioral therapy. These include the emphasis on empathy offered by self psychology (Kohut, 1971, 1977, 1984), the emphasis on hope offered by the positive psychology movement (Seligman and Csikszentmihalyi, 2000), and the emphasis on volition offered by the model of human occupation (Kielhofner, 2002).

3

The Psychological Complexities of Chronic Illness and Impairment

Chronic Conditions: Prevalence and Scope

Chronic conditions comprise both illness and impairments (Hoffman, Rice, and Sung 1996). They represent the leading cause of medical utilization, functional limitations, and death within the United States. A prominent public health concern since the 1920s, chronic illnesses explain 70 percent of all deaths and affect the quality of life of between 80 and 90 million people (Centers for Disease Control, 2004a; Hoffman, Rice, and Sung 1996; Pham, Simonson, Elnicki, Fried, Goroll, and Bass 2004).

Prevalence of Chronic Conditions

Research suggests that the prevalence of chronic illnesses is only increasing, so that by the year 2050, 167 million people are expected to have at least one chronic condition (Institute for Health and Aging, 1996). Among the most prevalent causes of impairment and death, approximately 3.5 percent of individuals living in the United States have some form of cancer (Surveillance, Epidemiology and End Results, 2001), 4.6 percent have coronary heart disease (American Heart Association, 2004), 6.3 percent have diabetes, 33 percent have some form of arthritis (1 percent with Rheumatoid arthritis) (National Institute of Arthritis and Musculoskeletal and Skin Diseases, 1998), and approximately 1.7 percent have had a stroke (American Heart Association, 2004).

Multiple Chronic Conditions

An additional reality facing health care and clients is the escalating number of individuals with more than one chronic illness. It has been estimated that 39 million individuals within the United States may have more than one chronic illness (Hoffman, Rice, and Sung 1996). Having more than one condition may only serve to increase the extant ambiguity and unpredictability of symptoms and their consequences. Having more than one condition may also cause the conditions to manifest themselves in unanticipated or uncharacteristic ways. The inherent confusion about the nature, severity, and cause of many symptoms of chronic illnesses may represent one variable that mediates feelings of anxiety, demoralization, or difficulties coping for some individuals.

The Challenge of Chronic Conditions

Chronic illnesses and impairments exert a significant and wide-ranging impact on health care systems worldwide (Friedman, et al., 1995). Within the United States, chronic conditions currently explain 75 percent of all health care expenditures (Cohen 1998), and estimates of total costs for people with chronic illnesses have reached as high as $659 billion (Hoffman, Rice, and Sung 1996). Researchers predict that these physical and economic burdens on health care systems will only continue in years to come, particularly as the population ages (Cohen 1998; Friedman et al., 1995). Despite this anticipated crisis, the understanding and management of chronic illness has received relatively little attention in undergraduate and graduate education in a wide range of disciplines (Cohen 1998; Pham et al., 2004). A growing number of studies suggest that today's physicians, in particular, may not be adequately prepared to assist their patients in navigating the complex medical and psychosocial challenges that accompany chronic illness and impairment (Blumenthal, et al., 2001; Grumbach and Bodenheimer 2002; Ogle, Mavis, and Rohrer 1997; Pham et al., 2004).

Moreover, patients' needs may be overlooked in cases where multidisciplinary treatment teams lack sufficient management and coordination. This dilemma is complicated by medical care customs and attitudes that are difficult to access and emphasize and reward the treatment of acute injuries and diseases over chronic conditions and impairments (Davis, et al., 2001; Griffith and Wilson 2001; Kutner 1978; Marple, Pangaro, and Kroenke 1994; Pham et al., 2004; White 2001). Health care systems throughout the world are moving toward more comprehensive systems of care, interdisciplinary treatment approaches, and shorter outpatient consultations and hospital stays. Many health care providers are expected to see large numbers of patients within increasingly short time frames, and many have limited time to address key aspects of chronic illness management, such as overall health promotion and prevention of secondary physical and psychiatric conditions (Sankar and Becker 1985; Steel, Musliner, and Boling 1995). Moreover, in this context health care can tend to focus on the physical and medical aspects of chronic conditions to the relative neglect of psychosocial aspects.

Importance of Psychosocial Issues in Chronic Illness and Impairment

When psychosocial aspects are not adequately addressed, clients may feel unsupported or even abandoned. Inattention to psychosocial aspects may mediate poor coping or other psychological difficulties that can accompany chronic illness.

One thing that has become clear is that psychological and behavioral variables have important roles to play in the cause, course, and prognosis of chronic illness (Taylor and Aspinwall 1990).

Mediators of Psychological Impact

A number of variables have been shown to mediate the psychological impact of a chronic condition (Atkinson, et al., 1991; Bombardier, D'Amico, and Jordan 1990; Erdal and Zautra 1995; Ebright, and Lyon 2002; Felton, Revenson, and Hinrichsen 1984; Holland et al., 1999; Hill, Beutler, and Daldrup 1989; Meijer, et al., 2002; Plach, Heidrich, and Waite 2003; Scharloo et al., 1998; Wider, Ahlstrom, and Ek 2004). These include, but are not limited to:

- Illness phase
- Coping styles
- Premorbid psychiatric status
- Level of available social support
- Religiosity
- Participation in psychotherapy

Health-Related Behaviors and Chronic Conditions

A number of studies suggest that the prevalence of chronic conditions is influenced by engagement in health-damaging risk behaviors coupled with a failure to engage in activities that promote health (Taylor and Aspinwall 1990). For example, the prevalence of coronary heart disease might be reduced by up to 20 percent in men between the ages of 35 and 55 if they reduced their weight by 10 percent (American Heart Association, 1984, Ashley and Kannel 1974; Taylor and Aspinwall 1990). Weight reduction can also lower the prevalence of heart attack, stroke, diabetes, some cancers, and degenerative arthritis (Taylor and Aspinwall 1990). Similarly, the elimination of smoking as a risk factor might reduce cancer deaths by 25 percent and it might prevent up to 350,000 premature deaths from heart attack (American Heart Association, 1988).

Relationship between Beliefs and Health-Related Behaviors

The cognitive psychology literature points to a close association between beliefs and health behaviors (Miller and O'Leary 1993). Research has shown that change in beliefs is central to health behavior change. A number of conceptual models are used to explain the relationship between the practice of health-promoting behavior and beliefs. Among the most widely utilized models are:

- Self-efficacy theory (Bandura 1986)
- The self regulation model (Leventhal, Meyer, and Nerenz 1980; Leventhal and Nerenz 1985)

- The health belief model (Rosenstock, 1974)
- The theory of reasoned action (Ajzen and Fishbein, 1977)
- Protection motivation theory (Rogers, 1984)

Taylor and Aspinwall (1990) have noted that there are a few important commonalities that can be observed across many of these models. Namely, an individual is more likely to stop health-damaging risk behaviors and engage in health-promoting behaviors if

- There is a significant threat to his or her health
- The likelihood of developing a chronic illness is high
- The person has a sense of self-efficacy, or a belief that he or she will be able to control or influence the condition through behavioral change

Response efficacy, or the degree to which an individuals' behavioral response is effective in overcoming a given threat, and behavioral intention, or the degree to which an individual intends to engage in health-promoting behavior, are additional variables that can influence health-related behavior. These findings are important because they can aid clinicians and researchers in identifying attitudinally based requirements for change (Taylor and Aspinwall 1990). For example, a four-year follow-up of individuals with rheumatoid arthritis and osteoarthritis illustrated that illness management training resulted in improved self-efficacy, and that high self-efficacy was associated with positive clinical and economic outcomes (Lorig, et al., 1989; Lorig, Mazonson, and Holman 1993).

It is widely accepted that change in beliefs, in itself, is a necessary, but likely insufficient requirement for the initiation and maintenance of health-related behavior change. Accordingly, cognitive behavioral therapy may offer a more sophisticated means of achieving behavior change because it emphasizes the complexities and significance involved in the relationships between cognitive, affective, motivational, behavioral, and physiological aspects of psychological and physical well being (Beck 1995, 1996). Moreover, it offers a structured, empowering, and time-efficient approach to psychotherapy, and clients can be educated to continue using the skills they acquire during therapy on an independent basis outside of therapy and following termination (Beck 1995). This can result in positive outcomes for clients and decreased medical expenditures.

Psychological Contributors to Chronic Illness Outcomes

Increasingly, health professionals from a variety of disciplines are coming to accept that the etiology, course, prognosis, and treatment outcomes associated with chronic illness are not solely determined by biology (Engel 1977). Despite the fact that some conditions are more easily diagnosed than others, rarely is it the case that there is a single cause, a predictable course, or a single treatment for any chronic condition (Smith and Nicassio 1995). Among other variables, research has shown that psychological stress can exert measurable and distinct effects on a wide range of physical health outcomes (Miller and O'Leary 1993) and on the practice of health-related risk behaviors, such as excessive food, alcohol, or tobacco intake (Friedman et al., 1995; Miller and O'Leary 1993).

Stress and the Course of Chronic Conditions

Humans, including individuals with chronic conditions, can be highly resilient to stress (Lichtenstein 1995). However, research indicates that bodily systems can break down at all levels, including molecular levels, when the mind and body are taxed or pushed beyond the limits of their ability to compensate (Kiecolt-Glaser and Glaser 1999). There is an extensive body of research and clinical literature that highlights the roles of acute and chronic stress in the cause and course of a wide range of chronic conditions (Friedman et al., 1995; Gatchel and Blanchard 1993; Kabat-Zin 1990; Glaser and Kiecolt-Glaser 1994). For example, stress can result in excessive and prolonged sympathetic nervous system activity, and this has been implicated as one potential contributor to the etiology of cardiovascular disease (Contrada and Krantz 1988).

It has been argued that the nervous system functions as one of the important command centers for the body. A number of additional bodily systems may become activated with sympathetic nervous system arousal. These include the autonomic nervous system, the immune system, and the neuroendocrine system (Friedman et al., 1995). For example, release of hormones from the neuroen-docrine system has been linked to states of chronic anxiety, social loss and disruption, and depression (Gitlin and Gerner 1986). Excessive activation of the hypothalamic-pituitary-adrenal axis, in conjunction with opioid activity, has been found to influence immune function and may be implicated in immune suppression.

It is now understood that the immune system is highly responsive to nervous system activity (Ader 2003). Research also indicates that the human body is not well-equipped to respond to states of acute and chronic distress and sustained states of negative affect, such as depression and anxiety (Kiecolt-Glaser, et al., Glaser 2002). Various states of stress and negative affective states have been implicated in the release of excessive amounts of potentially harmful cellular byproducts (Kiecolt-Glaser et al., 2002). This may be associated with a more significant process of chronic inflammation in some chronic illness conditions such as cancer (Kiecolt-Glaser, et al., 2002).

In summary, a substantial body of research illustrates multidirectional linkages between psychological functioning, the central nervous system, the immune system, and the neuroendocrine system in outcomes associated with a number of chronic conditions. These conditions include, but are not limited to, cancer, heart disease, HIV, frailty and functional decline in the elderly, and other infectious illnesses (Ader 1980; Gidron, et al., 2003; Jung and Irwin 1999; Keler, et al., 1994; Kiecolt-Glaser and Glaser 1996; Kiecolt-Glaser and Glaser 1999; Kiecolt-Glaser et al., 2002; Lichtenstein 1995; Prolo, et al., 2002). Other studies suggest that stress and negative affective states such as depression might alter DNA repair mechanisms (Kiecolt-Glaser, et al., 1985; Glaser, et al.,1985).

There is mounting evidence that stress and psychopathology may be implicated in the cause and perpetuation of a wide range of chronic conditions (Prolo et al., 2002). Because a comprehensive review of all existing literature explaining the relationship between stress and physiology is beyond the scope of this book, the next section will focus primarily on cognitive theories of the stress-physiology linkage and on the role of cognition in stress and physical health.

Stress, Cognition, and Chronic Illness

Cognition, or the appraisals, expectations, and beliefs about a given threat, affects all aspects of our experience and coping with stress (Miller and O'Leary 1993). Threats can be appraised in terms of their

- Likelihood of occurrence
- Immediacy
- Duration
- Consequences (degree of loss and value of the lost object)

Leventhal and colleagues (Leventhal, Meyer, and Nerenz 1980) developed a model (Leventhal's Self Regulation Model) that defines common themes or dimensions of how people with chronic conditions construe their illness experience. The most recently revised and widely utilized version of this model (Leventhal and Nerenz 1985) describes five dimensions of illness representation:

- Identity
- Timeline
- Cause
- Consequences
- Control/cure

Similarly, Lazarus and Folkman (1984) have outlined three types of basic appraisals, and these include irrelevant, benign-to-positive, and stressful appraisals. Stressful appraisals, or those in which an individual evaluates a situation as threatening, harmful, or involving loss, have been linked to greater experiences of stress and negative affective states (Frankenhaeuser 1986).

To illustrate the linkage between cognition and stress in chronic illness, let us consider two people recently diagnosed with hypothyroidism. The first person, a middle-aged professional, might find the diagnosis validating following many months of fatigue, pain, weight gain, and other mysterious symptoms. This reaction may be influenced by the individual's ability to understand the disease and its treatment, her ability to afford and access unlimited medical care, and her expectation that the recommended thyroid supplement will work – leading to improvements in symptoms and functioning. The second individual, a young single mother working full-time as a waitress, might find the diagnosis devastating due to her limited access to information about the disease and her expectation that she will not always be able to pay for the cost of her medication. As these examples illustrate, different people may have distinctly different reactions depending on how they appraise the diagnosis and depending on their experiences about the resources they have to manage an illness.

A number of studies support the likelihood that the different appraisals of these two individuals regarding the diagnosis of hypothyroidism will inevitably lead to several variations in outcome (Miller and O'Leary 1993; Murphy et al., 1999; Petrie et al., 1996). These include:

- Differences in acute and chronic stress reactions
- Different levels of self-care behavior
- Differences in overall psychological functioning
- Differences in the experience and severity of the illness

Two categories of psychological disorder have been presented as they relate to chronic conditions (Guthrie 1996). The first involves psychological reaction to physical illness, and the second involves somatic presentation of psychological disorder. Though the reality in clinical practice is such that some individuals vary between these two categories and it is sometimes difficult to determine the difference between them, the emphasis throughout this book will be on strategies to address the former category – the psychological role and consequences of chronic physical illness.

Psychological Consequences of Chronic Illness

Immediately and over time, chronic illness affects all aspects of life, including daily routines, level of independence in physical and cognitive functioning, employment, friendships, intimate relations, parenting, and emotional well-being. Chronic illness often involves fatigue, pain, or discomfort, economic expense, loss, and uncertainty about the future. These experiences can lead to feelings of disorientation or confusion, helplessness, isolation, abandonment, stigma, despair, and anxiety—even in the highest functioning individuals (Johnson and Webster 2002; Moorey and Greer 2002). An individual's personality and premorbid psychological history can play significant roles in adjustment to chronic illness, since the chronic illness itself inevitably functions as an additional source of stress (Taylor and Aspinwall 1990). Those with prior histories of trauma and psychopathology may be more vulnerable to developing an exaggerated emotional response to the illness or to engaging in maladaptive health behaviors (Taylor and Aspinwall 1990; White 2001).

Just as appraisal of stress can play a role in the causes and outcomes associated with chronic illness (Jung and Irwin 1999; Keler, et al., 1994; Kiecolt-Glaser and Glaser 1996; Kiecolt-Glaser and Glaser 1999), the way an individual appraises and copes with a chronic illness can affect his or her experience of stress, as well as a number of other aspects of psychological functioning (Lacroix, et al., 1991). An individual's economic resources and premorbid psychological resources, level of social support, perception of control over symptoms and illness course, illness severity, and even the amount of time that has passed between the time of initial diagnosis and the time of assessment, among numerous other variables, can affect an individual's psychological response to chronic illnesses (Affleck, et al., 1987).

Psychiatric Comorbidity

The exact prevalence of psychiatric comorbidity among individuals with chronic conditions is difficult to estimate due to methodological variation between studies, and subject to controversy depending on the condition being studied. Though many individuals adjust to the experience of chronic illness on their own, in research settings it has been estimated that roughly 15 to 39 percent of individuals with chronic illness also have clinically significant psychiatric overlay, depending on age, gender, sampling methodology, and diagnosis (Guthrie 1996). With respect to specific conditions, it has been estimated that adults with cancer are two to three times more likely than people without cancer to have a comorbid affective disorder, substance-related disorder, or an anxiety disorder (Honda and Goodwin 2004). The prevalence of depression in individuals with diabetes may be three times as high as it is in people without diabetes (Harris 2003). Among people living with HIV, rates of comorbid depression have been estimated to range from 22 to 45 percent (Krishnan, et al., 2002). These rates are similar in individuals with multiple sclerosis, congestive heart failure, and chronic fatigue syndrome (Krishnan et al., 2002; Patten, et al., 2003; Taylor, Friedberg, and Jason 2001).

Clinical Realities

In real-world clinical encounters, it is often the case that the psychological reactions and symptoms of an individual with chronic illness do not fit neatly into discrete diagnostic categories. In some cases, an individual's symptomatology may involve more than one diagnostic category, qualifying him or her for two or more diagnostic categories (e.g., major depressive episode, posttraumatic stress disorder, and borderline personality disorder). In other cases, symptoms may not meet criteria for any specific diagnostic criteria but instead they may be derived from a number of different diagnostic categories (e.g., mixed depression and anxiety, with occasional periods of psychotic anxiety). Experienced clinicians know that a complex, multilevel understanding of an individual offers the most reliable pathway to an accurate conceptualization of any presenting problem. This includes understanding the person's life narrative, cognitive, behavioral, emotional, and physiological experience (Beck, 1995).

Recognizing Client Heterogeneity

Individuals react to chronic conditions with tremendous variability. Recognizing and responding appropriately to psychological heterogeneity within and between clients is vital to a successful psychotherapy outcome. Fear, anxiety, sadness, hopelessness, anger, and rage are inevitable emotions that any client with a chronic condition faces during the course of his or her experience. However, the duration and degree to which these emotions become entrenched and affect overall psychological, interpersonal, occupational and health-related behavior and functioning varies considerably within and between individuals. For example, studies have shown that individuals with the same chronic condition can vary widely in terms of psychological response (Bombardier, D'Amico, and Jordan 1990; Lacroix, Martin, Avendano, and Goldstein 1991). Beck (1996) has acknowledged that there is a significant diversity in terms of the intensity of individuals' reactions to specific life circumstances over time, and there is also variation in terms of individuals' nonpathological psychological reactions to life events.

Individual Differences in Adaptation to Chronic Illness

Studies that have employed Leventhal's Self Regulation model (Leventhal, Meyer and Nerenz, 1980; Leventhal and Nerenz 1985) suggest that an individual's adaptation to illness is, in part, mediated by the appraisals, mental representations, or personal meanings that individuals derive from their illness in order to cope with and make sense of it (Bombardier, D'Amico, and Jordan 1990; Lacroix, Martin, Avendano, and Goldstein 1991; Leventhal, Nerenz, and Steele 1984). As indicated previously in this chapter, individuals can differ in terms of five dimensions that reflect how they think about their illness. They can differ in terms of illness identity, or their understanding of the disease and its symptoms; they can differ in terms of their perception of the illness timeline, or the course the illness takes; they can differ in terms of their perceptions of illness cause; and they can differ in terms of the impact or life consequences of the illness. The fifth dimension by which individuals can differ is in their perceptions of the controllability or curability of the illness. These dimensions have been shown to carry important implications for individuals' ability to cope with their conditions, their decisions to seek health care, their level of adherence to medical recommendations, and their ability to return to work (Hampson et al., 1990; Lacroix et al., 1991; Leventhal, Meyer, and Nerenz 1980). Adding further complexity to this issue, findings from one study suggest that the pattern of differences in illness representations observed between individuals may be disease-specific (Heijmans and deRidder 1998).

Leventhal's model (Leventhal et al., 1980; Leventhal and Nerenz 1985) is just one example of how individuals can differ in their response and adaptation to illness. Fennell has developed a four-phase model that also illustrates variation in psychological adjustment within and between individuals with chronic conditions (Fennell 1993). Studies that have evaluated this model indicate that it can be applied as one means of understanding that individuals can differ in terms of their psychological adjustment to illness (Jason, Fennell, et al., 1999; Jason, Fennell, Taylor, Fricano, and Halpert 2000).

Clinical experience teaches us that individuals in real-world clinical settings are highly unique in their response and adaptation to chronic illness, and it is likely that there are an infinite number of stages that can be described as capturing a given client's response and adaptation to physical illness. The following case example of Curtis, a married, 60 year-old African American furniture salesman with prostate cancer, illustrates two distinctly different psychological reactions to cancer exhibited by the same individual at two time points during the course of his illness.

Case Example
Curtis at Time 1: Two Weeks Post-Diagnosis. Curtis's general practitioner referred him to a urologist based upon a significant elevation in his Prostate Specific Antigen (PSA) blood test of 15 ng/ml and a report of frequent urination. The PSA test is used to measure an enzyme that reflects the number of cells (normal and cancerous) produced by the prostate that are released into the bloodstream. The higher the PSA, the greater the number of cancer cells present in the bloodstream. Following digital rectal examination and needle biopsy of the prostate gland, Curtis was diagnosed with Gleason 5 (average rate of growth) prostate cancer, stage T2c (tumor detectable on both sides of the prostate). The Gleason score, which is determined by a pathologist, indicates the rate at which the tumor is growing. The stage, which is initially determined by digital rectal examination and verified during surgery, describes the location of the cancer. All of these indicators describe disease severity and can be used as rough markers of prognosis.

The urologist explained to Curtis that these results were preliminary, but that they suggested that he had an above-average number of prostate cancer cells (normal PSA at age 60 = 2.5–4.0 ng/ml), his Gleason score of 5 suggested that his cancer was growing at an average rate, and his T2c staging meant that the urologist was able to palpate a lump on both sides of the prostate gland through digital rectal examination. In order to present the most optimistic scenario possible and to help Curtis maintain his motivation to receive treatment, the consulting urologist only made passing mention of the possibility that, in some patients, these cancer severity indicators can change following a more comprehensive evaluation of the prostate gland and its surrounding lymph nodes during surgery.

After a period of initial shock and confusion, Curtis reacted to his diagnosis with determination and resolve to gather as much information about treatment options as possible and to attack his cancer with the most aggressive forms of treatment available. After considering a number of different options, Curtis accepted his urologist's recommendation for a radical prostatectomy (surgical removal of the prostate gland and seminal vesicles, and reattachment of a severed urethra to the bladder). As a matter of hospital protocol and to maximize the likelihood that Curtis would be well prepared for surgery

Case Example

and what might be a difficult recovery, the urologist referred him for a routine psychotherapy consultation prior to surgery.

In terms of psychological functioning, Curtis described himself as an "upbeat" person that was "thankful that God had blessed [him] with a beautiful family and a job." When asked about problems or difficulties, Curtis only reported two, which included a mild level of realistic worry about how ill he might feel in the days following major surgery under general anesthesia, realistic worry about the anticipated outcomes of this type of surgery (his urologist informed him of the likelihood of incontinence and sexual dysfunction), and minor difficulty sleeping (sleep onset delay of approximately one hour for two nights within the past two weeks). When educated about the cognitive model, Curtis was resistant to exploring the possible presence of any other negative automatic thoughts and described himself as a "rational person [that does not] blow fears out of proportion." His assessments revealed an absence of any other symptoms of anxiety or depression, and he appeared optimistic that the surgery would cure his cancer. Curtis continued to work full-time and socialize with family and friends on weekends. Though the psychologist recommended that they schedule a "check in" appointment following the surgery, Curtis commented that he did not feel the need for therapy at this time.

Curtis at Time 2: One Month Post-Diagnosis. Surgery revealed that the consulting urologist and lab technicians had underestimated the extent of Curtis's disease involvement. Full exposure of the prostate and the surrounding pelvic lymph nodes during surgery showed that the largest portion of the cancer was located behind the prostate, and that the cancer had spread beyond the capsule (outside the prostate) and into most of the surrounding pelvic lymph nodes (new stage = T3). Because the cancer had spread beyond the capsule and into the lymph nodes, the consulting urologist estimated that it would only be a matter of time before the cancer would metastasize to other major organs. As a result, he changed his original plan to remove the cancerous prostate. Instead, the urologist took additional needle biopsies from multiple areas of the prostate to get a more accurate estimation of the Gleason score (i.e., rate of cancer growth). In addition, in an effort to slow the extent of metastasis, the urologist removed all of the surrounding lymph nodes in which the cancer was visibly present, and then sutured the patient and sent him to the recovery room.

Approximately 24 hours following surgery and once Curtis was fully oriented and had recovered sufficiently from the effects of the general anesthesia, the consulting urologist visited Curtis during his morning rounds. He informed Curtis that, because the cancer had penetrated the capsule and spread into the surrounding pelvic lymph nodes, it was inoperable and he chose not to remove his prostate gland in order to preserve his ability to control his urination and enjoy normal sexual functioning to the greatest extent possible. He also informed Curtis that hormone therapy and "watchful waiting" (i.e., PSA response to hormone therapy and periodic bone scans to screen for metastasis to the bone) would now be the most appropriate forms of treatment. Initially, Curtis reacted to this information by nodding his head, remaining silent, and appearing intensely sad.

Two days later, Curtis remained less talkative than usual and still appeared intensely sad. However, he denied feeling sad. His pain levels were more intense than would otherwise be expected, but there was no evidence of infection or other abnormalities. His appetite was poor, but he was able to walk and void on his own. His IV was removed and he was discharged from the hospital for continued recovery at home, with monitoring by his wife and daughter. Once home, Curtis continued to experience postoperative pelvic pain, some additional, expected bleeding, and difficulties controlling his urination. Possibly because of the pain, the bleeding, and the news he had received, he experienced a series of severe anxiety attacks during which he expressed a fear that he was dying. This was followed by nights characterized by insomnia, multiple awakenings, and nightmares of being assaulted by a masked man with a knife. Over the next few days Curtis's pain levels and ability to control his urinary functioning improved significantly, but his depressed and anxious mood appeared unchanged.

One week later, Curtis returned to the urologist for a follow-up appointment. Because he had maintained an interest in learning about all the details of his condition and prognosis, the urologist took time to draw pictures of the disease process for Curtis, to explain the process of capsule penetration, and to explain the implications of lymph node involvement (i.e., that there was a significant likelihood that the cancer would spread to major organs, such as the bones, kidneys, bladder, or brain, within the next six months to one year). The urologist also informed Curtis that he had removed all of the lymph nodes in hopes of delaying this process to the greatest extent possible. The urologist recommended that Curtis organize his financial affairs and plan to enjoy his life as much as possible in the coming months.

In terms of psychological functioning, Curtis now had more difficulty trusting his urologist and accepting his cancer diagnosis. He confronted the urologist by pointing out inconsistencies between the initial information he was provided regarding the average rate of his cancer growth (Gleason score = 5) and the location of his cancer inside the capsule (stage T2c) and the new information that was contained in his postoperative medical record (new Gleason score = 8, indicating rapid growing cancer; and new stage T3, indicating spread beyond the capsule). The urologist explained that Gleason scores, as well as cancer stage (location) can change in one-third to one-half of men following a more comprehensive surgical evaluation. Curtis then became angry and confronted the urologist regarding his recommendation to leave the prostate intact, to use hormone therapy to reduce the number of

Case Example Continued

cancer cells, and to maintain what the urologist labeled a "watchful waiting" approach through ongoing examination of PSA levels and periodic bone scans. Curtis accused the urologist of issuing him a premature "death sentence" and insisted that the urologist perform the operation they originally agreed upon in order to "remove all of the cancer that was inside of him." He had difficulty understanding the implications of capsule penetration and lymph node involvement, particularly given that the urologist had informed him that he removed all of the positive nodes. Based on observations of Curtis's affect and behavior, and considering Curtis's wife's report that he had been sleeping poorly and having nightmares and anxiety attacks, the urologist prescribed an antidepressant and referred Curtis back to psychotherapy.

Conclusion

Heterogeneity within and between patients is a key concept to keep in mind when seeing people with chronic conditions in psychotherapy. Heterogeneity becomes an important issue when using cognitive behavioral approaches because many of these approaches emphasize the role of errors or distortions in thinking. Individuals can and do vary in the extent to which they engage in cognitive distortion. Moreover, irrespective of the condition being studied, the literature consistently shows that there are a number of individuals with chronic conditions that never show evidence of a diagnosable psychiatric disorder.

Chronic conditions introduce a second level of complexity because variations in illness severity and course can introduce ambiguity in the extent to which any given cognition is realistic or unrealistic. The way in which a cognitive behavioral therapist evaluates and responds to a given cognition can have a significant impact on client retention and therapy outcomes. Cognitive behavioral approaches are well suited to accommodate changes in an individual's psychological functioning throughout the course of a chronic illness, because ongoing assessment is an inherent aspect of the psychotherapy process.

4

The Initial Assessment and Orientation to Cognitive Behavioral Therapy

Cognitive behavioral therapy is a highly structured and time-cognizant approach to therapy. It is generally performed according to an established set of events that take place in therapy, many of which are unique to this approach to practice. This chapter will cover nine steps that make up the beginning of cognitive behavioral therapy. These steps comprise what is generally known as the process of assessment and orientation to therapy. Ordinarily these nine steps are completed in the first therapy session. Alex, for example, was able to complete the nine steps in a single session. He was alert, focused, motivated, positive about receiving psychological help, and able to engage in the necessary cognitive tasks to complete the process. Because he did not have a complicated psychosocial history, he was able to identify a specific focal problem and corresponding goals for therapy relatively quickly.

However, for a variety of reasons, some persons with chronic conditions may require two or more sessions to complete these steps. One example is Nina. She required several sessions to complete the first nine steps for two main reasons. First, Nina had difficulty concentrating and found it hard to follow along with the more cognitively oriented tasks. Second, she was distrustful of health care providers in general after having a long series of encounters that were disappointing to her and that failed to lead to any improvement in her fatigue. As a consequence, her therapist decided to proceed more slowly. Proceeding more slowly allowed the therapist to build a stronger therapeutic relationship with Nina and it also allowed her to avoid over-functioning in therapy by overtaking Nina's share of responsibilities in the therapy process.

The Initial Sessions of Therapy

In this section, the structure and contents of the initial sessions of cognitive behavioral therapy are described in detail. In addition, common difficulties that therapists may encounter in structuring therapy sessions are introduced and suggestions for managing these difficulties are discussed. There are nine steps that should comprise the initial sessions of cognitive behavioral therapy for individuals with chronic illnesses or disabilities (Beck 1995; Moorey and Greer 2002). These include

1. Relationship building
2. Initial interview and assessment
3. Defining problems
4. Setting therapy goals
5. Determining client appropriateness and readiness
6. Teaching cognitive behavioral therapy
7. Educating the client about the role of cognitive behavioral therapy in the client's condition
8. Assigning homework
9. Summarizing the session and eliciting client feedback

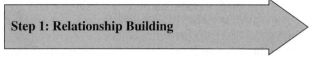

Step 1: Relationship Building

One of the central distinguishing features of the therapeutic relationship in cognitive behavioral therapy is that it asks the therapist to rely upon the client's interpretation of the meaning of his or her thoughts, behaviors, and experiences (Beck 1995). From a cognitive behavioral therapy perspective, this reliance on the client's interpretation

- Allows a client to assume an equal share of the responsibility for addressing his or her problems
- Facilitates open communication and feedback
- Empowers the client to act as the expert on his or her experience

In cognitive behavioral therapy, a strong, honest, and supportive therapeutic alliance with the client is an absolute (though not sufficient) requirement for a positive therapeutic outcome (Beck, Rush, Shaw and Emery 1979).

One of the fundamental processes involved in establishing this alliance is to assure that the client feels that

- His or her presenting problems are understood
- He or she is respected
- The therapist is responsive and genuinely cares about his or her well-being

Although it may seem natural for most therapists to achieve this kind of alliance with their clients, research suggests that this can be a challenging process for even the most capable and caring therapists. Irrespective of actual therapist behavior or intention, clients' perceptions of empathic failures and rifts in the therapeutic relationship are more often the rule than the exception. Chapter 11 includes more information about the theoretical underpinnings of empathy and how empathic understanding can be incorporated into therapy to aid in the resolution of rifts and to facilitate participation. Without establishing an alliance characterized by empathy, clients of cognitive behavioral therapy will not be prepared to adapt to the two additional fundamental ways of interacting within the therapeutic relationship. These two additional aspects of the therapeutic interaction are commonly referred to as collaborative empiricism and guided discovery (Beck 1995).

Collaborative Empiricism

In collaborative empiricism, the therapy process is viewed as an ongoing process of posing hypotheses and testing their validity and utility. The collaborative nature of this process is emphasized because the client is required to assume a fair amount of responsibility in defining problems and testing solutions, both inside and outside of therapy sessions. This approach allows a therapist to convey to clients that their belief systems make sense, while at the same time encouraging clients to treat a given belief as a hypothesis rather than an established fact.

Guided Discovery

Guided discovery is the second fundamental aspect of the therapeutic interaction. Guided discovery involves

- Questioning the client about what he or she believes
- Questioning the meaning of his or her beliefs
- Questioning the existing evidence available to support those beliefs

Questions serve as the central therapeutic tools in cognitive behavioral therapy. Questions are often posed in a Socratic style. Socratic questioning is an approach originally developed by Socrates to teach students of philosophy how to think critically about information. Adapted for use in a psychotherapeutic context, Socratic questioning involves asking clients questions that allow them to identify problematic cognitions and evaluate whether a given negative cognition is realistic or not realistic. The open-ended nature of the questioning allows therapists to ask these kinds of questions without judging or pressuring clients to automatically dispute their negative beliefs or assume they are wrong. The Socratic questioning method allows the client to make discoveries during therapy and to think about problems from many alternative perspectives. Socratic questioning can also be used to help a client synthesize information so that he or she can develop new ways of thinking or reacting to a given situation or crisis. More information about Socratic questioning and its central role in cognitive behavioral therapy is presented in Chapters 5 and 6.

Despite its open-ended and nonjudgmental nature, some clients will have difficulty responding to Socratic questioning in therapy. In these cases, empathic statements that convey understanding of a given belief can be used in alternation with Socratic questioning as a means of eliciting a client's full thinking about a given belief. Providing empathic support through summary statements that reflect understanding allows clients to synthesize all possible information related to a belief. It also allows clients to evaluate the belief in a more objective way without fear of being judged. More information about the use of this approach is presented in Chapter 11.

Step 2: Initial Interview and Assessment

Cognitive behavioral therapy views the entire therapy process as an ongoing assessment process. As therapy progresses, the client and therapist both uncover increasing amounts of information and detail pertinent to the client's cognitions, behaviors, and other emotional and physiological reactions to triggering events. However, it is important for the therapist to conduct a thorough initial interview and assessment at the beginning of the therapy process. Assessment serves a number of functions in cognitive behavioral therapy, but its main functions are to

- Aid in the identification of presenting problems
- Provide information for cognitive behavioral case conceptualizations
- Elicit various levels of maladaptive cognition
- Evaluate therapy progress and outcomes

Initially, assessment should facilitate the identification of presenting problems and goals for therapy. Initial assessment should also aim to provide the therapist with a general overview that includes

- Background information about the client's psychosocial and psychiatric history
- Current level of psychological functioning
- Living situation
- Available resources and social supports
- Access to and quality of health care
- Relationships with health care providers
- Physical health status

This information will aid the therapist in beginning to formulate a cognitive behavioral therapy case conceptualization. It will also assist the therapist in determining the client's level of readiness for cognitive behavioral therapy and the amount of time that will be required to socialize the client into the cognitive behavioral therapy process.

Importantly, for clients with chronic conditions, assessment should also allow the therapist to evaluate whether any accommodations or assistive technologies will be necessary to facilitate the client's full participation in therapy. In general, it is important to keep in mind that a therapist's approach to assessment should reflect the overall principles of a cognitive behavioral therapy approach. That is, it should be as structured and focused on present-day problems and symptoms as possible.

During the initial sessions of cognitive behavioral therapy, a therapist may use any number of approaches to assessment in order to gain an initial understanding of the presenting problems and therapeutic goals. As is true in any type of assessment, the more varied the approaches to gathering this information, the more valid the assessment will be. The approaches that are most commonly utilized by cognitive behavioral therapists during the initial sessions of therapy include clinical interviewing, a problem list, goal forms, and direct client observation.

Clinical Interviewing

Clinical interviewing is the most commonly utilized assessment method in cognitive behavioral therapy. Clinical interviews can be conducted either as an open-ended interview or by using a semistructured interview protocol. An open-ended approach is one in which the therapist derives his or her questions from what the client is reporting according to a spontaneous, minute-by-minute approach. The advantage to this approach is that therapists can ask questions that are most relevant to the client's reported problems and can then build upon those questions with the specific intention of gathering information for a later case conceptualization.

The disadvantage of this approach is that therapists newer to cognitive behavioral therapy may lack confidence and/or knowledge of content to ask clients. Moreover, they may lack experience in retaining the structure of the assessment process and in keeping the client focused and present-oriented in his or her responses. Sample interview questions that may be used in open-ended approaches to clinical interviewing with clients are provided in Table 1.

The way in which a client responds to these kinds of initial interview questions can provide a wealth of knowledge. It can illustrate, for instance, a client's priorities for treatment, his or her appropriateness for cognitive behavioral therapy, beliefs about self and others (including health care professionals), psychological

TABLE 1. Sample interview questions for clients with chronic conditions.

First I would like to get some information about what brought you here today, and I'll be making some notes as we go along.

— (If self-referred) What caused you to come to see me today?
— (If provider-referred) What do you understand to be the reasons that your doctor suggested that you come see me today? How valid do you think your doctor's concerns are?

1. Have you ever seen anyone for these problems before? (When? What worked/what didn't?)
2. If you could choose one problem from the list of things that brought you here today, what would you identify as your biggest problem right now?
3. How often do you think about this problem?
4. How does it affect other aspects of your life?
5. Is there anything specific that triggers you to think about it?
6. When are you most likely to think about it?
7. Would you tell me more about what this problem means to you?
8. When you think about this problem, how do you feel about yourself?
9. Would you tell me what kinds of thoughts or concerns pass though your mind when you are forced to think about this problem?
10. What emotions or feelings do you go through when you think about this problem?
11. Do you feel anything physically, in your body, when you think about this problem?
12. What do you do when you get these feelings?
13. What resources do you think are available to you to help you manage this problem?
14. Are there any people in your life whom you find particularly supportive right now?
15. How do you feel about your doctor's ability to help you manage this problem? What about other members of your health care team?
16. What do you know about how psychotherapy works?
17. Have you ever heard of cognitive behavioral therapy?

functioning, and potential ability to understand and accept the cognitive model of therapy. Questions 8-13 may be particularly helpful in preparing a client for the upcoming thought-analytic work of cognitive behavioral therapy. They will also provide the therapist with some preliminary information about a client's capacity for self-examination and ability to distinguish between beliefs, emotions, and behaviors.

For individuals with chronic illness or disability, gathering information about the history of the condition, its impact upon the client's life and functioning, and its meaning to the client is equally vital to the therapy process. The questions in Table 2 may be used to gather additional necessary information about a client's medical history, current illness and functioning, and beliefs about his or her illness.

A client's responses to the questions in Table 2 can provide the therapist with information that is critical to the cognitive behavioral therapy process. They provide information about

- History and origins of the condition
- A client's beliefs about the condition and its meaning
- Extent to which the condition has produced losses and disrupted the client's life
- Extent of a client's knowledge and interpretation of his or her symptoms and prognosis as compared against the opinions of his or her health care provider

TABLE 2. Supplemental health-related questions for clients with chronic conditions.

1. When did you first start experiencing symptoms of [your condition]? What were your first symptoms?
2. What did you do at that point?
3. When did you eventually get diagnosed with [your condition]? Who made the diagnosis?
4. What was your reaction to the diagnosis? Do you remember what thoughts passed through your mind?
5. What does is mean to you to have [your condition]?
6. In what ways does [your condition] make it difficult or impossible for you to do what you want to do?
7. How has [your condition] affected the way you feel about yourself?
8. How has [your condition] affected the way others perceive or treat you?
9. What consequences have occurred in your life as a result of having [your condition]?
10. What do you know about [your condition]? How did you get this information? What does your doctor say about it?
11. How have you and your health-care team managed your condition thus far? What treatments have worked? What haven't?
12. Have you done anything to manage the condition on your own? How successful have you been? How confident are you that you might develop additional ways to manage the condition?
13. Are there any symptoms that you think you can control just by virtue of what you do in your daily life?
14. Is there anything that you do or experience that you know makes your symptoms worse? (e.g., Overwork? Stress? Habits? Vices?)
15. Are you satisfied with your health care right now? Why or why not?
16. How would you describe your condition over time? Is it getting better? Worse? Waxing and waning? Staying the same?

These questions can also help assess whether the client can perceive any positive consequences that have emerged as a result of the condition, and the extent to which a client has a sense of control over his or her symptoms. Finally, these questions allow for the assessment of a client's feelings of self-efficacy, self-worth, and confidence in the ability to attain certain outcomes.

Semistructured Psychiatric Interviews

Semistructured psychiatric interviews, such as the Structured Clinical Interview for the Diagnostic and Statistical Manual of Mental Disorders – Version IV (SCID – First, Spitzer, Gibbon, and Williams 1995) may also be used. The SCID is particularly useful for individuals with chronic conditions. Its clinical overview section includes questions about the client's physical health and functioning. Moreover, it can be altered to include additional questions about these issues, when necessary. In addition, the SCID allows the clinician to decide whether a reported somatic symptom is attributable to psychiatric versus physical causes and, unlike many other structured psychiatric measures, it does not automatically presume that all somatic symptoms have psychiatric origins.

The advantage of using semistructured interviews like the SCID is that they help the therapist to maintain maximal structure during the assessment process and increase the likelihood that the therapist will be able to gather all the information. In addition, they provide newer therapists with the questions that would be relevant to the treatment process. The disadvantage of such interviews is that they are often lengthy and burdensome, particularly for clients with limitations in energy or concentration. For some clients, the questions contained in the interview may be irrelevant, causing the therapist to have to follow up with additional questions that are more relevant to a given client.

Step 3: Defining Problems

Problem List

In the initial sessions of therapy, a problem list can be generated to document all of the client's presenting problems. These include

- Problems that involve symptoms of his or her chronic condition
- Problems that are a direct result of the condition
- Problems in other areas of the client's life that appear unrelated to the condition

  The purpose of the problem list is to allow the client to

- Organize his or her thinking about the problems
- Identify priorities for treatment
- Begin to draw linkages between the identified problems and his or her beliefs, feelings, and behaviors

The problem list can be introduced at any time during the treatment process. It is most often introduced during the first session of therapy when the therapist asks the client to report on what brought him or her to therapy. Table 3 provides a scripted example of what a therapist might say when introducing the idea of a problem list to a client.

Distinct from psychotherapy clients without chronic conditions, many clients with chronic conditions may list certain physical or cognitive symptoms as their main concern, or they may list psychosocial concerns that appear to be a direct result of the condition. Once a client has identified problems for the list, a therapist should scan the list to see if there are any patterns or themes emerging from the list. For example, the therapist may ask:

- Did the client list only medical symptoms or problems that are a direct result of his or her condition?
- Did the client list problems in areas of his or her life that are completely unrelated to his or her condition?
- Did the client list problems that indicate difficulty coping?
- Did the client list problems indicating a loss of social support?

By scanning the list the therapist can better evaluate the client's desired approach to therapy. Moreover, the therapist can assess the quality and depth of the list as it reflects a client's level of self-awareness and/or willingness to self-disclose. The therapist can also make summary statements and solicit feedback from the client regarding his or her observations of the nature of the problems on the list.

Once the client and therapist have made a concrete list of the client's problems together, it will be easier for the client to identify his or her priorities for treatment. Using the problem list, the therapist can then ask the client to rank each problem on the list in terms of priority. If there are many problems, numeric ratings might be cumbersome, so a therapist may wish to use the following alphabetical system to help the client rate the importance of his or her problems.

A–level = high priority problem
B–level = moderate priority problem
C–level = lower priority problem

If a client reports numerous problems, a therapist may also wish to ask a client to restrict the number of problems he or she designates as "A-level problems" to one or two focal problems. An alternative for clients with cognitive

TABLE 3. Introducing an example approach to the problem list.

"Your reasons for coming in make good sense to me. The problems you have identified so far are very appropriate ones for us to work on and they are ones that many people facing your situation tend to have. Now that you have begun to identify some of the reasons that you came to see me today, I want to be certain that we list them all out so that I do not miss anything. It is also helpful to list out problems so we can return to examine them in more detail when you are finished. I will entitle this sheet of paper, problems, and I'll just start by summarizing what you have told me so far, okay?"

difficulties or for those with limited energy is to write each problem on a separate index card and ask the client to sort the cards into piles reflecting their importance level.

Troubleshooting a Client's Resistance to the Initial Assessment

In some cases (particularly during the first part of the initial session before a client is socialized into the cognitive behavioral therapy process), clients may have a difficult time understanding the relevance of the more structured assessment exercises used in cognitive behavioral therapy. If this is the case, then the therapist should interrupt the assessment process and question the client to gain a better understanding of his or her preferred style of approaching therapy, difficulties, or reasons for resisting a particular approach. The therapist should then work with the client to find a solution, with preservation of the therapeutic alliance being the first priority. One example of a client that had difficulty with the structured nature of the initial assessment is Nina. During the initial interview, Nina had difficulty remaining focused and often did not answer the therapist's questions directly. Instead, she digressed onto a different topic, or responded by asking the therapist why she felt a particular question was relevant to her treatment for fatigue.

Problems with the Problem List

If prioritizing problems appears to be the biggest dilemma, a therapist can ask the client questions that will clarify the extent to which a given problem is worth working on in therapy. According to Beck (1995), this determination can be made based upon the extent to which the problem is perceived as distressing, recurrent, chronic, and amenable to change. A problem is more likely to be amenable to change if a client is likely to be able to exert some degree of actual control over the problem, or, if it would be possible for the client to develop a sense of perceived control over the problem. For example, though it is clear that curing or eliminating an entire illness is not within a client's control, medical decisions regarding how a given condition should be treated are within the client's actual control. In addition, the day-to-day actions that a client can take to manage the symptoms of a given condition are within the client's control, and seeing tangible results of the actions will eventually lead the client to develop a sense of control over his or her symptoms.

Table 4 offers suggested questions that a therapist might ask in order to help determine whether a given problem should become a priority for treatment. Depending on the level of a given client's psychological mindedness and ability to grasp and buy into the cognitive model, these questions can be asked directly to the client or they can be assessed indirectly by the therapist through observation and based on the client's responses to other interview questions.

TABLE 4. Questions for determining whether a problem is a priority for treatment.

Emotional Arousal	• Do you find yourself worrying or becoming anxious about [this problem] a lot?
	• Does [this problem] cause you to feel unusually sad, down, or depressed?
	• Do you find yourself becoming angry or irritable more easily or more often because of [this problem]?
Frequency	• Has [this problem] happened more than once?
	• How frequently do you find yourself faced with [this problem]?
Chronicity	• How likely is [this problem] to go away on its own?
	• For how long have you been experiencing [this problem] – when did it begin?
Amenability to Change	• Do you think changing the way in which you think about [this problem] would help?
	• What do you imagine you might need to do to reduce the intensity of this problem or eliminate it altogether?

Many clients will struggle with the questions about amenability to change, and it is up to the therapist's judgment as to whether he or she should ask a given client these questions so early in the therapy process. Some might argue that if clients could answer these questions about a given problem on their own, they may not need a therapist's help in solving that problem. The alternative argument is that, although clients might be able to see the relevance of the cognitive model and be able to imagine the possibility of having more control over their problem by changing their thinking or behavior, they may require a good degree of therapist guidance and practice in actually addressing that problem

Criteria for Removing Problems from the List

In some cases, there will be reasons to eliminate problems from the list to be addressed in treatment. For instance, some clients will need to be made aware of problems on the list that they are likely to be able to manage or solve on their own. Generating this awareness may require a process of questioning, reassurance, or reminding. There will be other problems reflecting isolated events in time that are largely unrelated to a client's underlying thinking patterns and unlikely to reoccur.

Still other problems may be frequent, chronic, or amenable to change, but not significant enough to cause emotional arousal. Some research in the field of cognitive behavioral therapy that suggests that cognitive change is more likely if it occurs in the presence of affective arousal (Greenberg and Safran, 1987; Moorey and Greer 2002). Similarly, others have found that the ability to express emotion when coping with a chronic illness such as cancer implies active confrontation of thoughts and feelings and is positively correlated with hope (Stanton et al., 2000a; Stanton et al., 2000b). Thus, a certain level of emotional arousal/distress about a problem may be required for successful outcomes. Problems that are not currently emotionally distressing to a client because he or she has suppressed his or her emotional experience may be considered for treatment if the client and therapist determine that these problems are significant enough that they do have the potential for being emotionally distressing. Moorey and Greer (2002) offer a number of suggestions for how to elicit and assist a client in processing diffi-cult emotions if he or she is having difficulty sharing and emoting.

The Dilemma of Competing Problems

Clients that are referred for therapy by another health care professional, friend, or family member can be more likely to experience difficulties identifying their problems or feeling a sense of autonomy or investment in the therapy process. Though referring physicians, partners, or friends may be very clear about a client's problems, the client may not see the relevance of these problems or be able to own them on any significant level.

In situations like these, the therapist may wish to have clients create two prob-lem lists: one that clients make independently and one that clients make based on what they understand are the reasons others advised them to seek treatment. The two lists can then be compared to allow clients to be the final judge of which problems they want to focus on in treatment. This exercise will set a precedent for the client-directed sprit of collaborative empiricism that characterizes the thera-peutic relationship in cognitive behavioral therapy. To illustrate this approach, two problem lists with hypothetical priority ratings are presented in Table 5. One is a list of problems that a client, Paulette, has identified and the other is a list of problems that her referring physician identified.

In Paulette's case, she and her therapist were able to acknowledge that, although her physician felt that her anxiety and treatment-related fears were the greatest concern, her greatest concern was her pain. The fact that her therapist supported her perspective on the problem and agreed to focus on pain increased her invest-ment in the therapy process and eventually led to a greater degree of responsibility-taking on her part. Once Paulette learns to utilize the cognitive model to address her own treatment priorities, she can then begin to generalize her learning to other problems that are less of a priority for her.

Step 4: Setting Therapy Goals

Goal setting should follow naturally from problem identification. A client is most likely to adhere to treatment goals when they accurately reflect the client's main concerns. It is usually recommended that a client and therapist limit their goal set-ting to one or two goals that address the client's highest priority problems. This will increase a sense of control in both the client and the therapist and increase the likelihood that the goals are actually accomplished. In order to set goals, a client or therapist should specify both the problem behavior and the desired behavior in concrete and observable and measurable terms. In cognitive behav-ioral therapy (Beck 1995) goals should be concrete, behaviorally oriented, and easily attainable within a relatively short time frame.

TABLE 5. Two simultaneous problem lists.

Paulette's problems	Paulette's rating	Dr. X's problems	Paulette's rating
Pain	A	Appears anxious	C
Fatigue	B	Fears/rejects prescribed medications	C
Problems with partner	B	Fears/rejects physical activity	C

Types of Goals

Goals can generally be divided into three distinct types:

- Being goals
- Becoming goals
- Doing goals

Being goals are generally process-oriented and focus on issues like the essence of existence, or on a state of being in-the-moment. One example of a being goal for a client would be to "achieve a state of internal peace while in the presence of others." Becoming goals focus on issues of psychological or interpersonal development and reflect goals that are ongoing in nature but are less tangible than doing goals. One example of a becoming goal is "improve my relationships with others." Doing goals are concrete, very likely to be attainable, and outcome-oriented. An example of a doing goal is "increase social contact." This is contrasted with the becoming goal of "improving my relationships with others," which is less tangible, less subject to a client's direct control, and less measurable in terms of outcomes.

To facilitate clarity and communication around goal-setting, these examples may be shared with clients during the process of goal setting. As a general rule and particularly when clients are newer to the cognitive behavioral therapy process, clients and therapists are encouraged to set "doing" goals rather than "being" or "becoming" goals because "doing" goals are tangible, more easily attainable, and measurable in terms of outcomes. Accomplishing "doing" goals will automatically lead to increased feelings of perceived control and a sense of hope. Other examples of doing goals for a client with a chronic condition might include

- Complete my thought record once a day
- Walk outdoors for at least 10 minutes in the AM and PM each day
- Go to bed and wake up at the same times each day

Time Frames of Goals

Goals can be broken down into three categories:

- Immediate goals
- Short-term goals
- Long-term goals

Examples of each of these types of goals are given in Table 6.

As a general rule, immediate or short term goals that can be completed in one or two steps are recommended as a good starting point for clients newer to cognitive behavioral therapy. The steps should be described in concrete, behavioral terms so that outcomes can be easily rated. If a therapist is concerned that a client may lose motivation if he or she is prevented from also setting long-term goals, such as "reduce pain," then the therapist can create two columns within the goal form – one to reflect the long-range goal and one to reflect objectives, or the immediate, concrete steps a client can take toward accomplishing that goal. An example of a goal form is provided in the Appendix.

Readers will observe that the goal form contained in the Appendix also contains a "confidence rating" column based on an approach used by Lorig, Mazonson and Holman (1993). In this column clients can rate the degree to which they feel confident about their ability to attain a given step or goal within a specified time frame. Goals with confidence ratings below a set number (e.g., 8 on a scale of 1 to 10, where 10 is highly confident) can be reexamined and problem-solved during the next session to determine whether the goal should be abandoned, put on hold, adjusted in some way, or if additional resources are needed to facilitate goal attainment. Though cognitive behavioral therapy recommends that therapists work with clients to set easily attainable goals, particularly in the initial stages of therapy, failure to attain even the easiest of goals is sometimes inevitable. It is possible that clients with chronic conditions are at higher risk for failures in goal attainment due to the ever-changing nature of their health and physical and mental capabilities. Prior to setting goals, all clients should be psychologically prepared to drop or alter a goal if an unanticipated circumstance arises or if signs indicate that a change is needed.

Caveats in Goal Setting

A caveat is that goal setting assumes people are hopeful about the possibility of change or improvement. Therapists working with individuals with chronic conditions will discover that clients will vary in the degree to which they are hopeful about change, particularly as it applies to the more significant and

TABLE 6. Time frames of goals.

	Immediate goals	Short-term goals	Long-term goals
Steps	1	2–3	More than 3
Time Frame	Can do in present time	Accomplished within 1 month	Time frame less clear
Outcome	Concrete	Concrete	Abstract
Example	Do hand exercises 3 times per day	Evaluate and test pain-related cognitions by completing thought records and trying behavioral experiments	Reduce pain

chronic problems in their lives. A client's level of hope may vary according to the course of illness or based upon other events and circumstances in the client's life.

There is some debate as to whether goal setting is appropriate for clients in crisis, for those with fewer resources, or for those whose cultural backgrounds may reflect less of a future-orientation in thinking (Kielhofner and Barrett 1998). Table 7 outlines some potential individual differences in approaches to goal setting. The categories in this table should not reflect literal categories into which clients can be neatly placed, but rather a clustering of myriad possible permutations of combinations of characteristics that would reflect a client's ability to engage in goal setting at any given time.

Troubleshooting in Goal Setting

Clients most likely to respond positively to goal setting

- Are somewhat hopeful or optimistic about change
- Have a sufficient degree of self-esteem to believe that they can accomplish a goal
- Have had past experiences of mastery and competency from which they can draw confidence
- Are sufficiently insight oriented to be able to see the link between problems and their own behavior
- Have sufficient material and interpersonal resources available to meet their basic survival needs
- Live in a safe, supportive, or facilitative environment that is free of barriers or obstacles to goal attainment

In circumstances where clients are having difficulties with goal setting the therapist may utilize the questions in Table 8 to increase a client's investment in the process of goal-setting, his or her motivation to pursue and stick with a given goal, and his or her sense of autonomy and control.

Once a goal has been proposed, together the client and therapist can evaluate the quality of the chosen goal and the likelihood of attainment. The selected goal can be evaluated in terms of six dimensions:

TABLE 7. Client characteristics affecting goal orientation.

Goal-irrelevant	Goal-uncertain	Goal-oriented
Not hopeful	Cautiously optimistic	Hopeful/optimistic
Low self-esteem	Some challenges to self-esteem	High self-esteem
Few mastery-competency experiences	Inconsistent mastery-competency experiences	Consistent mastery-competency
Too much/too little insight	Inconsistent insight	Insight-oriented
Lacking resources	Inconsistent resources	Resources
Environmental barriers	Inconsistent environment	Facilitative environment

TABLE 8. Questions to facilitate goal setting.

- What would you say is your greatest worry or difficulty right now?
- What would need to happen in order to overcome that difficulty?
- Is there a role you could play in helping to overcome this difficulty?
- What do need most today?
- What would you like to gain from our work together?
- What are some of your hopes for the future?
- Would you [visualize, write, draw, or describe] your goal for me?

- Relevance to the presenting problems
- Intrinsic versus extrinsic motivation
- Measurability
- Resources required
- Estimated completion time
- Steps required for completion

Table 9 contains suggested questions for a therapist and client to consider when evaluating a selected goal along these dimensions.

Step 5: Determining Client Appropriateness and Readiness

A growing body of health psychology research has demonstrated that many, but not all, individuals with chronic conditions will benefit from cognitive-behavioral approaches to psychotherapy. A client's response to cognitive behavioral intervention may, in part, depend on a number of variables, including such factors as

- The degree to which a client is psychologically distressed by his or her condition
- The time point during the course of the illness or disability that cognitive behavioral therapy is introduced
- A client's readiness for change
- The degree to which a client possesses the psychological resources necessary to participate in therapy

TABLE 9. Questions for evaluating goals for therapy.

Relevance to Presenting Problem	How likely is it that this goal will reduce or eliminate my major concern?
Intrinsic/Extrinsic Motivation	How important is it to me to attain this goal? How important is it to others?
Measurability	How will I know when I have achieved this goal?
Resources	Do I have the resources I need to attain this goal?
Estimated Completion Time	How much time will it take to achieve this goal?
Steps for Completion	What steps will I need to take to achieve this goal?

Moorey and Greer (2002) contend that most studies of cognitive behavioral therapy confirm its effectiveness in improving psychological symptoms (e.g., reducing symptoms of depression or anxiety) of individuals with various forms of cancer. Based on their review of the literature, Moorey and Greer (2002) also argue that cognitive behavioral therapy may render the most positive outcomes for clients who also demonstrate psychological symptoms or distress about their illness.

Some studies suggest that the timing of entry into therapy may be an issue for many individuals with chronic conditions (Edgar et al., 1992; Moynihan et al., 1998). In a study of men with a recent diagnosis of testicular cancer, Moynihan and colleagues (1998) found that many of the men did not wish to receive psychotherapy. Men in the immediate treatment group who did not wish to receive therapy demonstrated little benefit in contrast to the men in the delayed treatment group who waited one year before receiving therapy. Similarly, Edger and associates (1992) found that waiting for a seven-month period following initial diagnosis produced better results than administering therapy within three months of onset.

Based on these findings Moorey and Greer (2002) have raised the possibility that intervening too early in the onset of a chronic condition may be ineffective and could lead to iatrogenic or other negative outcomes. For some, introducing cognitive behavioral therapy too early after initial diagnosis may thwart or complicate people's natural coping processes and may actually interfere with their sense of personal control (Moorey and Greer 2002). It is also possible that the problem-focused nature of traditional approaches to cognitive behavioral therapy may actually cause some individuals to dwell too much on their physical symptoms and bodily functions. For these reasons, the incorporation of complementary strategies from other psychotherapy orientations (discussed in Chapters 11–13) may be appropriate when conducting therapy for individuals with chronic conditions who may not consistently fit the ideal as candidates for cognitive behavioral therapy. Returning to Nina, it was necessary in her therapy to pay careful attention to issues of trust. Therefore, the therapist used empathically based strategies (discussed in Chapter 11) to develop a therapeutic alliance with her. Once this necessary relationship-building work was completed, therapy could continue more along the lines of traditional cognitive behavioral therapy.

There are a number of other variables to consider when assessing a given client's readiness for cognitive behavioral therapy (Safran and Segal 1996; White 2001). For individuals with chronic conditions, a therapist may wish to pay particular attention to evaluating the following client capacities:

- Acceptance of mind-body linkages
- Responsibility-taking
- Interpersonal resources
- Cognitive, educational or intellectual resources:
- Psychological-mindedness

The significance of each is discussed below.

Acceptance of Mind-Body Linkages

Therapists should assess a client's initial willingness to accept that there is a relationship between emotions, beliefs, behavior, and health outcomes. It can be expected that some clients will have difficulty accepting the notion of mind-body linkage and understanding all of the aspects of these linkages proposed by the cognitive model. Figure 1 presents a simple diagram of the two pathways of mind-body linage, or means by which beliefs can affect health outcomes.

The first pathway shows how a client's beliefs can have conscious effects on decision-making about health-related behaviors and medical treatment options. The second pathway shows how a client's beliefs can have unconscious effects on his or her mood, stress levels, and physiological reactions. Clients resistant to the idea of mind-body linkage can be queried about which of the two pathways, if any, resonate most with their own beliefs or experiences.

Responsibility-Taking

A client should exhibit some degree of willingness to take responsibility for his or her psychological reactions to the illness and to participate actively in a therapeutic process that aims to address the psychological management of a given symptom or health-related behavior. Clients that expect a therapist to engage only in interventions involving caretaking, listening, or soothing will have difficulty with cognitive behavioral therapy. Clients that expect the therapist to be available by telephone or in person at an unrealistic level may not be able to take responsibility for the change process and will require additional coaching in this regard. Clients that only want or expect to be cured of their symptoms with medication or other medically based interventions will have more difficulty accepting the cognitive model and participating actively and constructively in the therapy process.

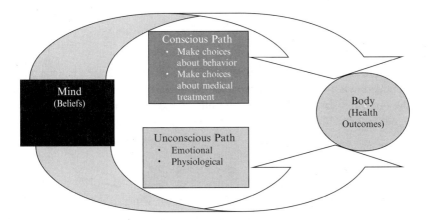

FIGURE 1. Two Pathways of Mind-Body Linkage in Cognitive Behavioral Therapy

Interpersonal Resources

A client should demonstrate a basic capacity to actively participate in an open and trusting relationship. For clients with a long history of interaction with health-care providers, this capacity for relating may be biased by past negative interactions. If so, these biases will need to be assessed and actively addressed. Other interpersonal capacities include the

- Ability to provide the therapist with essential feedback about what is and is not working in therapy
- Ability to adhere to the structure of therapy
- Ability to follow the therapist's lead, in the initial stages of therapy, with respect to cooperating with therapeutic tasks and completing homework assignments.

Cognitive, Educational or Intellectual Resources

A client must possess sufficient cognitive and intellectual resources to

- Understand the cognitive model
- Complete tasks such as thought diaries and homework assignments
- Understand the relevance of the cognitive model to symptoms

For full participation in cognitive behavioral therapy, clients should be able to read (or use Braille/understand audio-translations), write (or communicate in writing with the assistance of a computer), and comprehend abstract relationships to some degree. With guidance, a client should demonstrate some ease in identifying and differentiating between his or her emotions, beliefs, and behaviors. More involved approaches to cognitive behavioral therapy, such as differentiating between core beliefs, intermediate beliefs, and automatic thoughts, will require a greater degree of intellectual ability and may also require some psychological sophistication on the part of the client.

Psychological-Mindedness

To participate in therapy, clients will need some minimal capacity for insight so that they can learn to identify problematic cognitions and understand their consequences. Therapists may gain some preliminary information about a client's level of psychological-mindedness based upon the number of therapists the client has seen in the past and the outcomes of those past therapy contacts.

When a client initially appears inappropriate for a traditional cognitive behavioral therapy approach, a therapist may want to review some of these criteria with the client. This can serve to more concretely determine whether a client is willing to work toward readiness for therapy. In addition, a therapist may wish to offer the client a trial period of two or three sessions during which the therapist can work to better prepare the client for participation in cognitive behavioral therapy and continue to assess his or her progress (White 2001). In these cases, a therapist may have to dedicate extra effort to establishing an empathic understanding of the presenting problem (as discussed in Chapter 11), to educating the client about the empirical support for and relevance of the cognitive model, and to socializing the client to the cognitive behavioral therapy treatment process.

Step 6: Teaching Cognitive Behavioral Therapy

One of the most fundamental aspects of cognitive behavioral therapy involves socializing the client to the unique philosophy, structure, and practices of this approach to therapy. A study of individuals with depression underscores this point. Fennell and Teasdale (1987) found that acceptance of the cognitive model predicted cognitive behavioral therapy outcomes. Clients that responded more rapidly to therapy were more likely to report positive reactions to the explanation of the cognitive model of depression in the first session and were also more likely to have a positive response to the first homework assignment.

Once clients understand the rationale behind this approach, they will be more likely to actively participate and follow the therapy process in subsequent sessions. They will also be better prepared to apply what they have learned to other problems once therapy has ended (Beck 1995). All clients should be taught the basic principles and practices of cognitive behavioral therapy as early as possible. Nonetheless, the timing will vary depending on the characteristics and readiness of each client.

The first step in the process of socializing a client into cognitive behavioral therapy involves assessing a client's existing knowledge about the therapy process (Beck 1995). A client should be asked what he or she already knows about cognitive behavioral therapy, and his or her response should be corrected or supplemented with a brief description of the therapy process and of the cognitive model.

All clients should be taught that cognitive behavioral therapy is characterized by five required practices:

- A collaborative relationship
- Setting and following a weekly structure and agenda
- Answering questions and providing feedback
- Completing weekly homework assignments
- Learning to become one's own therapist

Clients may be informed that these required practices should be followed as closely as possible, unless there is some complicating variable or crisis that demands a slower and less structured approach. In these cases, the change or necessary accommodation that deviates from the regular practices of cognitive behavioral therapy should be made explicit to the client and the original structure should be returned to as soon as the client is ready (White 2001).

The Cognitive Model

The cognitive model explains how beliefs play a determining role in an individual's emotional, behavioral, and physiological reactions to a given health event trigger. As discussed in Chapter 2, beliefs are conceptualized at three levels (see Figure 2).

Automatic thoughts or images, represented at the top of the triangle, are the most shallow and least developed level of beliefs. They are situation-specific and easier to identify than the other types of beliefs. Because they are more readily available to consciousness and more immediately identifiable, the automatic thoughts are generally viewed as the surface-level mediators of an individual's reactions to stressful health events.

Intermediate beliefs act as an underlying influence on a person's automatic thoughts. Intermediate beliefs are composed of implicit rules for living or assumptions about the way the world functions. They generally occur across –different situations and can present themselves as either conditional or unconditional. Conditional intermediate beliefs usually reflect "if-then reasoning" (e.g., "If I do everything my partner asks, then she will be able to accept my illness"). Unconditional intermediate beliefs usually reflect "should" or "must do" thinking (e.g., "Every partner should be able to accept a chronic illness").

Core beliefs are the second underlying influence on automatic thoughts. Core beliefs reflect the content of schemas, which are deep cognitive structures within the mind (Beck 1964). Generally these beliefs are global, rigid, and absolutistic. They exist in all individuals regardless of the presence of psychopathology. According to the cognitive model (Beck 1995), core beliefs that influence a person in negative ways may emerge very early in development in relation to

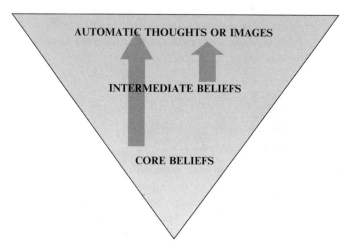

FIGURE 2. Three Levels of Beliefs in the Cognitive Model

a significant trauma or chronic issue. Problematic core beliefs of individuals with chronic conditions can be conceptualized in terms of four categories:

- Core beliefs about the self (e.g., "I am a burden to society")
- Core beliefs about others (e.g., "Others are uncomfortable around me")
- Core beliefs about the condition (e.g., "Crohn's Disease is always fatal")
- Core beliefs about health care or health-care professionals (e.g., "Doctors are only interested in making money")

Role of Automatic Thoughts Meditating Reactions to Triggering Events

An individual's automatic thoughts about a given event will determine his or her emotional, behavioral, and physiological reactions to that event, as depicted in Figure 3.

Health event triggers are the potentially stressful events related to an individual's chronic condition. According to the cognitive model, these health events can trigger negative automatic thoughts, which are a product of underlying dysfunctional belief systems (i.e., intermediate and core beliefs) (White 2001). In turn, these thoughts or belief systems lead to aversive emotional, behavioral, or physiological reactions. The following are some examples of health event triggers:

- A physician orders additional testing due to suspicion of a chronic condition
- A client receives confirmation of the diagnosis
- A client learns that his or her condition does have fatality rates associated with it
- A client is told for certain that his or her condition is terminal
- A client is faced with the necessity to tell others about his or her condition
- A client is forced to bear witness to the negative reactions of others that learn about his or her diagnosis (e.g., worry, anger, or sadness)

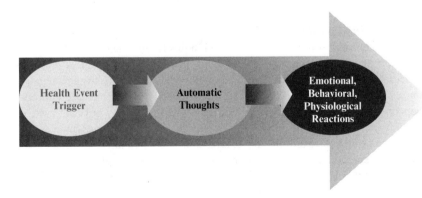

FIGURE 3. Pathway of Triggers Affecting Automatic Thoughts and Emotional, Behavioral and Physiological Reactions

- A client learns that he or she must undergo a painful and time-consuming diagnostic test or medical procedure
- A client experiences a flare-up or an acute exacerbation of symptoms
- A client is hospitalized
- A client is forced to alter his or her work commitments or must resign from work completely
- A client is faced with the realization that he or she is no longer able to complete all of his or her basic responsibilities as a parent
- A client learns that he or she can no longer engage in a cherished activity or hobby
- A client learns that he or she has developed a secondary or additional health problem
- A client is mistreated, made unnecessarily anxious, or treated in an insensitive manner by a health-care professional
- A client is forced to change to a new health-care provider

Thus, the cognitive model specifies that triggering events, such as those listed above, ignite a client's underlying belief system, and depending upon the nature of a client's beliefs, a client can experience a negative or positive reaction. Rarely is a reaction neutral.

A client may experience the reaction

- At an emotional level (e.g., anxious preoccupation, grief, or rage)
- At a behavioral level (e.g., avoidance of others, changes in sleep patterns, or changes in activity levels)
- At a physiological level (e.g., heart racing or pounding, shortness of breath, fatigue, exhaustion)

The strongest reactions will involve the client's experience at all three levels.

A Cognitive Model for Individuals with Chronic Conditions

Figure 4 presents a complete illustration of the cognitive model for use with individuals with chronic conditions. As depicted in this figure, the effects of stressful medical events on a person's emotional, behavioral, and physiological reactions are mediated by a person's automatic thoughts. Health events trigger negative automatic thoughts, which are influenced by underlying intermediate and core beliefs of the four types discussed above. In turn, these thoughts or belief systems lead to aversive emotional, behavioral, or physiological reactions. Immediately and over time, these reactions can exert acute and cumulative effects on the immune system, and arguably upon an individual's overall health status (as discussed in Chapter 3).

The therapist is advised to move very slowly when teaching the cognitive model, explaining each aspect of the cognitive model in chunks and prompting the client to repeat his or her understanding of the model in his or her own words

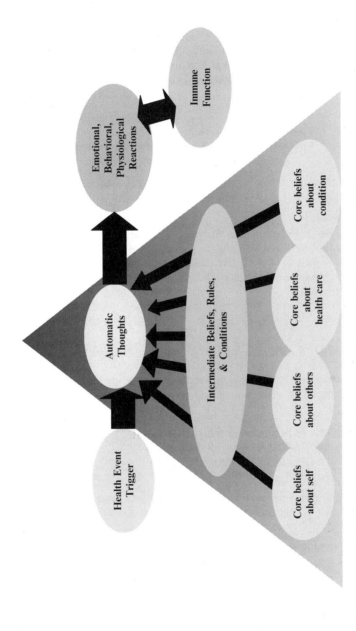

FIGURE 4. The Cognitive Model for Individuals with Chronic Conditions (adapted from Beck 1995)

until full understanding is reached (Beck 1995). As a starting point, the client can be encouraged to provide an example of a health event trigger that has led him or her to feel a significant degree of emotional distress. The client is then asked to describe his or her emotional reaction to the event and also any change in behavior or physical sensations that may have accompanied that reaction. Finally, the client is asked to recall any thoughts that may have run through his or her mind after the health event trigger, and the therapist elicits as much detail as possible about the various levels of belief in the cognitive model. Clients are again reminded of the power of thinking and beliefs in determining their reactions to given life events.

Making it simple

According to the cognitive model, only one symptom category can be addressed at any given time. For example, if a client wishes to learn how to cope with and manage his or her fatigue levels, fatigue must be the symptom category of focus and the client should not attempt to work on the management of gastrointestinal symptoms simultaneously. The rationale for this is to keep the approach to therapy as straightforward and understandable to the client as possible. In the later stages of therapy, once clients have learned how to use the cognitive model, they can begin to be taught to generalize what they have learned and apply it to other physical symptom categories or to psychiatric symptoms.

Making it concrete

When teaching the model, a therapist should typically draw or show detailed pictures of the various aspects of the cognitive model with examples from the client's own life experience and cognition. Figures 1–3 provided in this chapter can serve as models for these illustrations made by the therapist, or they may be shown directly to the client. Once the client understands these basic aspects of the model, he or she can be presented with a full diagram of all aspects of the cognitive model shown together (i.e., Figure 4). The reason for the diagram is to teach the clients the powerful role of beliefs within the entire network that links life events, an individual's deeper levels of beliefs, and his or her emotional, behavioral, physiological (and immunological) reactions.

Making it specific

Once the client has a basic grasp of the cognitive model, the client and therapist can then begin to apply the model to the client's circumstance. One way to do this is to work together to fill in the spaces within the cognitive model that apply to the client's specific life circumstances and cognitive approach. A case conceptualization worksheet is contained in the Appendix to this chapter for this purpose. When doing this the therapist should guide the client to focus on only one symptom. At this point clients should be discouraged from trying to dispute or fix their beliefs, even if they are quickly able to recognize that they are dysfunctional.

Adapting to fit the client

The degree of information and detail in the cognitive model can be down-graded for clients that are initially resistant or vulnerable to excessive self-blame, and for those with severe mental fatigue, attention or concentration difficulties, or other cognitive difficulties. For example, Alex was able to take in a great deal of information on the model in his first session. Moreover, he was interested in doing some reading on his own based on his therapist's rec-ommendations. Curtis, on the other hand, wanted a straightforward expla-nation and was satisfied with a basic presentation by his therapist. Nina questioned the cognitive behavioral model constantly, raising new questions that required her therapists to revisit the model explaining different aspects of it on different occasions.

Expectations and Time Frames

The final step in socializing a client into cognitive behavioral therapy involves eliciting and correcting, if necessary, the client's expectations for therapy (Beck 1995). Clients with chronic conditions may be particularly vulnerable to holding unrealistically low or unrealistically high expectations of the therapist and the therapy. Other clients may hold a view that psychotherapy is an abstract, spiritual, or highly complex and incomprehensible process by which positive outcomes are produced. After a therapist fully educates a client on the process of therapy and on the cognitive model, one means by which he or she can evaluate a client's understanding and responsibility-taking is by asking the client how he or she expects to improve. If at this point a client does not understand that therapy will involve a process of education about how to manage his or her own symptoms and active participation in the change process, the therapist should clarify these issues and reassess the client's understanding. During the first session the therapist should also try to provide the client with a general time frame for therapy (e.g., between 1-1/2 and 4 months) (Beck 1995). In part, this time frame will be based on the complexity of the client's difficulties as well as his or her time and access to economic resources.

Step 7: Educating the Client about the Role of Cognitive Behavioral Therapy in the Client's Condition

Clients are generally reassured and more likely to follow through with therapy if a therapist also takes the time to educate them about their presenting problem and about the efficacy of the cognitive and behavioral techniques that are typi-cally used to treat their presenting problem. For example, a therapist might educate a client with fatigue about the research indicating that cognitive behav-ioral interventions emphasizing graded exercise training have been found to be associated with reductions in fatigue severity levels.

Clients may also be provided with copies of research studies or consumer brochures that point to the efficacy of a particular cognitive or behavioral approach in treating a given symptom. Any concerted effort that a therapist can make to educate clients about the empirical evidence for the efficacy of a treatment approach for a given condition will increase the likelihood of a client's ownership of his or her symptom and active participation in the corresponding treatment approach.

Step 8: Assigning Homework

According to White (2001), cognitive behavioral therapy is a process that must be *lived* in order to be effective. The only structured means by which cognitive and behavioral strategies can be practiced intensively is by extending this practice outside of the session through weekly homework assignments (Beck 1995). Beck et al. (1979) maintain that homework in cognitive behavioral therapy is not optional. Research has found that clients who complete their homework assignments regularly demonstrate more improvement on symptoms than clients that do not adhere to their homework on a regular basis (Niemeyer and Feixas 1990; Persons et al., 1988).

During the initial session, clients should be fully educated about the necessity of homework completion as part of their involvement in therapy. A therapist should clearly explain Beck's (1995) rationale for completing homework regularly, potential obstacles to completing homework should be explored up-front, and any doubts about the capacity to do homework or about its efficacy should be addressed in the initial session (Beck 1995). Initially, therapists develop and set homework assignments for clients but they quickly move toward a model in which clients are asked to assume an increasing role in setting their own assignments (Beck 1995).

Clients will vary greatly in their preferences for some therapy tasks over others. Because of this inevitable individual variation, therapists should become accustomed to using and assigning a wide range of homework assignments, and homework should be individually customized and relevant to a client's main symptom or problem. This is often challenging for therapists, as the more likely inclination is that therapists will tend to utilize the same homework assignments repeatedly because they are familiar with them or because they have worked in the past. In addition to these issues, it is important to remember that homework should reflect the steps that the therapist has outlined as being required to meet the client's therapy outcome goal. Chapter 5 provides a number of examples of homework assignments that are commonly utilized with clients with chronic conditions.

Troubleshooting Problems with Homework

Though follow-through on homework assignments can be a problem for any client, clients with chronic conditions may be particularly vulnerable to problems in this area because of real limitations in attention, concentration, time, and energy. It is important to provide clients with a sense of control over homework assignments. Once a client becomes familiar with an array of typical homework assignments, control can be enhanced by having the client begin to select the assignment and participate in modifying the assignment, when necessary. Soliciting a client's feedback about the assignment, which is typically initiated in the first session, is another means of increasing his or her sense of control.

In addition to being cognizant of common reasons for lack of follow-through with homework, therapists treating individuals with chronic conditions must also be aware of the need to make reasonable accommodations to homework assignments based on a client's performance capacity. For example, there will likely be times when a homework assignment will need to be completed during a therapy session because a client was simply too ill to do anything the prior week. On other occasions, a homework assignment might be abbreviated.

Assistive devices may be needed to facilitate homework completion, such as calendars, alarm clocks, or handheld computer devices with alarm-type prompts. Some clients may use an audiotaping device, rather than paper and pencil, to play and record their participation in a homework assignment. Others may require the use of a computer with voice-activated software. Some clients may be able to rely on devoted and responsible partners, family members, or other in-home care providers to provide reminders to complete homework or to assist the client in completing a given assignment. Helpers must be trained and supervised by the therapist on an ongoing basis and must be taught to understand the value of empowering the client to become his or her own therapist to the greatest extent possible.

If a therapist is unsure whether a client will be able to complete an assignment, assignments can be introduced in the format of a behavioral experiment. This will preserve the client's motivation and sense of efficacy should he or she fail to complete it or find the assignment unhelpful. Chapter 5 discusses additional strategies to facilitate completion of homework assignments.

Step 9: Summarizing the Session and Eliciting Client Feedback

At the end of the initial session the therapist makes a comprehensive summary statement about what occurred during that session. Typically, the therapist will review the presenting problems, the therapy goals, and the most important elements of the cognitive behavioral therapy process (e.g., collaborative relationship, setting and following a weekly structure and agenda, answering questions and providing feedback, completing weekly homework assignments, and learning to become one's own therapist). The therapist will then remind the client that the homework assignment is due next session and asks if he or she has any questions about it. Finally, the therapist asks the client for his or her reflections and feelings about the initial session.

Cognitive Behavioral Therapy and the Importance of Structure

The structure of the cognitive behavioral therapy treatment process is fundamental to successful therapy outcomes (Beck 1995). As a general rule, cognitive behavioral therapy seeks to make the therapy process as transparent and understandable to the client as possible. In part, this is accomplished through adherence to a predictable and reliable sequence and format so that a client knows what to expect from therapy, understands his or her role and responsibilities in the process, and also understands the therapist's role (Beck 1995).

One of the most fundamental aspects of "getting structure right" in therapy is to determine a client's preferred need for guidance versus autonomy (directive versus nondirective behavior on the part of the therapist). The traditional way of thinking in most approaches within the larger field of cognitive behavioral therapy is to begin therapy with a highly directive approach and to encourage the client to assume increasing levels of autonomy and control over time. The ultimate goal is to teach and empower clients to become their own therapists. However, time and the course of therapy do not always determine a client's preference and readiness to assume autonomy and control in therapy. Any client's need for a directive versus nondirective approach may vary based upon the life circumstances or medical issues he or she is facing at any given time. A skilled cognitive behavioral therapist assesses these issues and adjusts his or her level of directiveness accordingly, while still maintaining an ultimate objective of client empowerment in the back of his or her mind.

Troubleshooting a Client's Problems with Structure
Some clients will inevitably have a more difficult time adapting to the structure of cognitive behavioral therapy than others. There will be times when a client that otherwise seemed to have no difficulty with the structure of therapy may unexpectedly resist conforming to the structured aspects of a given session. When structural problems arise, the therapist should

- Interrupt the session
- Tell the client that he or she has observed the client's difficulties with the structure
- Explore the client's level of awareness of his or her difficulties
- Problem-solve with the client
- Reeducate the client about the role of structure in the therapy process, if necessary.

In most cases, clients may encounter difficulties adhering to the structure only on an occasional basis due to a crisis or increased symptoms, or they may struggle consistently with only an isolated element of the session, such as providing the therapist with feedback about therapy.

In some cases, a client's diffic[...]ervasive and may affect all aspects of the [...] may be linked to underlying errors in thi[...]out therapy or the therapist's style (Beck [...]a symptom of a broader problem for wh[...]y (White 2001). In other cases difficulties [...]be attributable to unrecognized attitudes [...]ne use of structured approaches to psychot[...] number of possible explanations for more global problems maintaining structure during therapy. These and other potential explanations that have emerged from the author's observations are described below.

- **A client has not been socialized to the cognitive behavioral therapy process adequately.** For example, the client may not have been taught the importance of structure to the therapeutic relationship, the therapeutic process, and to therapy outcomes. For many clients, a simple review of the cognitive model and of the rationale for session structure will suffice.

- **A client has had prior experience in psychotherapy and is more accustomed to a less structured or nondirective approach.** In these cases, a therapist may find that he or she has to place extra emphasis on providing the client with a rationale for each aspect of the cognitive behavioral therapy session and on educating the client about the importance of structure to the change process. The therapist will need to make explicit to the client that cognitive behavioral therapy involves unique and distinct roles and expectations within the therapeutic relationship. A therapist might prepare a client for this new way of relating by explaining up front that these roles and expectations may seem unfamiliar or challenging at first, particularly if a client is not accustomed to ongoing, mutual interaction with the therapist that involves providing the therapist with critical feedback and assuming an assertive, autonomous, and active role during therapy.

- **A client prefers a less structured (or conversely, a more structured) approach due to cultural differences or other intercultural communication issues arising from issues of human diversity.** In some cases a client simply expects the therapist to assume the role of expert. For such clients, the structure of cognitive behavioral therapy can be maintained while lowering the expectation for the client to be active, assertive, or directive within the relationship. Alternatively, in cases where a client may wish the therapist to be less active and directive, the structure of cognitive behavioral therapy can still be maintained if the client buys into the rationale and evidence for the importance of retaining each part of the therapy process. Moreover, this structure can be maintained while at the same time giving the client more control over the process and content of therapy. In other cases, if a client is interested in learning a new style of relating that is different

Continued

from his or her cultural preference, he or she can be socialized into responding and relating according to the traditional expectations of cognitive behavioral therapy. This requires close attention to making interpersonal dynamics and expectations concrete and understandable to the client. Preserving the therapeutic relationship as well as a client's own sense of identity and integrity is paramount. Clients that are not interested in learning new ways of relating should not be pressured or forced to do so. When indicated, their cultural preferences should be respected and incorporated into a somewhat revised approach to the structure of cognitive behavioral therapy.

- **A therapist may fail to guide and remind the client who is not familiar with the usual structure of cognitive behavioral therapy.** Thus, the therapist may have unrealistic expectations that the client will remember to provide an update at the beginning of each session, report on his or her homework assignment, and remember that an agenda for each session is typically set in an organized and brief manner. Moreover, the client may be unaware of the therapist's expectation that he or she will provide the therapist with ongoing feedback, be able to reflect upon and summarize session content, and complete his or her weekly homework in a timely and consistent way.

  Many therapists find that, in order for the structure of cognitive behavioral therapy to be maintained, they must gently remind and teach their clients to adhere to each of the different structural aspects of therapy each session, while continuing to provide a rationale for the importance of each of the session's parts. Some clients may need to be prompted to make the shift before each new aspect of the therapy process. Others may only need to be reminded about a single aspect, such as the importance of completing homework assignments.

- **A therapist may be unaware of his or her own resistances or concerns about structuring the therapy session.** Therapists may have concerns that manifest in the following questions. Will the client feel too controlled? Am I robbing the client of his or her independence or empowerment? Will I miss important content by limiting the client's opportunities to bring up new problems? Will the structure lead to a lack of understanding of this client from a more holistic perspective? Will the client perceive the structure as cold or routinized? Will structuring the session make me appear rigid or less intelligent to the client? If a therapist finds that he or she is having difficulty with these kinds of concerns, he or she can seek consultation from someone with expertise in cognitive behavioral therapy. Alternatively, he or she can attempt to evaluate and test his or her beliefs by completing a thought record and by testing these beliefs with a behavioral experiment (Beck 1995).

- **A therapist may behave in an overprotective way toward a client because of insufficient knowledge about the chronic condition or because of dysfunctional beliefs about chronic illness or impairment.** As a result, therapists may not set as many limits with their clients as they should. Moreover, they may be at more risk for allowing their clients to deviate from the recommended structure of therapy. If this becomes apparent, a therapist can seek consultation to assist him or her in making more accurate estimations of the amount of structure that a client with a particular chronic condition or disability can tolerate.
- **A therapist may approach structure in an overly enthusiastic way.** When this is the case, a therapist may have difficulty appropriately matching his or her approach to a given client's level of tolerance for structure. Alternatively, a therapist may believe that structure is more important than other aspects of therapy. For example, a therapist may be so focused on structure that he or she forgets to seek empathic understanding at key moments within the therapeutic relationship. The following are typical reactions of clients to feeling overwhelmed or threatened by an overly rigid application of structure. The client has inconsistent attendance to therapy sessions, appears resistant, or provides ongoing feedback to the therapist that he or she is incorrect in his or her interpretations, asks too many questions, seems invasive or critical, or does not really understand his or her problems or situation.

  In these instances, a therapist should rethink the approach to structure and place greater emphasis on achieving an empathic understanding of the client. In some cases, clients that resist the structure of therapy may actually be resisting other aspects of the therapist's approach to the relationship. These issues are discussed further in Chapter 11.
- **A client may have difficulty adhering to the structure of cognitive behavioral therapy because he or she is in a true state of physical or emotional crisis.** When a client is in an acute state of crisis that is not reflective of any more chronic or ongoing pattern, the emergent issue should become evident rather quickly. If it is a physical issue, such as a sudden increase in pain or an unexpected symptom, the therapist should ask a client if he or she would prefer that the session be terminated or end early for the day so that he or she can seek medical attention or go home and recover. Alternatively, if the symptom is a familiar one, the therapist can facilitate the client's coping with the symptom in the moment by utilizing attention diversion, distraction, or relaxation/meditation techniques (covered in Chapter 9).

  Similarly, if the client is in a state of emotional crisis, the therapist should always deviate from the usual structure of therapy in order to assist the client in addressing the issue at hand. Brief crisis counseling generally involves assessing the client's safety and the safety of others, providing

Continued

support, reviewing facts and circumstances of the crisis, and assisting the client with practical planning and problem solving.

- **A client may have difficulty with structure because of a personality disorder or other significant limitations in the interpersonal domain.** In cases where resistance to structure arises from an interpersonal issue (e.g., dysfunctional or distorted cognitions about self or about the therapist), broader approaches to cognitive behavioral therapy that emphasize empathic understanding and dialectical reasoning may be required (e.g., Linehan 1993a,b; Sperry 1999).

Conclusion

This chapter provided an overview of the nine steps that comprise the initial assessment and orientation to cognitive behavioral therapy for clients with chronic conditions. As noted earlier, these steps may not be completed in a single session with the client who has a chronic illness or impairment. The therapist should pace the assessment and orientation according to the client's ability to understand and tolerate the process.

The next chapter will discuss how to structure the therapy sessions that follow. Readers will notice that some of the steps covered in this chapter will automatically be incorporated into the regular structure and process of the subsequent therapy sessions of cognitive behavioral therapy. This consistency in approach provides an easy transition into the main working sessions of therapy and maximizes the likelihood that clients will learn enough about the structure and process of cognitive behavioral therapy that they will be able to apply it to themselves following treatment.

Appendix

	Confidence	Objectives (realistic steps I can take to
Goal(s) Target Date	Rating (1–10)	achieve goal)

Goal 1:

Target date:

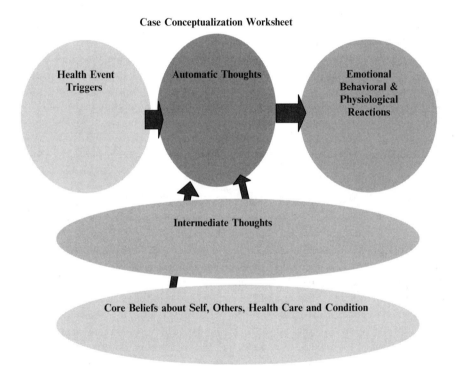

Case Conceptualization Worksheet

5

The Subsequent Sessions of Cognitive Behavioral Therapy

As with the initial assessment and orientation sessions, which were discussed in the previous chapter, subsequent therapy sessions are highly structured. There are nine general steps that should comprise these sessions (Beck 1995; Moorey and Greer 2002):

- Brief Update on Therapy Goals and Symptom Check
- Feedback and Homework from Last Session
- Setting the Agenda for Today's Session
- Working through Today's Agenda
- Ongoing Assessment and Socratic Questioning
- Therapist's Periodic Summaries and Summary Statements
- Setting New Homework
- Client's Final Summary of Today's Session and Feedback about the Session
- Relapse Prevention and Preparation for Termination

These steps will each be described in more detail in the following sections. Before proceeding it is important to note that the steps are considered important to include in every therapy session. How much time is spent on each step within the session depends on the client's needs. However, the therapist must be sure to structure the session so that all the steps can be fit into the therapy session. For the experienced therapist, this process will become second nature. However, the therapist beginning cognitive behavioral therapy may wish to use the cognitive behavioral therapy session checklist, which is located in the Appendix.

Step 1: Brief Update on Goals and Symptom Check

This initial part of the session involves two elements, which are updating goals and doing a symptom check. The goal update involves

- Revisiting the client's goals
- Reviewing the steps he or she took toward those goals since the last session
- Troubleshooting any difficulties that arose

The symptom check involves gathering a brief update on the client's condition and focal symptom for therapy. It also involves a check-in to determine whether the client has pursued any new treatments of which the therapist should be aware. The symptom check also involves a brief inquiry about psychological symptoms and about any relationships that the client may have perceived between his or her mood or stress levels and the severity of his or her physical symptoms in the past week.

Step 2: Feedback and Homework from Last Session

In step two, the therapist asks the client to provide any feedback about the prior session and to reflect upon his or her overall progress in therapy. On some occasions, a therapist might ask the client his or her opinion as to what has been most beneficial about therapy so far and what has not worked so well so that adjustments can be made, when necessary. At this time the therapist also requests that the client provide his or her homework assignment from the last session. Results of the assignment are reviewed and client feedback about the homework process is solicited.

Step 3: Setting the Agenda for Today's Session:

Step three involves determining whether any emergent issues or new problems identified during the update should be added to the client's main therapy goals, or whether the therapy should continue to focus on the problems and goals of the prior session or sessions. In the initial stages of therapy, the therapist sets the agenda for each session as it corresponds to a client's presenting problem and goal. As clients become more socialized to cognitive behavioral therapy, they can begin to set the agenda for each session.

If a client raises a new problem that has not been identified as a priority for treatment, the therapist should first gain an empathic understanding of that problem. The therapist should also determine whether it might relate in any way to the focal problems or current work of therapy. If the problem appears to be an isolated and unrelated incident, a crisis, or something that is outside of the client's immediate control, the therapist should assist the client in gaining some resolution or perspective on it.

The therapist should make it explicit to the client that he or she is intentionally deviating from the usual structure of therapy. Once the client is stable, the therapist should try to return to the main structure and agenda of the session as soon as it is appropriate. The amount of time or number of sessions it may take to return to the usual structure of therapy will vary depending on nature of the client's new problem or crisis and on the therapist's judgment. For example, the sudden death of a friend might take several sessions to process, while an argument with a friend might take less than five minutes to process.

Step 4: Working through the Session's Agenda

Working through the agenda for each session typically involves planning the continued steps that the client will need to take toward goal attainment in the following week. It can also involve discussing or working on any additional issues or tasks that the therapist and client have identified as likely to be helpful in facilitating cognitive and behavioral change. This might include, for instance:

- Reviewing the cognitive model
- Identifying and responding to negative automatic thoughts in response to a symptom
- Identifying errors in thinking about the chronic condition
- Exploring and restructuring dysfunctional intermediate and core beliefs
- Engaging in a behavioral experiment during the session
- Providing immediate symptom relief by teaching distraction techniques or by practicing relaxation or meditation exercises with the client

These and other procedures are reviewed in greater detail later in this book.

Step 5: Ongoing Assessment and Socratic Questioning:

Assessments most commonly used following the initial therapy session or sessions commonly include, but are not limited to:

- Self-report measures of physical and psychological symptoms
- Goal forms
- Thought records
- Activity diaries

Descriptions and examples of some of these measures are provided later in this chapter and in subsequent chapters of the book.

Another key form of assessment is Socratic questioning; a strategic and disciplined approach to asking clients questions. The purpose of Socratic questioning is to allow clients to examine their thinking from a more objective and logical standpoint and to test the validity of their ideas. Socratic questioning may also allow the client to engage in dialectical reasoning, and this can facilitate a client's consideration of different points of view.

The Socratic questions (Paul and Elder 2002) that are recommended for use in cognitive behavioral therapy with individuals with chronic conditions include:

- Origin or source questions
- Questions that probe evidence
- Questions that probe assumptions
- Questions about viewpoint
- Questions about consequences

Examples of questions according to each category are provided in Table 1.

The Socratic approach to questioning can be utilized by therapists in a wide range of therapy activities. It can be used to gather evidence to support or disconfirm an automatic thought. It can reveal intermediate and core beliefs. It can be used to plan a behavioral experiment. Finally, it can be used as a part of preparing for termination.

Step 6: Therapist's Periodic Summary Statements

In addition to the frequent use of key comments that reflect a therapist's empathic understanding of the client (as discussed in Chapter 11), cognitive behavioral therapists periodically make summary statements that reflect their understanding of a critical problem or achievement in therapy. These are sometimes referred to as "capsule summaries" (Beck 1995) and they serve a number of functions, including:

- Assisting the client in clarifying problems,
- Organizing a client's thinking,
- Reinforcing a key point in therapy, or
- Celebrating a significant insight or other therapy achievement.

TABLE 1. Socratic questions for use in cognitive behavioral therapy for chronic conditions.

Origin or Source Questions:	How did you first get the idea that [a brain tumor] is always fatal? Does your doctor feel otherwise?
Questions that Probe Evidence	What do you already know that supports your idea that you [cannot conceive]?
	Do you believe this constitutes enough evidence?
	Are there any alternative explanations for your [reproductive pain]?
	What has led you to believe that your doctor is not telling you the truth?
Questions that Probe Assumptions	Let's assume for the moment that your belief [that your husband no longer finds you physically attractive] is true. What does this say about you?
	In order to conclude that [you will never be able to think as clearly as you once did], what must you assume?
	Do you think someone else would make this same assumption?
Questions about Viewpoint	It sounds like you believe that you are being punished for [your affair].
	Why have you chosen to explain [your heart disease] from this perspective?
	How might someone else that [has had an affair] explain the fact that she also has [heart disease]?
Questions about Consequences	If you decide not to [have surgery], what positive consequences might be involved? What negative consequences might be involved?
	What are the likely short-term consequences of [skipping your medication to drink alcohol]? What long-term consequences might be involved?

Step 7: Setting New Homework

As noted earlier, homework is considered an indispensable step. Generating homework assignments that are relevant and attainable is a major challenge. Table 2 provides a summary of tips that therapists can use to facilitate completion of homework for clients with chronic conditions as well as tips for when clients

TABLE 2. Tips for facilitating completion and resolving problems with homework assignments.

Tips for Facilitating Completion of Homework Assignments	• Always provide the client with a rationale for why the assignment is predicted to help
	• Be certain that the task is relevant to the client's central problem and goal
	• Begin the assignment in the company of the client during the session
	• It is better that an assignment be too easy, rather than too difficult, for a client
	• Concretize the assignment by having a client document or record his or her activity, regardless of whether the activity is cognitive or behavioral in nature
	• Always review the client's homework in the next session, solicit feedback, and reinforce the client for his or her effort
	• Provide client with a sense of control in choosing and structuring his or her assignments
	• Make the assignment pleasurable and attractive to the client, when possible and appropriate. This may involve some creativity on the part of the therapist (e.g., laminate the client's coping cards, use bright-colored paper or art to enhance written assignments, use or provide the client with physical objects with which to complete assignments, when appropriate).
	• Anticipate potential obstacles and prepare the client for a possible negative outcome
Tips to Use for Clients with Homework Difficulties	• Say something positive about a client's effort, even if the assignment failed
	• If an assignment has failed, ask the client to identify at least one thing about it that he or she learned or found useful
	• Therapists should consider accepting responsibility for a client's failure on an assignment, particularly if it is apparent that the client made some effort and the therapist may not have selected the best assignment
	• Always find a way to gently explore why a client did not do the homework. Never allow failure to even make an effort to go overlooked, since this has implications for the therapeutic relationship
	• Therapists should explore their own cognitions about assigning and reinforcing the necessity of homework
	• If a client made an effort but was unable to complete the assignment, use the therapy session to allow the client to complete the assignment
	• Recruit the assistance of a housemate (under appropriate conditions)
	• Be certain not to pressure or make a client feel guilty for not completing his or her assignment. Instead, explore and problem-solve with the client to increase the likelihood that assignments will be completed

are having particular difficulty completing homework assignments. Some of these tips have been recommended by Beck (1995).

With time and experience a therapist will develop a wider range of assignments and be increasingly facile in generating new assignments as the client's situation demands.

Table 3 contains examples of traditional cognitive behavioral therapy homework assignments (Beck 1995) as well as new and modified homework assignments that may be particularly relevant for use with individuals with chronic conditions. Other chapters in this book contain additional homework assignments that may be used in addition to the central approaches described on the following pages. Behavioral experiments are the last form of homework listed in Table 3. Additional information about behavioral experiments is contained in Chapter 9.

TABLE 3. Examples of homework assignments.

Completing a Weekly Goal Form	If brevity and focus are of high importance, one of the most effective ways to structure the course of therapy within and outside of sessions is to ask clients to complete a weekly goal form. For this assignment, clients are asked to simply document or verify that they have completed one or more concrete, behavioral steps toward accomplishing the central goal of therapy.
Reviewing Coping Cards	Coping cards (Beck 1995) are usually made during sessions for review outside of sessions as a type of "homework task." Coping cards are tangible flash-card-type devices (or audiotaped statements in the therapist's or client's own voice) that are easily carried with the client wherever he or she goes. They may contain reminders about various distraction, relaxation, or pain-management techniques and other coping strategies (to be described in more detail in this chapter). Coping cards may be particularly useful to clients during times of change, challenge, or crisis (e.g., before a diagnostic test or during a medical procedure).
Listing Positive Activities	For clients that are demoralized, have difficulty with self-care, or demonstrate a cognitive bias that involves excessive negative focus, a client can be asked to make a daily list of positive self-statements, self-care activities, accomplishments, or examples of obstacles overcome each day (e.g., "I went to the health club to swim today despite feeling depressed this morning"). This list involves relatively little effort and can be recorded in a client's daily calendar. The number of positive activities can be summed each day. These tallies can then be reviewed in session so a client can begin to learn self-care and recognize his or her accomplishments. Clients may also learn to see connections between their efforts and other characteristics, such as symptoms and mood.
Making a List of Positive or Humorous Memories	Often it takes clients time to conjure up memories of positive or humorous occasions in their lives, and this can be done in between sessions to address goals related to emotion regulation and mood improvement. Many clients view this task as pleasurable, but some clients may find it painful to reflect on what they may perceive as happier times in their lives. In these cases, clients are encouraged to focus more on present-day positive or humorous moments. If client feedback indicates that the list was helpful in accomplishing these goals, future homework assignments can involve periodically reading or expanding this list.

TABLE 3. *Continued*

"Bad Day" Letter	Clients with chronic difficulties coping with conditions that involve relapses, flare-ups, or other symptoms that appear to wax and wane unpredictably can be instructed to write themselves an uplifting or nurturing letter that they can read on "bad days" (Dolan 1998; Johnson and Webster, 2002). This "bad day" letter can serve as a reminder to the client that his or her circumstances will change and the condition or symptoms will improve again. The letter might also contain a list of self-care activities, pleasurable activities, and gratifying activities that the client knows will bring comfort. Clients may also want to add personal affirmations, self-coaching statements, problem-solving strategies, or a reminder to make contact with favored people. It might also contain a list of accomplishments that the client has made in therapy thus far. Some clients may also wish to add a description of a current activity that they are able to do or a food that they are able to eat on "good days" so that they can look forward to doing that activity or to eating that food when they are feeling better. (Clearly, this aspect of the letter should not be encouraged for clients with rapidly progressing, terminal conditions.) Clearly, the letter should be written on a "good day" or after a sufficient progress has been made in therapy such that the client possesses a sufficient number of resources to be of help to him- or herself on a "bad day." This exercise is often a useful activity for clients to engage in when approaching termination because it allows them to consolidate what they have learned in therapy.
Reviewing Notes/ Audiotapes of Important Sessions	Clients are encouraged to integrate and review what they have learned in therapy (Beck 1995). This can be accomplished by listening to an audiotaped recording of a particularly helpful session or by reviewing notes or assignments completed during the session.
Reviewing the Cognitive Model	Clients can be encouraged take a copy of their personalized "cognitive model diagram" home so that they can review the hypothesized linkages between triggering events, beliefs, and reactions.
Relaxation, Breathing, and Meditation Assignments	Clients who adapt readily to practicing relaxation, breathing, or meditation exercises during sessions and find them helpful may be encouraged to practice these exercises several times a day within the home setting and to collect data on physical or emotional symptoms before and after engaging in an exercise.
Comfort Kit	Many clients with conditions that involve difficult or uncomfortable physical symptoms (e.g., pain, nausea, severe exhaustion, fever) will benefit from various basic supplies and objects that may bring them some degree of comfort. Clients can be assigned to prepare in advance a "comfort kit" that contains medications that are prescribed only-as-needed, a selection of favorite, comforting music, cans of ginger ale, a comforting picture, or a certain pillow or blanket, for example.
Self-Education Assignments	These assignments are designed to increase a client's understanding of his or her condition, available medical treatments, available approaches to rehabilitation (including cognitive and behavioral strategies), and available assistive technologies. Knowledge about one's own condition maximizes the opportunity for informed participation in treatment decisions and self-advocacy in medical settings, increases knowledge about available resources for independent living, and can dispel any myths or dysfunctional beliefs a client may have. Assignments may consist of reading consumer-oriented literature (for some clients, scientific journal articles) or viewing/hearing educational videotapes.

Self-Advocacy Assignments	Clients can be provided with the names and telephone numbers of agencies and contact people that can provide linkage to available community-based resources, including access to specialized transportation options, personal care assistants, housekeepers, and home delivery of food. These resources are often available by calling one's local mayor's office to inquire about public resources for individuals with disabilities, or by contacting disability advocacy organizations (e.g., Centers for Independent Living) or self-help organizations (e.g., The National Multiple Sclerosis Society) for information.
Provider Questions	Clients can be encouraged to develop a list of questions about their condition, its symptoms, or its treatment to present to their health care provider (usually a physician). Clients can be encouraged to read this list aloud to their providers and audiotape responses. Many clients become overwhelmed and confused by rapid and abundant amounts of information provided by their physicians, and audiotaping a question-and-answer session can structure the interaction and allow a client to review the information later in a nonstressful setting.
Completing a Thought Record	Once they are introduced to the thought record during a therapy session, clients may be encouraged to continue to complete it as homework. Thought records allow clients to evaluate and respond to negative automatic thoughts, and they may be of particular aid to clients during times when they are feeling anxious, depressed, or experiencing a given physical symptom. Thought records are described in detail in chapters 6 and 7. Thought records should only be assigned as homework under the condition that clients can demonstrate that they are able to effectively respond to negative automatic thoughts on their own. Instructing clients to simply monitor negative automatic thoughts when experiencing symptoms without providing them with alternative ways of thinking can lead to discouragement, somatic preoccupation, or increased distress in some individuals.
Activity Diaries	Activity diaries or assignments are often a fundamental aspect of therapy homework for individuals with chronic conditions, particularly if overactivity, underactivity, or a lack of balance in activities are potential contributors to symptoms. These diaries allow both the client and the therapist to monitor, assign, or downgrade a client's levels of physical activity or to increase participation in more desired types of activities.
Behavioral Experiments	Behavioral experiments are often assigned as homework to allow clients to test dysfunctional thoughts and beliefs about a given activity or situation. Behavioral experiments are broadly defined because they can be introduced at any level of involvement and can involve any range of recommended therapy tasks. For example, a behavioral experiment might be used to address a client's fears or doubts about the value of completing a homework assignment (Beck 1995). This might at least activate a resistant or fearful client to try the assignment. More entrenched beliefs can also be tested through behavioral experiments.

Because behavioral experiments are designed to allow people to overcome significant barriers to acting in their own best interest, and are often very difficult for clients to attempt, therapists should do their best to make provisions to ensure that the assignment will be successful. In addition, therapists should always be honest with their clients about the possibility that their engagement in an experiment might lead to a confirmation of their fears or concerns, rather than to a disconfirmation. In some cases it may be appropriate to make plans in advance in preparation for the possibility of failure. Chapter 9 contains examples of behavioral experiments that can be used with clients with chronic conditions. Behavioral experiments involving food or medication intake or changes in the nature or degree of activity, for example, should be approved by the client's physician before prescribing them. Physician approval should be solicited even if a therapist is convinced that a client's fears are irrational and health-damaging.

Step 8: Client's Final Summary of Today's Session and Feedback

The first time this step is done or until the client is able to take over, the therapist gives a summary. In subsequent sessions, clients are asked to make a summary statement about what they have learned and understood to have occurred at the end of each session. During this summary, the therapist's only role is to listen to be sure that the client has understood the key events of the session.

Following the summary, therapists also ask clients to report on what they found effective about the session and what they found ineffective. A therapist might ask if there was anything that he or she may have misunderstood or whether there was anything that he or she said that upset the client (Beck 1995).

Step 9: Relapse Prevention and Preparation for Termination

As a general rule, cognitive behavioral therapy is time-structured. Following the initial assessment, the therapist typically provides the client with an estimate of how long the therapy will take and an expected termination date is set. In each session, the therapist should assist the client in planning actively for how he or she might address the problem or symptom that was the focus of the session's agenda in the future and outside of the therapy context. A rationale for this planning should be provided to the client in the context of relapse prevention and preparation for termination. As clients demonstrate increasing capacity to manage symptoms independently, they should be reminded periodically of the planned date of termination and informed that the ultimate purpose of therapy is to guide them to become their own therapists over time.

Unless setting or payment constraints make it impossible to do so, the planned termination date can be adjusted if new complications arise or if a therapist and client decide that more time is needed. Adjustments in termination dates are relatively common in work with people with chronic conditions because unanticipated medical issues can often complicate the process and usual progress of therapy.

Conclusion

This chapter has reviewed the basic structure of the cognitive behavioral therapy sessions that follow the initial assessment and orientation session(s). In cognitive behavioral therapy, each session is generally characterized by gathering a brief update from the client on recent symptoms and progress toward goals, discussing feedback and reviewing the assigned homework, determining the agenda for the day, discussing issues or working through cognitive and behavioral exercises on that agenda, setting new homework, and soliciting a final summary and feedback from the client. In addition to these fundamental tasks, each therapy session is characterized by ongoing assessment and Socratic questioning, periodic summary statements, and reminders about relapse prevention or termination, when appropriate.

Clients will vary in the degree of coaching and structuring needed to ensure that each step is covered. In addition, the speed at which they are able to memorize and intuitively follow these steps on their own will vary between clients. Some clients may require several reminders and a fair amount of limit-setting throughout the therapy process in order to ensure that all steps are followed. Others may require coaching and limit-setting in the first session or two, but will quickly learn to follow the process in the sessions thereafter.

Alex is one example of a client that learned to follow the general structure of cognitive behavioral therapy relatively quickly over time. During his second session of therapy, Alex was well prepared with an agenda and had completed his homework assignment from the initial session. He responded well to prompts and reminders from the therapist to move from step to step within the overall structure of therapy. When it was time for him to provide a summary of the second session and to provide the therapist with feedback, he summarized the session well and was very comfortable telling the therapist that he liked "being told to move along from step to step" because it made him feel that he was "accomplishing something." Other clients do not respond as well or as naturally to prompting or limit-setting. As discussed in chapter 4, these clients may take longer to learn to follow and adhere to the steps of therapy, forcing the therapist to move more slowly and rely more upon the incorporation of empathy and other areas of related knowledge.

Appendix

Cognitive Behavioral Therapy Session Checklist

Brief Update on Therapy Goals and Symptom Check	• revisit the client's goals, • review steps taken toward those goals since the last session • troubleshoot any difficulties • briefly update client's condition and focal symptom
Feedback and Homework	• feedback on last session (and therapy progress so far) • review results of assignment and solicit client feedback about the homework process
Set Agenda for Today's Session	• should any emergent issues or new problems should be added to main therapy goals, or should therapy should continue to focus on the problems and goals of the prior session?
Working through Today's Agenda	• planning the continued steps for goal attainment • working on any additional issues or tasks to facilitate cognitive and behavioral change
Ongoing Assessment and Socratic Questioning	
Periodic Summaries and Summary Statements	
Set New Homework	
Client's Summary and Feedback about the Session	• key events of the session. • what was effective and ineffective.
Relapse Prevention and Preparation for Termination	

6

Introduction to the Techniques of Cognitive Behavioral Therapy

The previous two chapters covered the structure of cognitive behavior therapy, discussing what goes on in the assessment and orientation phase and presenting the typical structure of subsequent therapy sessions. This and subsequent chapters address the techniques of cognitive behavioral therapy.

The Rationale for the Techniques Cognitive Behavioral Therapy

Cognitive behavioral therapy argues that the beliefs one holds about a situation, rather than the situation itself, are what determine an individual's resulting emotional experience, behavioral reactions, and physiological response (Beck et al. 1979; Beck, 1995). Individuals with chronic conditions are forced to experience real-world situations that would be interpreted as negative or frightening by almost anyone. When this is simply the case, cognitive behavioral therapy approaches aimed at restructuring cognition are not indicated.

Dysfunctional Thinking and Beliefs

The circumstance of having a chronic condition can be accompanied by repeated experiences of rejection, alienation, exclusion, discrimination, loss, or failure at once-valued activities. Vulnerable individuals are at risk for developing dysfunctional thinking and beliefs over time. These maladaptive cognitive patterns include

- Errors in thinking
- Preoccupations

Individuals with psychiatric overlay may not only bring dysfunctional thinking and beliefs into the experience of having a chronic condition, they are also likely to react to its stresses with increased tendencies toward cognitions that worsen their situation.

Persons with maladaptive cognitions will inevitably exhibit negative emotional, behavioral, and physiological consequences. For some individuals with chronic conditions, maladaptive cognitions may manifest themselves in the misinterpretation of otherwise neutral medical events or in the development of exaggerated concerns about health and functioning.

Common Errors in Thinking

Automatic thoughts, intermediate beliefs, or core beliefs typically cluster together in patterns that reflect cognitive distortions or errors in thinking. Figure 1 shows an example of a cluster of cognitive distortions that transects the three levels of cognition.

Beck and associates (1979) described a number of different cognitive distortions that lead to negative affective states and maladaptive behavior. During therapy, these distortions are typically identified by listening to the client's automatic thoughts and attempting to identify the specific type of error that that client seems to be making (Beck, 1995). The client can then be educated to identify his or her

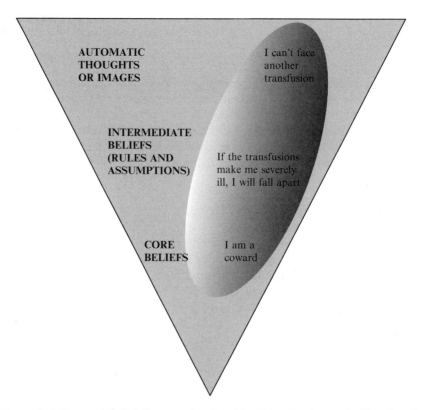

FIGURE 1. A Cluster of Beliefs Representing Cognitive Distortion Across the Three Levels

errors in thinking independently. Typically, the cognitive distortions of any given client will form distinctive clusters and patterns, and a client will tend to manifest similar distortions on a repeated basis. Table 1 lists 12 of the common cognitive distortions and provides examples of how they might manifest in the automatic thoughts and intermediate and core beliefs of clients with chronic conditions.

These patterns may be reflective of underlying core beliefs (Beck, 1995). For this reason and because too many distortions can overwhelm a client, it is important to present clients with only the distortions that are relevant to his or her cognitive tendencies (Beck, 1995).

Preoccupations

Other individuals may never develop illogical ways of thinking but may become preoccupied by realistic negative cognitions about their health and functioning. Though their cognitions are real, logical and well-founded in terms of evidence, the fact that they are preoccupied with these thoughts becomes problematic. These preoccupations are unhelpful to clients. They are also usually accompanied by difficult emotions, problematic behaviors, or aversive physiological reactions. Hence the person without distorted thinking, whose preoccupations reduce functioning or quality of life, can also be a candidate for cognitive behavioral therapy.

TABLE 1. Common cognitive distortions involving chronic conditions (Adapted from Aaron T. Beck and Judith S. Beck).

Distortion	Definition	Example
Black-and-white thinking	A client views a situation in an overly simplistic and dichotomous way – considering only two extremes rather than the "shades of gray" or all of the possibilities in between.	"I've been in bed for three days. I just know my condition is only going to get worse from here."
"Shoulds" and "musts"	A client has rigid or overly idealistic expectations for his or her own behavior as well as for the behavior of others. A client is inappropriately judgmental or dooming if a given expectation is not met.	"Health care professionals should always be positive and optimistic when they discuss health matters with a patient."
Personalization	A client blames him- or herself for negative circumstances or for the negative behaviors of others rather than considering more likely, alternative explanations for their behavior.	"Dr. Harvey seemed so down today. It must be really depressing for him to have to treat people like me."

TABLE 1. *Continued*

Distortion	Definition	Example
Tunnel vision	A client can only perceive the negative characteristics of him- or herself or of a given event.	"I can't do these behavioral experiments. I'm too afraid of a flare-up and I'm basically just a coward anyway."
Emotional reasoning	A client assumes his or her belief is true merely based upon his or her feeling about it rather than based upon the objective reality.	"I know my cancer is back, I can just feel it."
Overgeneralization	A client forms a sweeping and negativistic belief about a situation that extends well beyond the facts or actual characteristics of that situation.	"That last infusion was really painful. I know this new drug is going to be even worse."
Jumping to conclusions	A client believes in a negative future regardless of other possibilities or alternatives.	"My back hurts again. There must be something wrong with my kidneys."
Magnification/minimization	A client exaggerates the negative aspects of a given situation and downplays the positive aspects.	"They say the surgery went well, but I don't think so because I am not healing as quickly as they said I would. Something else must be wrong."
Mind reading	A client believes others are thinking about him or her in a negative or judgmental way in situations where there is no evidence and it is likely not the case.	"My boyfriend is disgusted by my catheter."
Ignoring the positive	A client chooses to focus only on the negative aspects of him- or herself, of a situation, or of his or her performance. The positive aspects are discounted or ignored.	"People say I'm courageous, but they would say that about anyone who is forced to face something like this."
Mental filter	A client selects one negative detail about his or her appearance, performance, or a given situation and ignores all other aspects of the situation as a whole.	"That nurse was so curt, I bet this is not a good medical practice."
Labeling	A client ascribes a single, rigid label to self or others without considering other strengths or positive characteristics	"I am a coward."

Therapeutic Considerations Pertaining to Different Thinking Patterns

It is useful for therapists, and often for clients, to distinguish between distorted thinking (invalid thoughts) and valid thoughts that constitute preoccupations. These two different thought patterns have different implications for the type of cognitive behavioral techniques for addressing them (i.e., distorted thinking is best addressed through cognitive techniques that seek to correct the thinking pattern, whereas realistic preoccupations are often best addressed through coping skills and symptom management training). Beck (1995) recommends that it is helpful for clients to subclassify and evaluate their automatic thoughts in terms of their validity and utility. Many times thoughts about their condition may be valid but not particularly useful or health-promoting (White 2001).

The therapist should be vigilant to identify whether a client tends to have predominantly one or both thinking patterns (i.e., distortion and/or preoccupation). The therapist will also need to consider if and when it is necessary to engage the client in a process of distinguishing thoughts into realistic and unrealistic and into helpful and unhelpful categories.

If the client has predominantly distorted thinking, then it is not necessary to sub-classify thoughts. If the client has predominantly preoccupations, it will be useful to examine the extent of their utility. If the client has a pattern of both, then it may be helpful to distinguish which are realistic and unrealistic and which of the former have utility.

A Continuum of Cognitive Behavioral Interventions Relevant to Chronic Conditions

Cognitive behavioral therapists practicing with persons who have chronic illness and impairment have a number of potential techniques available to them. Because it is beyond the scope of this book to cover all of these techniques, this chapter will focus on those that are most relevant to individuals with chronic conditions and on those that show greatest promise in terms of available empirical support.

The interventions to be discussed in the subsequent chapters can be conceptualized as falling along a continuum that ranges in emphasis from more cognitively oriented approaches to more behaviorally oriented approaches. Extremes of the continuum can be utilized together or separately provided that the therapist and client always conduct therapy according to the issues outlined in an underlying cognitive case conceptualization. Figure 2 illustrates the continuum of techniques that will be discussed.

Techniques that are most cognitive in nature are those most suited to address distortions of thinking. These include

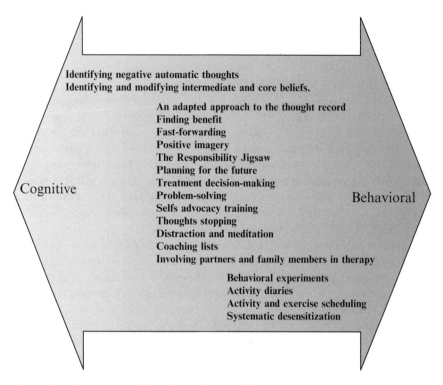

Figure 2. A Continuum of Cognitive Behavioral Techniques

- Identifying negative automatic thoughts in therapy
- Teaching the client to respond to negative automatic thoughts using thought records
- Identifying intermediate and core beliefs
- Teaching the client to modify intermediate and core beliefs

These techniques are presented and discussed in Chapter 7.

Techniques that are in the middle of the continuum are those that are most suited to addressing maladaptive cognitions that do not involve distortions of thinking. These include:

- An adapted approach to the thought record
- Finding benefit
- Fast-forwarding
- Positive Imagery
- The Responsibility jigsaw
- Planning for the future
- Treatment decision-making
- Problem-solving
- Self-advocacy training

- Thought-stopping
- Distraction and meditation
- Coaching lists
- Involving partners and family members in therapy

These techniques are presented and discussed in Chapter 8.

Finally the techniques which are primarily behavioral in nature are discussed in Chapter 9. They include:

- Behavioral experiments
- Activity diaries
- Activity and exercise scheduling
- Systematic desensitization

Although these interventions are discussed separately in the following three chapters, the clinician should integrate them as needed for each client. The extent to which the therapist employs strategies that are more cognitive versus behavioral in nature depends on the nature of the client's maladaptive cognitions and on the client's preference for and response to different techniques.

7

Techniques for Addressing Maladaptive Cognitions That Are Unrealistic

Chapter 6 emphasized the importance of distinguishing between maladaptive cognitions that are unrealistic and those that are realistic when working with individuals with chronic conditions. This chapter describes the techniques of cognitive behavioral therapy that most closely address unrealistic maladaptive cognitions. These include:

- Identifying negative automatic thoughts in therapy
- Teaching the client to respond to negative automatic thoughts using thought records
- Identifying intermediate and core beliefs
- Teaching the client to modify intermediate and core beliefs

In the sections that follow these three main techniques will be explained and exemplified.

Identifying Negative Automatic Thoughts

As discussed in earlier chapters, automatic thoughts occupy the lowest and most concrete of the three cognitive levels. Automatic thoughts are brief, spontaneous thoughts that are just barely in conscious awareness (Beck, 1964). They commonly reflect a client's underlying intermediate and core belief systems (Beck, 1964; Beck, 1995). Negative automatic thoughts are verbal self-statements and/or mental images that are characterized by:

- Distortion of reality,
- Emotional distress, and/or
- Interference with the pursuit and attainment of life goals (Beck 1995).

"Hot thoughts" (i.e., automatic thoughts characterized by emotional experience) are the most essential automatic thoughts to work with in psychotherapy (Beck 1995; Greenberger and Padesky 1995). Some argue that a prerequisite for change is that emotional experience must be attached to automatic thoughts targeted for change (Moorey and Greer 2002). Before cognitive change can take place, automatic thoughts must be elicited and identified. The primary method of identifying automatic thoughts is sequential questioning.

Sequential Questioning to Identify Automatic Thoughts

Clients new to cognitive behavioral therapy tend to be more able to identify negative emotions or physical sensations than the negative automatic thoughts themselves (Beck, 1995). Thus, the therapist engages in a process of questioning that teaches the client how to successfully identify hot thoughts on his or her own. Differentiating emotional or bodily experience from thinking is often the best starting point for both clients and therapists when beginning work with automatic thoughts. The most effective way to allow for this differentiation is to ask the client four specific questions, which are indicated in Table 1 (Beck, 1995; White, 2001). Experience with most clients with chronic conditions indicates that it is most effective to ask these four questions in the order that they are listed. Consequently, the process of asking these questions will be referred to as "sequential questioning." Sequential questioning begins with eliciting the nature of an individual's emotional experience, or accessing an individual's experience of pain. This allows patients and therapists to arrive at a basic level of understanding before identifying the automatic thought that is associated with that emotion or pain.

The use of Question 2 is left to the therapist's judgment because the utility of this question may depend on a number of variables. Question 2 is typically useful with clients that tend to use intellectualization as a defense when they are having difficulty describing their emotional experience. Question 2 is also useful with clients who tend to somatize in situations in which it is clear that the client is unable to distinguish his or her somatic symptoms from his or her thoughts and feelings.

Therapists may not find Question 2 helpful for clients that are able to identify their emotions and do not tend to locate them within their body. These clients do not typically somaticize their feelings and do not typically report increased physical symptoms with emotional distress. In these cases, Question 2 may risk inducing physical symptom-focusing and somatization, rather than alleviating it.

Helping the client to identify what he or she is feeling will generally make it easier for the client to later distinguish and identify an automatic thought or image. Nonetheless, this process can be challenging. There will be some clients that are not accustomed to identifying and discussing feelings. When asked to discuss feelings, they may shut down or they may become confused about their feelings.

TABLE 1. Sequential questions to elicit automatic thoughts.

- What are you feeling right now?
- Where in your body do you feel it? (optional)
- What thoughts or pictures pass through your mind as you feel this?
- Which thought or picture makes you feel the worst?

In these circumstances, a therapist may wish to ask only the third and fourth questions. To avoid the emphasis on emotional experience, the third question can be modified as: "What thoughts or pictures come to mind right now?" As soon as a client becomes more able to identify feelings and more comfortable sharing them in therapy, the therapist should return to using all of the sequential questions in the order that they are recommended.

Still other clients may intellectualize what they are feeling and may only be able to articulate interpretations of their thoughts and feelings (e.g., "I'm probably just worrying too much about things I cannot control"). These more guarded clients can be coached to identify their feelings and their more spontaneous cognitions (i.e., automatic thoughts) through modeling and Socratic questioning. For example, if a client reports rather flatly that her partner of five years, whom she loves deeply, wants to break up with her now that she has cervical cancer, and she has difficulty expressing or identifying her feelings about this, a therapist might begin the sequential questioning in the following way:

"Examples of feelings that someone could have in this situation are sadness, despair, anger, and fear .... Do any of these feelings match what you feel?"

or

"How do you think another person such as one of your friends, might feel, if they learned that their partner wanted to break up with them?"

Initiating Sequential Questioning.

An important judgment on the part of the therapist is when to begin or how to initiate the process of sequential questioning. There are two common ways that a therapist can initiate sequential questioning:

- Taking advantage of a spontaneous observation of a critical change in the client's affect
- Asking questions to generate examples of past stressful life events

The following sections discuss these two strategies.

Observed change in the client's affect

One of the most effective circumstances for using sequential questioning to elicit an automatic thought is when the therapist observes the client

- Experiencing or expressing a difficult emotion or
- Describing a difficult experience (Beck, 1995).

In order to be aware of such opportunities, the therapist should listen for unusually difficult content and watch for sudden changes in posture, facial expression, or voice (Beck, 1995). When the therapist becomes aware of such data, she/he proceeds with the sequential questioning presented in Table 1.

Asking questions about past experiences

Another strategy for initiating sequential questioning is to ask a client to think up an example of a difficult experience, recount the story in narrative form, and then respond to the sequential questions. This method is typically used when there is not any readily apparent in-session content from which to derive automatic thoughts. This approach allows the therapist an opportunity to teach a client the process of identifying automatic thoughts for future exercises within and outside of therapy.

Responding to Negative Automatic Thoughts: Thought Records

As the client is being taught to take over the therapy process, sequential questioning is gradually replaced with a self-report process that also incorporates response to automatic thoughts. A fundamental milestone for clients of cognitive behavioral therapy is to learn how to identify their own automatic thoughts so that they can actively explore and respond to them. The primary means by which this is accomplished is through having clients complete a "thought record."

The purpose of the thought record is to allow the client to identify and respond to automatic thoughts. Once automatic thoughts are identified, they must be addressed. Otherwise clients are left vulnerable to focus on and possibly dwell on their negative or dysfunctional thinking without resources to address it. This can backfire and lead to iatrogenic outcomes and therapy dropouts. Thus, it is important that when the thought record is given as a homework assignment, a client must know not only how to identify, but also how to respond to automatic thoughts.

To this end, when the therapist first gives the thought record as homework assignment it is advised that the assignment be initiated in the company of the therapist during the session so that the therapist can coach the client through the process. Also, before sending the client home to complete homework with the thought record it is important to make sure the client understands the instructions for evaluating and responding to those thoughts.

What Is a Thought Record?

Thought records offer one of the most effective and commonly utilized means of teaching and habituating clients to restructure their dysfunctional thinking. Numerous examples of various types of thought records exist in the literature (e.g., Beck 1995; Greenberger and Padesky 1995; Seligman 2002; White 2001). Traditional approaches to thought records focus on exploring the validity of a thought through multiple targeted questions.

Individuals with medical issues may have energy limitations, difficulties with attention, concentration, or other aspects of cognitive functioning, and limited frustration tolerance during periods of increased symptoms. Therefore, thought records need to be designed with a focus on ease of use and efficiency. At the same time, the thought record should address all aspects of the cognitive model with sufficient sophistication so as not to lose the fundamental value of this intervention approach. For this reason, the author developed a "response record" for use with individuals with chronic conditions who have distorted cognitions (see Figure 1). The response record was inspired by existing thought records and approaches derived from Beck (1995), Greenberger and Padesky (1995), Seligman (2002), Ellis (1962), Michenbaum (1977), and White (2001). This thought record is unique in that it considers issues that are specific to individuals with chronic conditions.

A client can be provided with as many copies of the record as the therapist and client decide would be necessary or useful.

Using this record, the client is guided through each of the essential aspects of the cognitive model as he or she describes and reacts to a given triggering event. Many clients with medical issues will tend to experience negative events related to their

Response Record				
Date:	Health event trigger (or other triggering event):			
What am I feeling right now? (Circle all that apply.)	panicked	numb	sad	angry
	hopeless	worried	other:	
What thoughts or pictures are passing through my mind?				
Which of these thoughts or pictures makes me feel the worst? (circle one above)				
What are the emotional, behavioral, and physical consequences of thinking this way?				
Emotional:		Behavioral:	Physical:	

- What do I already know that supports this belief?
- What do I already know that does not support this belief?
- What might someone else think about this situation?
- What advice would I give to a friend if he or she was in this situation?
- What is the best possible outcome of this situation?
- What is the worst possible outcome of this situation?
- If (the worst outcome) were to happen, what could I do to minimize its impact?
- Given what I know so far, how likely is (the worst outcome) to happen?
- How do I benefit from keeping this belief?
- What negative consequences go along with keeping this belief?
- Is there anything else that could explain this situation?

FIGURE 1. Response Record

condition or health as triggers to dysfunctional thinking. Those with other psychosocial issues and those with psychiatric overlay will also experience other daily life events unrelated to health that serve as triggers to dysfunctional thinking.

As is typical of many thought records (Beck 1995), the response record challenges the client to consider alternative ways of thinking and viewing his or her situation. When the therapist decides to use the response record, clients should also be trained and socialized in how to ask themselves the questions contained in the response record shown in Figure 1 as well as other questions that are consistent with the Socratic method (Beck, Shaw and Emory, 1979; Beck, 1995; Moorey and Greer, 2002) if they are found to be helpful to the client.

One example of a completed response record is presented in Figure 2. This response record was completed with the client Paulette, who has rheumatoid arthritis. In this case Paulette had experienced a flare-up of her arthritic symptoms, which led her to anticipate that she might be unable to attend her niece's wedding. She began to feel anxious, had difficulty sleeping, and resorted to overeating to manage her increased anxiety. When Paulette reported this the next day in therapy, the therapist worked with her to complete the response record. As shown in Figure 2, Paulette identified her feeling as "worried" and noted four thoughts that passed through her mind. She circled "my family will think I don't care about them" as the thought that made her feel the worst. Her responses to the response record questions are also shown in the form. Paulette reported that completing the response record reduced her anxiety significantly. Following the therapy session she called her sister to explain that she might not be able to attend the wedding. Her sister reassured her that while she would be missed, everyone would understand.

Tailoring the thought record process

Aspects of doing the response record can be tailored to meet a client's more specific needs. It may require more than one session to work through examples of the response record with a client until he or she fully understands and becomes invested in the process. Therapists new to this exercise should always work through personal examples first before trying this with a client (Beck, 1995).

In some instances where the degree of distortion is not great or when it is difficult or impossible to change the cognition, the therapist may wish to consider another approach to the thought record, which is discussed in the next chapter. This approach focuses not on changing the cognition but on guiding the client to engage in an activity that reverses the consequences of the cognition.

Identifying Intermediate and Core Beliefs

According to Beck, (1995), intermediate and core beliefs are "the deeper, often unarticulated ideas or understandings that patients have about themselves, others, and their personal worlds which give rise to specific automatic thoughts"

Response Record				
Date: Nov. 3	**Health event trigger (or other triggering event):** Symptom flare-up			
What am I feeling right now? (Circle all that apply.)	panicked	numb	sad	angry
	hopeless	(worried)	other: (pain)	

What thoughts or pictures are passing through my mind?

I won't be able to attend my niece's wedding;
I will be letting my family down;
(My family will think I don't care about them;)
Maybe I won't be missed, anyway.

Which of these thoughts or pictures makes me feel the worst? (Circle one above.)

What are the emotional, behavioral, and physical consequences of thinking this way?		
Emotional: Feel more anxious	Behavioral: Eating too much	Physical: Increased pain, can't sleep

- What do I already know that supports this belief?
That my mother considers it rude to miss family events.
- What do I already know that does not support this belief?
My niece and brothers know me better than that and know
I would attend if I could.
- What might someone else think about this situation?
My brother knows what it is like to have to miss out on
activities because he had to miss my parents' anniversary when
he was dealing with depression.
- What advice would I give to a friend if he or she was in this situation?
Take care of yourself and explain your situation.
- What is the best possible outcome of this situation?
I could let them know how much I care by making it clear that
I really hate to miss this event.
- What is the worst possible outcome of this situation?
My mother will call me up and make me feel selfish and guilty.
- If the [worst outcome] were to happen, what could I do to minimize its impact?
I could send a message they could read or call them on a cell
phone during the event.
- Given what I know so far, how likely is [the worst outcome] to happen?
Likely, but that's ok.
- How do I benefit from keeping this belief?
I don't - I just feel guilty and sad.
- What negative consequences go along with keeping this belief?
Worry and sadness
- Is there anything else that could explain this situation?
I'm projecting my own insecurities onto the situation, but I
really doubt that knowing my mother.

FIGURE 2. Paulette's First Response Record

(p. 137). As discussed in previous chapters, the cognitive model theorizes that an individual's cognition is organized according to a distinct hierarchy in which core beliefs serve as the foundation for intermediate beliefs, which manifest in terms of attitudes, assumptions, or rules for living and acting in the world (Beck 1995). Automatic thoughts then reflect an individual's intermediate and core beliefs (Beck 1995).

Like automatic thoughts, intermediate and core beliefs that reflect dysfunctional thinking must be brought to consciousness, recognized by the client, and restructured. The primary means by which these more entrenched beliefs can be brought to consciousness is through a very specific sequence of questioning that allows the client to probe progressively deeper levels of consciousness. This strategy was introduced by Burns (1980) and it is also referred to as the "downward arrow technique."

The strategy proceeds as follows. Once the therapist has identified a hot thought (i.e., one characterized by an emotional experience and likely to have been prompted by an underlying dysfunctional belief system), the therapist then temporarily assumes the hot thought is true and questions the client as to the meaning of the hot thought.

Depending on the client and the nature of his or her "hot thought," other questions that target meaning might be utilized to elicit intermediate and core beliefs. Generally, questions that identify intermediate beliefs ask a client what a given thought, situation, or action means to them or means about their worldview, about their value system, or about the way the world works. In many cases, therapists will have to restate what the client is saying so as to articulate a given assumption, rule, or condition in the form of an intermediate belief.

For example, a client is asked: "What does it mean to you to use a scooter at the grocery store?" and he responds, "That I am exaggerating my illness." A therapist should then help the client identify his intermediate belief by articulating it for him: "ok, to make sure I understand, you have a belief that says if you use a scooter at the grocery store it means you are exaggerating your illness?"

If the client states or agrees with the therapist's phrasing of an intermediate belief, the therapist would then proceed to probe the core belief. This is done by asking the client "And if you were to exaggerate your illness, what would that say about you as a person?" As covered in Chapter 4, there are four types of core beliefs that apply to work with individuals with chronic conditions:

- Core beliefs about self
- Core beliefs about others
- Core beliefs about the health care system
- Core beliefs about the chronic condition.

Following this structure, the therapist would ask the client what a given thought, situation, or action conveys about

- Him or her as a person
- Other people in general

- Health care or health-care professionals in general
- His or her health condition

The following is an example of the process of identifying a core belief. As illustrated in Figure 3, Paulette's dilemma over whether to attend a family wedding generated the automatic thought, "My family will think I don't care." By posing questions about what her automatic thought meant about the way the world works, the therapist enabled Paulette to identify her intermediate belief as, "People should show they care at any cost." Finally, by using the framework above, the therapist posed the question, "If it were true that people should care at any cost, what would not going to the wedding say about you?" This question allowed Paulette to identify that her core belief was that "[she] is a selfish person." In discussing this core belief the therapist and Paulette were able to identify that it stemmed from relevant early childhood experiences of being told she was selfish each time she challenged her mother or failed to meet her mother's needs. Understanding core beliefs in the context of relevant childhood data can be important in cognitive conceptualization for many clients with chronic condi-

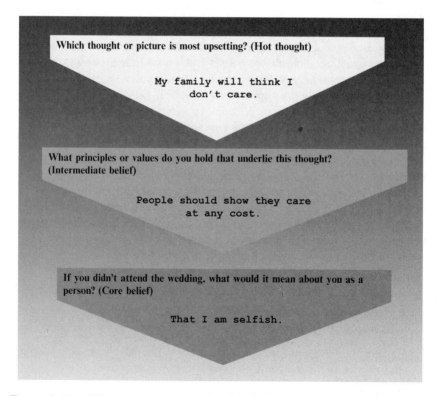

FIGURE 3. Use of Downward Sequential Questioning to Access Intermediate and Core Beliefs

tions (Beck, 1995). It also leads to an empathic understanding of the client in the context of his or her broader psychological development.

Modifying Intermediate and Core Beliefs

Just as it is important to teach a client to respond to his or her automatic thoughts, it is equally imperative to work with a client in order to modify and restructure his or her intermediate and core beliefs. In so doing, intermediate and core beliefs that represent firm convictions or strong beliefs must be distinguished from inter-mediate and core beliefs that the client only partially believes (Beck 1995). Sometimes it is difficult to get a client to a point where he or she is willing to admit that a particular belief is a firm conviction, particularly when he or she has insight into the fact that the belief is dysfunctional and is also aware that the ther-apist or others see that the belief has disadvantages.

Under these circumstances, empathic understanding can be used to assist clients in being truthful with themselves about the degree to which they endorse a given belief. In addition, the belief can be evaluated in terms of its relevance to the case conceptualization and in terms of its overall impact on quality of life and function-ing. Because intermediate and core beliefs are more likely to have been present since childhood and are more likely to be considered a key part of an individual's worldview, they are very difficult to modify. Consequently, therapists must take special care in gaining a full understanding of a client's cognition through observa-tion of cognitive patterns and by continually checking the accuracy of the case conceptualization through questioning and by soliciting feedback.

Once a firmly held intermediate or core belief is identified, a number of meth-ods can be utilized to assist a client in modifying or restructuring that belief. Some clients will have some insight or level of awareness that their belief is not adaptive. In this case Socratic questioning (discussed in Chapters 4 and 6) alone may allow the client to talk him- or herself into a more moderate or adaptive belief.

In other cases more structured exercises might be required. There are numer-ous ways to teach a client to evaluate the advantages and disadvantages of a given belief and to formulate new, more moderate and adaptive beliefs. These have been reviewed extensively by Beck (1995). The methods that will be considered in this text and that are most likely to be helpful for persons with chronic conditions are:

- Reframing the past
- Using the "Practicing Moderation in Beliefs" worksheet

These methods will be discussed below.

Reframing the Past

Clients with dysfunctional core beliefs can be asked about their first memories of having each belief (Beck 1995). Often these first memories date back to child-hood. Some clients, particularly those with previous experience in psychotherapy or those with highly difficult childhoods, will have numerous examples of how their negative core beliefs originated and how they were sustained throughout the course of their development. These clients can be guided backwards in time to think of personal examples that disconfirm the negative core belief during each developmental period. A time line is often helpful when pursuing this exercise with a client in therapy. To illustrate how such a time line works, we will consider Paulette once again. When asked to reflect on situations that led to her feeling unlovable, Paulette identified five incidents/situations spanning her childhood up to the present, which are shown in Figure 4. The therapist then helped Paulette to identify other circumstances/events occurring at the same time that contradicted her belief that she was unlovable. These are also reflected on Figure 4. By recording and reviewing these two sets of events/circumstances Paulette was able to reframe her belief that she was unlovable. Instead, she could see that others could respond to her in a variety of ways and that whether or not others approved of, cherished, or regarded her with affection was not linked to some trait or traits that made her unlovable.

Practicing Moderation in Beliefs

One of the most effective means of allowing a client to modify or restructure these more entrenched beliefs is to utilize the "Practicing Moderation in Beliefs" worksheet found in the Appendix of this chapter. Using this worksheet, a single core belief is selected during therapy and worked on by the client using a variety of examples that surface in his or her automatic thinking. In the arrows on the left-hand side of the worksheet, the client (and therapist, if necessary) fill in each

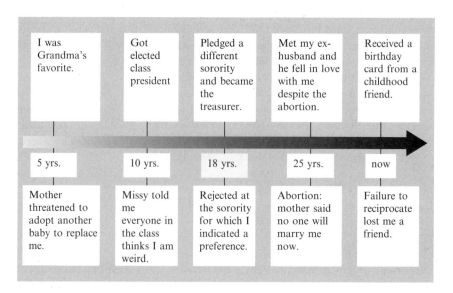

FIGURE 4. Reframing the Past: Paulette's Time Line

of the client's levels of dysfunctional cognition (i.e., the negative automatic (hot) thought, the intermediate belief, and the core belief). They then work together to identify more moderate or adaptive beliefs within each category. For many clients, the identification of more moderate and adaptive beliefs can be accomplished with the use of questions such as:

- Now that you have identified the worst outcome and the best outcome, what might be an outcome that is in-between?
- Can you think of a more moderate way of viewing this situation?
- Would you provide an example of how someone might cope with or adapt to this situation?
- What might someone with a more moderate viewpoint believe?
- Is there any middle ground between those two ideas?
- Do you think this is true all the time or is it more likely to be true when you are having a relapse?
- Do you think everyone has the same attitudes about disabled people?
- Can you think of anyone you know who is not impatient and uncaring?
- Have you ever known anyone that was capable of loving others even if the relationship was not very reciprocal? Do you believe such people exist?
- Have you ever had any other kinds of experiences with doctors and hospitals?
- Have you had any neutral experiences that do not stick out as having been so bad?
- Have you ever known someone who recovered from breast cancer?
- Have you ever had an experience where you took a medication and it worked?
- What do you make of the fact that the literature says that many people with your condition live into their 80s?

In the beginning stages of therapy, a therapist may need to provide the client with an alternative, more moderate or adaptive belief rather than relying solely on questioning. As therapy progresses and a client achieves more insight into his or her core beliefs and also has more experience working with them, questioning can be utilized more frequently and the client can be coached to revise his or her own maladaptive beliefs.

An example of the use of such a worksheet with Paulette, who has a core belief that involves her own lack of lovability, is provided in Figure 5. This first worksheet was completed in therapy. Paulette identified a disconcerting automatic thought that she was not as helpful to others as she had been in the past before her arthritis had progressed. Using Socratic questioning her therapist was able to help her identify that her underlying intermediate belief was, "I must be useful in order to be loved." As they explored together the underlying core belief, Paulette first stated it in terms of no one wanting to be around an ill person like herself who could offer little in return. Her therapist pointed out to her that this appeared to be the same belief they had identified earlier—i.e., that she was unlovable. Paulette agreed. With minimal coaching Paulette was able to come up with the revised thoughts that are shown in Figure 5. She felt a great deal of relief after completing the worksheet. Her therapist used this example to illustrate to Paulette

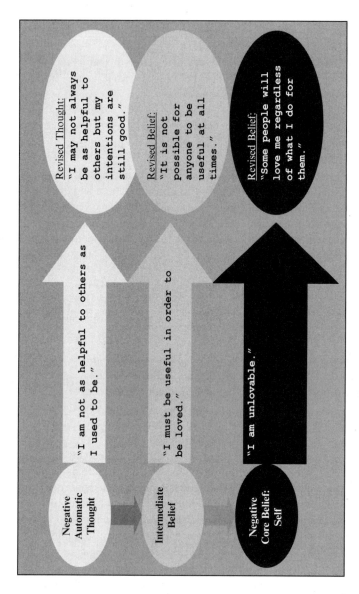

FIGURE 5. Paulette's Practicing Moderation in Beliefs Worksheet

how she could repeat the "Practicing Moderation in Beliefs" worksheet in the future to modify her cognitions and feel better.

Other Techniques for Addressing Unrealistic/Distorted Cognitions

In addition to the methods discussed above there are a number of other cognitive approaches to unrealistic/distorted cognitions. The final two methods that will be discussed in this chapter are:

- Imagining the extreme
- Finding positive examples

These methods can be used to address any or all of the three levels of cognition (core beliefs, intermediate beliefs, or automatic thoughts). These are not core parts of cognitive behavior therapy but are best considered ancillary techniques.

Imagining the Extreme

Clients that are working on negative beliefs about themselves or others that are not only negative but also unrealistic on some level can be asked to imagine someone else that represents the extreme version of that negative image (Beck 1995). For example, in working with Paulette's core belief that she is not lovable because she is disabled, the therapist would ask her to imagine a person (real or imagined) that would represent the most unlovable person alive. If necessary, Paulette might be coached to imagine an individual that is constantly hostile, rude, loud, and obnoxious regardless of the situation or person with whom she is interacting. This image might be offered to Paulette deliberately because it represents an individual with a personality and characteristics very different from her own.

Finding Positive Examples

Clients that are demoralized or having difficulty seeing themselves, others, or their health care workers in a positive light can be encouraged to think of positive examples of others facing similar circumstances. For example, consider the instance of a client that believes that "all health care professionals are burned out and do not care." Such a client might be encouraged to recall a positive example that they or one of their family members have encountered when ill. If they can't recall this, they might be coached to recall or imagine examples they have read about or seen on television or in a movie.

Another example is client that believes that "if you tell people you have a chronic illness, they are immediately made to feel uncomfortable." Such a client may benefit from learning about advocacy-based organizations that view illness and disability as a neutral human difference and normal part of life. This client might also be encouraged to be vigilant to watch for people who don't react with discomfort or to look for other, positive reactions that persons might have in addition to any discomfort they might display. Such a client might discover, for example, that while many people are uncomfortable and don't know quite how to respond to the news that one has a chronic condition, most will make an attempt to say or do something positive once they know.

Conclusion

This chapter described cognitive behavioral methods that are likely to be most effective in addressing the client with a chronic condition who has distorted thinking. These techniques have a common characteristic of aiming to change the cognition in some way. For clients who have cognitive distortions, it is important to address and, when possible, alter the cognition. The next chapter addresses those situations in which the cognition is mostly based in reality but is still maladaptive in some way.

Appendix

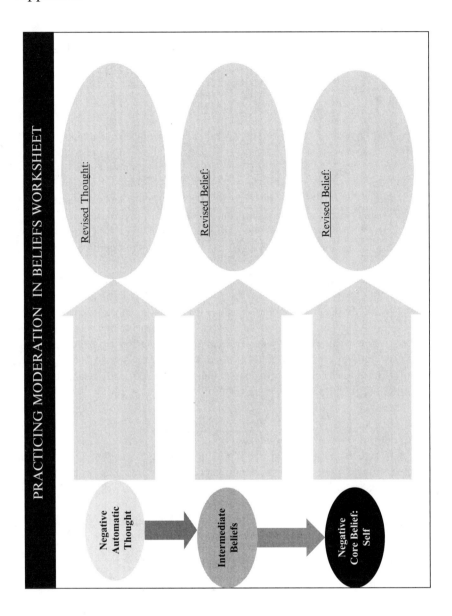

PRACTICING MODERATION IN BELIEFS WORKSHEET

Revised Thought:

Revised Belief:

Revised Belief:

Negative Automatic Thought

Intermediate Beliefs

Negative Core Belief: Self

8

Techniques for Addressing Realistic but Maladaptive Cognitions

As noted in Chapter 5, persons with chronic conditions can have maladaptive cognitions that do not involve distortion of reality. In these cases, clients may be plagued with realistic worries and anxieties. These negative cognitions can become preoccupations that increase stress, hinder positive coping and interfere with doings that matter to the client.

It is not appropriate to challenge or try to correct the beliefs of clients who report negative thoughts that are valid based on their experience and well grounded in reality (White, 2001). For example, clients with advanced cancer who worry that their chemotherapy might not be successful or are concerned about what will happen to their partners if they die are well justified in having these concerns. Therapists working with individuals with chronic conditions must be continually aware of times during which their clients' beliefs are realistically negative versus when their beliefs reflect errors in thinking.

Research has found that people's appraisals of negative life events are not static, nor is their adjustment to chronic illness (Moorey, 1996). Sometimes the adjustment process will be complicated by psychiatric overlay and other times it will not. When adjustment to chronic illness or disability is characterized by usual and expected reactions, therapists should validate those reactions, work to understand the meaning of a client's beliefs, and work to facilitate a client's emotional adjustment to his or her circumstances (Moorey, 1996).

In the initial stages of therapy, many clients with chronic conditions, and particularly those with long-standing illness, may appear to hold only realistic negative cognitions. Later in therapy as they become more comfortable with disclosure and as the therapist becomes more familiar with the client's general cognitive style, a therapist may begin to detect some distorted beliefs in addition to realistic negative cognitions.

However, regardless of what the future of therapy might bring, when a client appears to report only realistic negative cognitions, initial socialization to the cognitive model should always teach the client that his or her beliefs are not always incorrect and will not always need to be modified, even if they tend to be negative. The therapist should then inform the client that in these cases the therapy will focus on teaching the client how to manage his or her negative thoughts so that they do not completely restrict his or her functioning and well-being. (Moorey, 1996; Moorey and Greer, 2002 book; White, 2001).

A number of cognitive behavioral techniques can be useful with individuals with chronic conditions who have maladaptive cognitions that do not involve cognitive distortion. These include

- An adapted approach to the thought record
- Finding benefit
- Fast-forwarding
- Positive imagery
- The responsibility jigsaw
- Planning for the future
- Treatment decision-making
- Problem-solving
- Self-advocacy training
- Thought-stopping
- Distraction and meditation
- Coaching lists
- Involving partners and family members in therapy

Each of these methods will be discussed in this chapter.

Adapted Thought Record

Because many individuals with chronic conditions may have realistic, yet negative cognitions, it is important to shift the emphasis of the thought record intervention toward prompting clients to take some kind of action aimed to reverse the maladaptive mood-related or behavioral consequences of their thinking. To this end the author has adapted the thought record to create a "reversal record" (see Figure 1), which emphasizes how to manage the painful or interfering cognition.

Instead of focusing on challenging the cognition, the reversal record emphasizes recognition of its consequence and choosing a reversal activity to alter the mood-related and behavioral consequences of negative thinking. The reversal record was inspired by the work of Beck (1995), Greenberger and Padesky (1995), Seligman (2002), Ellis (1962), Michenbaum (1977), and White (2001).

The Reversal Activity

Most fundamental to the Reversal Record is that a client is required to select a "reversal activity." The reversal activity can consist of any one of the following categories of activities:

- Coping mechanisms
- Self-care activities

Reversal Record				
Date:	Health Event Trigger (or other triggering event):			
What am I feeling right now? (Circle all that apply.)	Panicked	Numb	sad	angry
	hopeless	worried	other:	
What thoughts or pictures are passing through my mind?				
Which of these thoughts or pictures makes me feel the worst? (circle one above)				

What are the emotional, behavioral, and physical consequences of thinking this way?

Emotional:	Behavioral:	Physical:

	Are there alternative ways to view this situation or picture?	____ Yes, I can think of the following alternative:
		____No, this is a realistic belief ⬇

Highly useful	1 2 3 4 5 6 7 8 9 10	**Not at all useful** ⬅	How useful is this belief:
Reversal activity:			

FIGURE 1. Reversal Record

- Gratifying activities
- Distraction exercises
- Pleasurable activities
- Motivating activities
- Goal-oriented activities

The literal definition of a reversal activity is one that aims to reverse the mood, behavioral, or physiological consequence of the maladaptive thought. Typically these are empirically validated exercises or activities that correspond to reducing the given consequence (e.g., walking to alleviate anxiety) and they are designed to facilitate coping, emotion regulation, or engagement in activity. However, because some clients may feel constrained by limited choices and may prefer to develop and discover their own additional activities, the meaning of a reversal activity can be adjusted to encompass motivating activities, self-care activities, and activities that a client finds pleasurable or gratifying.

The Appendix at the end of this chapter contains a list of reversal activities that can be provided to the client to generate ideas. Reversal activities would typically be selected by the therapist and client prior to the thought record exercise, and they would be refined and added to as therapy progresses. It is a good idea to support each client to prepare and maintain a list of personalized reversal activities.

The process of choosing and enacting reversal activities can sometimes be challenging. As noted earlier, it is useful to help the client to create a personalized list of reversal activities which are carried or kept handy along with the response record. Activities can be listed on an index card or in other formats that are tangible and accessible to the client.

Since completion of the record is usually assigned as homework, it is part of the therapy session structure to check the homework and identify any difficulties the client has following through on reversal activities. When there are difficulties, the therapist and client should problem-solve about how to remove barriers, identify more realistic and motivating activities, and otherwise assure that the client can choose and enact the activities.

The following is an example of use of the reversal record. Curtis was referred to therapy shortly after his initial surgery and the news that his prostate cancer had spread into the surrounding pelvic lymph nodes and was inoperable. During the initial assessment, Curtis reported to the therapist that he originally experienced a series of severe panic attacks associated with the fear that he was dying. He also reported insomnia and nightmares. He indicated that the depression and anxiety had lessened somewhat since he began taking the antidepressant medication his physician prescribed. However, he noted that he still had "minor panic attacks" at times when he thought about his diagnosis, and his sleep difficulties had become worse, rather than better. When questioned further about his thoughts, Curtis indicated that they had to do with the fear of dying. Curtis's fear was not unrealistic, since there was a significant likelihood that the cancer would spread to major organs, such as the bones, kidneys, bladder, or brain, within the next six months to one year. It appeared as though Curtis's recurrent thoughts about dying were interfering with his desire to make the most of the time he had remaining.

Based on this information, the therapist recommended that Curtis might find the reversal record a helpful tool. Curtis agreed that he would be willing to try anything that might help him control his anxiety and fear and focus on living in the here and now. Figure 2 shows the reversal record that Curtis completed in therapy.

In completing this reversal record, Curtis recalled that whenever he was reminded of his illness by receiving a bill from the hospital, a notice from his insurance company, or a call from the pharmacy or doctor, which happened almost daily, he had a tendency to become sad, anxious, and unable to sleep in the evening. He described his feelings as being "paralyzed" and "unable to do anything but stare into space and worry." During this particular session, he indicated that this had occurred earlier in the day when the mail came and he had received what appeared to be a hospital bill. He had planned to go out and work in the garden and went to pick up the mail first. Then, when he saw the envelope, he was overwhelmed

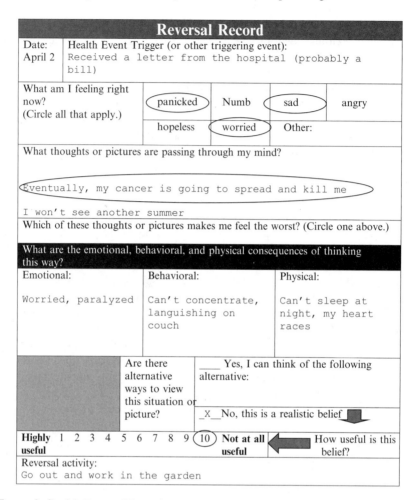

FIGURE 2. Curtis's Reversal Record

by negative emotion and sat for an hour thinking about how he probably would not be around next summer to work in the garden.

The therapist supported Curtis in his concern about the possibility that the cancer could progress and take away his ability to work in the garden next year. At the same time, the therapist reminded Curtis that he could prevent the cancer from taking away his ability to work in his garden in the present time by testing the possibility that doing work in his garden would be enjoyable to him now. Curtis's belief that he couldn't control the cancer was validated. At the same time, the therapist reminded him that he could control the decision as to whether he went outside to work in the garden today. Curtis agreed that that next time he got a letter or other reminder of his health condition, he would immediately force himself to go out and spend some time in the garden.

The next week Curtis reported that on two occasions he had received letters reminding him of his condition and on each occasion he went out to work in the garden and found not only that it reduced his anxiety and sadness but that he actually enjoyed being in the garden. He was even able to make the following humorous comment, "I guess the more of those letters I get, the better our garden is going to look."

Using reversal activities in association with negative moods and behaviors in the absence of clear triggers or automatic thoughts

Some clients with chronic conditions report mood or behavioral symptoms (e.g., depression, anxiety, isolative behavior) that wax and wane chronically and do not appear to correspond to specific antecedent health-care triggers and automatic thoughts. In these cases, thought records may be reformatted to elicit specific information about other temporal, situational, or environmental covariates. For instance, when a client is feeling a negative emotion (e.g., anxious or depressed) and can't identify any thoughts going through his or her mind or any precipitating events, the client can be coached to ask questions such as:

- Where am I right now?
- Am I alone or with others? Whom am I with?
- What am I doing now?
- What time of day or night is it?

This process has been referred to as "information gathering" and its aim is to generate insights into circumstances that surround negative emotions (Moorey and Greer, 2001).

For example, Curtis reported that he also experienced waves of anxiety that did not appear linked to any specific triggering event. By carefully recording the times that his anxiety was at its worst, Curtis identified that he tended to be most anxious in the mornings when eating breakfast. Once this was discovered, future homework assignments focused on having Curtis select more active reversal activities during or immediately following breakfast. He decided to reinstate the subscription he had to a favorite newspaper and read it at breakfast, and he started taking a short walk immediately after breakfast. This had the effect of reducing his anxiety during this time and it increased his level of perceived control over his symptoms.

Benefit-Finding: The Good and the Bad

Benefit-finding is the process of finding examples of how a life event, such as a chronic condition, has been associated with positive changes or positive outcomes in one's life. Individuals facing a variety of life circumstances, including bereavement (Davis, Jason, and Banghart, 1998), bone marrow transplant (Fromm, Andrykowski and Hunt, 1996), cancer (Antoni et al., 2001), childhood sexual abuse (McMillen, Zuravin, and Rideout 1995), heart attack (Affleck,

Tennen, Croog and Levine 1987), fibromyalgia (Affleck and Tennen 1996), HIV infection (Updegraff, Taylor, Kemery and Wyatt 2002), infertility (McLaney, Tennen, Affleck, and Fitzgerald 1995), lupus (Katz, Flasher, Cacciapoglia and Nelson 2001), multiple sclerosis (Mohr, Dick, Russo, Pinn, Boudewyn, Likosky, and Goodkin 1999), rheumatoid arthritis (Tennen, Affleck, Urrows, Higgins, and Mendola 1992), and motor vehicle accidents (Joseph, Williams and Yule 1993) have been found to report positive outcomes associated with these events.

The ability to engage in benefit-finding has been linked with positive quality of life outcomes and lower distress and depression in a number of studies (Davis, Nolen-Hoeksema, and Larson 1998; McMillen, Smith and Fisher 1997; Revenson, Wollman, and Felton 1983; Taylor 1983; Taylor, Lichtman, and Wood 1984; Thompson 1985; Tomich, and Helgeson 2002). Carver and Antoni (2004) recently found that benefit-finding within one year following breast cancer surgery predicted lower distress and depression four to seven years later (controlling for initial levels of distress and depression). In addition, benefit-finding has been emphasized in some cognitive behavioral interventions (e.g., Antoni et al., 2001).

In a study of women with breast cancer, Antoni and associates (2001) found that women with breast cancer who participated in cognitive behavioral therapy were more likely to be able to identify benefits related to having had breast cancer than controls. Some of the benefits that were identified included: "Breast cancer has led me to be more accepting of things," "Breast cancer has brought my family closer together," "Breast cancer has shown me that all people need to be loved," and "Breast cancer has helped me become a stronger person, more able to cope effectively with future life challenges." Sears, Stanton, and Danoff-Burg (2003) found that 83 percent of women with breast cancer were able to identify at least one benefit from their experience with breast cancer. The most common benefit involved improved relationships with others.

Despite these findings, not all studies would suggest that benefit-finding is associated with positive outcomes. Directly asking clients to search for personal examples of how their condition has contributed positively to their lives may not be helpful or welcomed (Lehman et al., 1993; Park, Cohen, and Murch 1996; Sears, Stanton, and Danoff-Burg 2003). The author's clinical experience working with clients with chronic conditions would support this argument. Some clients will feel highly invalidated, personally offended, or resentful if asked to identify benefits of having a chronic condition, particularly if their primary experience is that the condition has only led to a series of painful losses.

It is important to recognize that clients will react differently to having a chronic condition depending on their stage of adjustment to the illness and a number of other variables. Individuals with prior experiences of life trauma, greater negative affect, and greater disease severity have been found to perceive greater benefits of chronic illness (Tomich and Helgeson 2004). Sociodemographic characteristics have also been found to explain differences in benefit finding. Low socioeconomic status and being a member of a numerical minority group, which may be related to having different religious beliefs and coping styles, have been linked to a greater ability to engage in benefit-finding in a study of women with breast cancer (Tomich and Helgeson 2004).

Sears, Stanton, and Danoff-Burg (2003) suggest that interventions that aim to increase benefit-finding and positive reappraisal coping (as defined by responses to the positive reappraisal subscale of the COPE – Carver, Schier, and Weintraub, 1989) may not be universally helpful to clients and should be approached carefully in clinical practice. Therapists should never impose a goal or suggestion that a client should try to find benefit in their experience (Sears et al., 2003).

Rather, they should question clients about their general tendency and coping styles when faced with stressful situations. Alternatively, they can administer the COPE (Carver et al., 1989) to get a better sense of a client's general coping style and then examine the client's responses to the positive reappraisal subscale. If it becomes evident that a client "always tries to find something positive in a bad situation," therapists can then help clients make active use of these coping strategies.

The Fast-Forwarding Technique

The strategy of fast-forwarding involves guiding a client to think about or picture him/herself in a future point in time that is fundamentally different from the present time. This technique is most useful for clients that are anticipating an upcoming stressful event, such as a major medical procedure. These clients can be guided to think about or picture themselves having successfully completed the procedure and recovery period. This technique is also very useful for clients experiencing a relapse or flare-up of symptoms who are also feeling stuck, demoralized, and hopeless in their current situation.

Reminding clients with chronic conditions that are relapsing and remitting that change is inevitable in life, that you have witnessed they have better periods, and that tomorrow (or two weeks from now) can bring an entirely different experience than what they are currently facing can be very reassuring. Clients who respond that the future might be worse than the present should be reminded that no matter how bad the future is, change in that future will also be inevitable, so positive circumstances are bound to occur in life.

Positive Imagery

Positive imagery encompasses a number of brief or more involved meditation exercises. One technique commonly used in cognitive behavioral therapy involves "coping in the image" (Beck 1995). This approach is used when a client reports a negative experience with which he or she had a difficult time coping, and it can also be used when a client is anticipating difficulties coping with an upcoming stressful event.

In this approach, the therapist guides the client to imagine the event and imagine him- or herself coping effectively with that event. In some cases, the therapist may need to tell the client what effective coping might look like before beginning the imagery exercise. Similarly, clients with unrealistic images can be coached through a process of changing the image or the anticipated sequence of events in their minds (Beck, 1995).

Positive imagery can also be a fundamental part of a structured relaxation or meditation exercise. For example, with the use of a script a client can be guided to envision him- or herself visiting his or her real or imagined "favorite place" and taking in the sights, sounds, weather, and memories associated with that place.

Responsibility Jigsaw

The responsibility jigsaw is an adaptation of the "pie technique" (Beck 1995) and the "responsibility pie" (Greenberger and Padesky 1995). The responsibility jigsaw is recommended for use with clients that are struggling with issues related to anger, guilt, or shame. These more difficult emotions are often linked to dysfunctional cognitions involving blame. There are times during a chronic illness or new-onset disability when clients may struggle with these feelings as they relate to circumstances surrounding the onset of their illness or impairment, unexpected difficulties with the course of treatment, or as they relate to the functional and social losses associated with their condition. Issues of guilt and shame may also emerge for some clients with terminal illness who may examine their relationships, their behaviors, and their lives as a whole as they anticipate their death.

For example, Curtis, a husband and father, expressed tremendous concern that he would die before he could pay off his debts, leaving his family in a financial crisis. Curtis blamed this circumstance entirely on himself and felt incredibly shameful for "not having planned more effectively." To assist clients like Curtis in seeing that negative life circumstances are often multifactorial and not solely the fault of a single individual, event or behavior, this exercise asks the client to fill in all of the "pieces of the puzzle" that had a role in the negative outcome. This helps diffuse the sense of self-blame that an individual might carry as a result of limitations or losses imposed by a chronic condition. Curtis's jigsaw, which is presented in Figure 3, allowed him to recognize that a series of interconnected events (including other persons' decisions) actually contributed to his family's current financial crisis. This led to some relief of his self-blame and shame.

Planning for the Future

For clients with realistic concerns about the future who can tolerate the anxiety involved in problem-solving and planning, this strategy can be used to ultimately

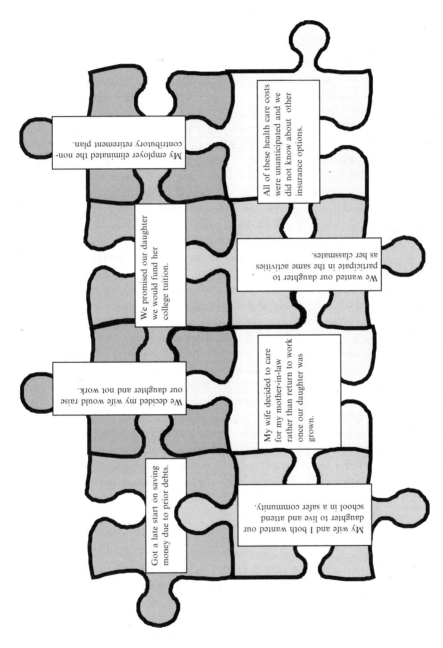

FIGURE 3. Curtis's Responsibility Jigsaw—*Situation: Financial Crisis*

alleviate anticipatory anxiety. The planning for the future exercise is best used with individuals that

- Are aware that their conditions are progressive or terminal,
- Are emotionally stable,
- Do not use denial as a coping mechanism.

Clients who anticipate that they are going to require increased assistance with functioning can be coached to problem-solve about what resources they will require to function as independently as possible. These resources may range from having an in-home personal care assistant, to hiring a housekeeper, to renovating the home for greater accessibility, to obtaining a motorized transportation device. Occupational or physical therapists specializing in home modification and assistive technologies should be consulted to assist clients with the more pragmatic aspects of this planning.

Clients with terminal illness who are concerned about the welfare of loved ones can be assisted in listing unresolved business in their lives and in anticipating the potential ways in which their death would affect the lives of others. They can then be assisted in problem-solving about ways to reduce negative outcomes.

For example, if a client is worried about the well-being of others for whom he or she is responsible as a caretaker (e.g., children, a partner, or a disabled parent), a plan can be constructed to try to maximize the likelihood that these individuals will be taken care of in his or her absence. If a client expresses a wish for assistance in planning for his or her anticipated death, suggestions can be made regarding constructing a will, contacting a financial planner, arranging for a disabled parent to enter a care facility, and selecting and notifying a close friend or family member to serve as a guardian for children. A client may also wish to prepare letters, audiotapes, or videotapes of messages, thoughts, advice or stories he or she wishes to leave behind for children, partners, and other loved ones.

Though clients report that these exercises in closure can bring a degree of relief and peace, therapists and clients who undertake this task should be prepared for the emotional pain that often accompanies the process of planning to say good-bye to loved ones. To decrease feelings of isolation and fear, clients may wish to engage in this planning only at specifically scheduled times or when in the presence of the therapist.

Treatment Decision-Making

Chronic conditions are often complex and in many cases there are no easy answers about how best to treat them. Though many physicians still attempt to make treatment decisions for their clients by strongly recommending one treatment over another, some are increasingly making more options available to their patients. Though this may be overwhelming, the greater the role a client has in his or her treatment decision-making the more likely he or she will be to attempt and stick with a given treatment option.

Throughout the course of managing their illness, many clients with chronic conditions are faced with very difficult decisions. These decisions can involve such things as deciding which medication option to pursue, deciding whether or not to undergo surgery, and deciding which doctor's advice to follow. Decisions about medical care are unique in that they often involve eliminating the "worst of the evils" rather than having the privilege of selecting an appealing option.

Clients may also have difficulty making decisions about issues in their lives that are secondary to the chronic illness or impairment, such as whether to remain employed, how much to rely on friends for assistance, and whether and when to tell others about the diagnosis. If not addressed, difficulties with decision-making can have serious implications. This is particularly so if they delay or interfere with a recommended course of treatment. Difficulties with treatment decision-making are often evident in avoidant or noncompliant behaviors. At times, difficulties with treatment decision-making can be masked by what initially appears to be denial or apathy. For these reasons, clients that do not spontaneously report issues related to decision-making but appear to be avoiding recommended treatments should be asked directly about these issues.

Once a problem with decision-making has been identified, therapists can construct worksheets, like the one presented in Figure 4, to assist clients in organizing their thinking and in weighing the advantages and disadvantages of a given action. Depending on their intellectual, cognitive, and educational capacities, some clients can be encouraged to search the Internet and medical journals to begin to complete the table. Others will do this naturally on their own. In all

Treatment	Description and purpose	Success rates for my stage/type of cancer	Risks & side effects	Long-term consequences of pursuing this treatment	Long-term consequences of not pursuing this treatment

FIGURE 4. Weighing Medical Treatment Options: Curtis's Worksheet

cases, a client will need to consult his or her physician to determine whether the research and information he or she has used to complete the table is accurate, and to provide additional medical information required to complete the decision matrix. Many clients will want to obtain second and third opinions regarding the accuracy of the information contained in the matrix, and they should be encouraged to do this if they so desire. Therapists should never allow clients to make treatment decisions based on information that has not been approved by a physician.

Figure 4 shows the type of worksheet that clients can be provided. The worksheet has spaces for patients to list their various treatment options and the likely outcomes, including risks of going forward or not pursuing the treatment. The worksheet is often helpful for clients to record the information they receive from their physician(s). It allows them to see all the information in one place and to make comparisons of the different treatment options that are available.

As illustrated in Figure 4, in the first column of the worksheet the treatment option should be listed. In Column 2, the procedures and purposes of that form of treatment are described. Column 3 lists the anticipated success rates for that treatment option. It is important that the success rates account for the particular subtype of the illness condition. For example, cure and survival rates associated with radical prostatectomy, or the removal of the prostate gland and seminal vesicles, will vary greatly depending on whether the cancer cells have penetrated the capsule or not. Column 4 includes risks and side effects of a given treatment (including side effects of medications and their expected duration). Column 5 includes long-term consequences of pursuing the treatment and Column 6 includes the long-term consequences of not pursuing the treatment.

As clients complete worksheets it is important that they verify with their physicians that the information in the worksheet is accurate. Ultimately the purpose of the worksheet is to organize information that is often difficult for a client to remember and that, sometimes, the client does not receive. The role of the therapist is not to lead a client toward a particular treatment decision but to assist the client to gather and organize all the necessary information to make an informed decision in consultation with the physician.

Problem-Solving

Problem-solving has been written about extensively in cognitive behavioral therapy (e.g., D'Zurilla and Goldfried 1971; D'Zurilla and Nezu 2001; Turk and Salovey 1995). It has been found to be particularly useful to individuals managing chronic conditions. Turk and Salovey (1995) have recommended a set of general guidelines for therapists to consider when teaching clients with chronic illness problem-solving skills. Therapists who use problem-solving techniques regularly will find their detailed guidelines helpful. Their guidelines, in part, are reflected in the worksheet presented in Figure 5. This worksheet is designed to coach clients to take more initiative in problem-solving.

Problem-Solving Worksheet					
Problem:				Date:	
Goal:					
Steps I can take					
Potential consequences of these steps					
What will I do?					
Alternate action if it does not work					
What did I do?			Was it effective?	__Yes	
				__No	
What happened?					

FIGURE 5. Problem-Solving Worksheet

Readers may notice some similarities between this worksheet and the goal form presented in Chapter 4. Problem-solving (and use of this worksheet) can be efficiently accomplished by building it into a client's weekly goal-attainment reporting. Therapists can begin by providing clients with some examples of suggested ways to solve the problem and by asking the client for feedback about the predicted efficacy of those approaches. Quickly thereafter, the therapist can begin to ask the client to brainstorm and evaluate potential solutions on his or her own.

The following is an example of the use of the problem solving worksheet. Curtis was feeling that his urologist was not competent because his prediction of the outcome of the initial treatment turned out to be wrong. As shown in Figure 6, Curtis decided to undertake a series of steps to identify a new urologist covered by his insurance. After making an appointment and seeing the new urologist, Curtis received feedback that his original urologist had taken the appropriate course of action and that the information he gave Curtis was accurate given what was known

Problem-Solving Worksheet					
Problem: Difficulty finding a competent urologist				**Date:** 5/6/02	
Goal: Find a competent urologist					
Steps I can take	List what is important to me in a doctor.	Internet search of top urologists in my State.	Check whether the doctor accepts my insurance.	Call hospitals or offices and ask nurses to provide their opinions about nominated physicians.	
Potential consequences of these steps	Time and energy to find a good doctor, but I might find a good doctor.				
What will I do?	Follow all the steps in sequence.				
Alternate action if it does not work	Use the same process to develop a new list of doctors. Consider traveling to see a urologist and expanding the search to other states or regions of the country.				
What did I do? Followed all the steps			Was it effective?	X Yes __No	
What happened? I identified three potential doctors and I made an appointment with the one that was closest to my home.					

FIGURE 6. Curtis' Problem Solving Worksheet

at the time. As a result of this, Curtis's decided to retain his original urologist. The importance of this process was that it restored Curtis's sense of confidence in his urologist and allowed him to work more effectively with this physician.

Self-Advocacy Training

Often referred to as "assertiveness and communication training" within the cognitive behavioral literature, self-advocacy training involves teaching and empowering clients to act in their own best interest when interacting with health care professionals, employers, friends, family, partners, and others. Self-advocacy training can assist clients in reestablishing positions of esteem and in reinvoking former roles within family and work settings (Turk and Salovey 1995). It can also facilitate clearer and more useful communication with health-care professionals.

Self-advocacy training is most typically approached by role-playing difficult interpersonal scenarios with clients, modeling assertive interpersonal behavior, and providing clients with feedback if they should demonstrate nonassertive behavior or difficulties with communication. Self-advocacy training can also be accomplished with the assistance of peer mentors at centers for independent living. These centers, which number approximately 500 nationwide, are organized by and for individuals with disabilities to address issues of inclusion, advocacy, and public policy for people with disabilities.

Thought-Stopping

Thought-stopping involves teaching a client to actively clear his or her mind of verbal messages or visual images that are negative or painful (Beck and Emery 1985; Davis, Eshelman, and McKay 1988). Thought-stopping (or image-stopping) is best used as a means of coping with an acutely difficult situation. Thought-stopping is accomplished by instructing a client to say "stop," picture a barricade or stop sign in his or her mind, and/or snap a rubber band around his or her wrist when a negative thought or image comes to mind.

The negative thought is then arrested by one of two techniques:

- Actively substituting it with a soothing or positive alternative
- Using distraction techniques (described below) to arrest the negative thinking.

Therapists should keep in mind that this technique is not recommended for long-term use in controlling intrusive thoughts and images, since research has found that thought suppression can lead to an increase in intrusive thoughts or images, rather than a decrease.

Distraction and Meditation

Attention, distraction and meditation techniques have been shown to be effective in managing anxiety related to chronic illness and painful medical procedures (Kabat-Zin 2005; Papageorgious and Wells 1998).

The method of distraction is most often prescribed as a means of managing acute anxiety and pain states, such as those experienced during medical procedures. Meditation offers another means by which clients with chronic conditions can manage their symptoms and stress levels and also learn to cope with acute crisis situations. Kabat-Zin (1990, 2005) has made some significant contributions to the literature in this area.

Before describing any of these techniques to clients, therapists should first explain to clients the powerful influence that attention can have on perception (Turk and Salovey 1995). Clients can be informed that, typically, people are able to focus their attention on only one thought, feeling, or sensation at a time. Clients should also be informed that, although it may be difficult in times of intense pain, it is possible to exert some control over what one chooses to pay attention to (Turk and Salovey 1995).

Some examples of distraction and meditation techniques recommended for use with individuals with chronic conditions are described in Table 1. These have been adapted from techniques used by Johnson and Webster (2002) and Kabat-Zin (1990, 2005).

Coaching Lists

Clients can be encouraged to observe situations, people, and environments that are stress reducing and stress promoting. They can be encouraged to make lists of those situations so that they will remember to either increase or decrease their interactions with those situations, people, or environments in the future. Examples of such lists might include: "A list of people who cause me stress," "A list of quiet and uncrowded restaurants with good food," "A list of situations that zap energy," "A list of situations that cause me stress or frustration." Clients can also be educated about the importance and need for ongoing self-encouragement. Statements that reflect what is commonly referred to as "positive self talk" can also be listed by clients.

Involving Partners and Family Members in Therapy

The emotional and psychological effects of chronic conditions are not limited to the clients who have them. Intimate partners, close friends and family members also undergo an adjustment process. For many, the chronic condition can lead to disorganization within the family system, role changes, financial losses, and other unanticipated stressors.

Intimate partners may become overwhelmed, anxious, or depressed by new caretaking responsibilities or by feelings of abandonment or anticipated loss of their loved one. Many partners will struggle with mixed or ambivalent feelings. Some may feel that relationships or entire households now revolve around medical issues or around the needs of the ill client. This may lead to feelings of resentment and anger in partners and family members. Children may be expected to take on new responsibilities and caregiving roles within the family. Some of these role changes may be inconsistent with Western standards for age-appropriate behavior. When parents are less available, children may spend more time alone and may also feel abandoned or less supported to pursue their academic responsibilities and extracurricular activities on their own.

These and other emotional and psychological reactions will become more exaggerated within an already-stressed family system or in one that is dysfunc-

TABLE 1. Distraction and meditation techniques

Technique	Indication	Procedure
Observational Thinking Distraction Technique (Johnson and Webster 2002)	To decrease intrusive thinking, reduce anxiety, and situate a client in a state of neutral, present awareness	1) Client is seated comfortably but is not permitted to turn head. 2) Client is asked to report one thing that he or she sees in his or her field of vision, one thing that he or she hears, and one bodily sensation that he or she feels. 3) Client is asked to report two new things he or she sees, hears, and feels. 4) Client is asked to continue this practice, each time adding one more to the number of things required to see, hear, and feel.
Favorite Place Distraction Technique (Johnson and Webster 2002)	Recommended for clients who need to distance themselves from a present painful, fearful, or uncomfortable situation.	1) Client is asked to imagine his or her favorite place – one that represents comfort, safety, or pleasure. This is labeled the "inside world." Client is then asked to turn his or her attention back to the present, which is labeled the "outside world." 2) Client is asked to name three things that he or she sees in his or her "outside" field of vision. 3) Client is asked to name three things that he or she sees in his or her "inside" field of vision. 4) Client is asked to name three sounds from the "outside world." 5) Client is asked to name three sounds from the "inside world." 6) Client is asked to name three bodily sensations from the "outside world." 7) Client is asked to name three bodily sensations from the "inside world." 8) Client is asked to continue this practice by either increasing or reducing the number of things he or she sees, hears and feels. 9) With time, all the therapist has to say is "outside" or "inside" in order to cue the client to switch his or her awareness from the outside to the inside world.

TABLE 1. *Continued*

Technique	Indication	Procedure
Breathing Meditation (Johnson and Webster 2002)	Best used in acute situations, such as when a client is in severe pain, feeling panicked, or undergoing a medical procedure.	1) Client is taught diaphragmatic breathing and instructed to breathe in through the nose, watching the lower abdominal area rise, and to breathe out through the mouth. 2) Once a comfortable breathing pattern has been established, client is asked to close the eyes while inhaling in and to open the eyes while exhaling. 3) Once this pattern has been established, the client is instructed imagine himself or herself breathing in a color, substance, or object that he imagines as being soothing, comforting, or purifying. He or she can then be instructed to breathe out a color, substance, or object that represents waste, negative energy, or toxicity.
Walking Meditation (Kabat-Zin 1990)	Used to alleviate preoccupation with negative thinking and to ground clients in present awareness. This can also be modified to encompass other physical activities. For example, clients that enjoy water can be encouraged to practice "swimming meditation" in which they focus on a single aspect of the swimming process.	1) The exercise is designed to train clients to selectively attend to the process of walking itself. 2) It is best performed in the smallest environments (i.e., pacing in lanes or walking in circles) to reinforce the need to focus on walking. 3) Any pace is appropriate, but the pace should be chosen to maximize the client's attention on the process of walking. Beginners should begin at a slow pace if possible. 4) A set time frame for walking should be chosen. Ten minutes is appropriate for beginners if it is well tolerated. 5) To calm the mind, walkers are to focus only on a single aspect of the walking process and should not shift their attention to any other aspect of walking. If a person chooses to focus on the sensations and movements of the feet, then this is where his or her attention should remain.

tional and thus more vulnerable to stressors associated with a chronic condition. Some partners or family members will attempt to involve themselves in a client's therapy, whereas other clients may wish to involve their partners or family members in therapy. Other clients may be unaware of the need for their partners or family members to be involved in therapy, or they may feel that they are solely to blame for the family problems.

During the course of treatment, a therapist will often face decisions about whether to involve certain family members in a client's treatment, whether to refer the entire family for family therapy, whether couples' therapy is indicated, or whether individual family members should be referred to undergo their own psychotherapy. A recent meta-analytic review of the general literature on psychosocial interventions for chronic illness revealed that interventions that include intimate partners have positive effects on clients' levels of depression and, in some cases, on mortality (Martire et al., 2004). Positive effects were also observed among family members themselves, and these included decreased caregiver burden, depression, and anxiety levels. The strongest effects were observed when the family member was provided with individual psychotherapy on a separate basis and when the intervention focused on addressing relationship issues (Martire et al., 2004).

As a general rule, family members should be involved in individual approaches to a client's cognitive behavioral therapy only if a client wishes for the family member to be involved, and only if the therapist determines that involvement of the family member will support the client in achieving his or her goals for therapy. Like clients, family members must be socialized to the cognitive model and must understand the importance of structure, homework, etc. before participating. In many cases, and particularly when dysfunctional systems are involved, a therapist may decide that partners and family members should be referred to another therapist for treatment because the risk for sabotaging a client's current work in therapy is too great.

Conclusion

This chapter discussed a number of methods which can be used to address maladaptive cognitions that do not involve distortion. While these methods have been discussed in this context, they may be also be used effectively with clients who do have distortions, when the aim is to manage the emotional and behavioral consequences of cognitive distortions while they exist and cause problems for the client.

Appendix

Examples of Reversal Activities

1) Listen to music or favorite radio program
2) Take a warm bath
3) Get favorite food or beverage
4) Listen to books on tape
5) Watch a movie or favorite television program
6) Read a book
7) Get a new hairstyle
8) Get a massage
9) Get a manicure or pedicure
10) Go to a museum or gallery
11) Go shopping just to browse
12) Attend a musical or theatrical event
13) Take a class to learn a new skill
    a. Learn advanced meditation or yoga
    b. Learn fly fishing
    c. Learn pottery
    d. Learn woodworking
    e. Learn welding
    f. Learn flower arranging
    g. Learn how to draw or paint
    h. Learn how to make stained glass
    i. Learn to sew or knit
14) Do a hobby you already know how to do
15) Form or join a group or club
    a. Book reading club
    b. Movie club
    c. Poetry group
    d. Support group
    e. Political club
    f. Debate club
    g. Religious club
16) Host a gathering of friends or have a party for yourself or someone else
17) Do something physically active
    a. Walking
    b. Boating
    c. Swimming
    d. Yoga
    e. Tai Chi
    f. Pilates
    g. Cycling

9

Behavioral Approaches

The previous two chapters examined therapeutic approaches which were predominantly cognitive in nature and which address problems associated with maladaptive cognitions. This chapter examines approaches which are more behavioral in nature. These include:

- Behavioral experiments
- Activity diaries
- Activity and exercise scheduling
- Systematic desensitization

These behaviorally oriented approaches are generally useful in addressing both kinds of maladaptive cognitions (i.e., those with and without distortion). Each is discussed below.

Behavioral Experiments

Behavioral experiments are actions or activities recommended by the therapist in order to allow a client to test the validity of his or her beliefs directly. Behavioral experiments are most appropriate for use with individuals with dysfunctional cognitions and behaviors that do not involve realistic cognitions but instead reflect systematic errors in thinking or excessive fears. These experiments should never be used as a means of invalidating a client's appropriate emotional reaction to a negative life event. However, they can sometimes be useful for a client to examine whether the extent of his or her preoccupation with certain concerns is necessary.

Because they represent a kind of "ultimate test" of the validity of a client's thoughts, great care should be taken in recommending behavioral experiments. They should only be recommended when the therapist is nearly 100 percent certain that the outcome of the experiment will be positive and will disprove the client's faulty belief (or allay the level of a client's preoccupation/concern). According to White (2001), behavioral experiments are most appropriate for the client with chronic conditions when:

- The client is at least partially open to considering that a given belief might not be valid and is willing to test its validity
- Attempts to change behavior through education or cognitive work alone are not working
- The therapist wants to teach a client a new way of coping with a difficult medical procedure or a new way of managing a given physical symptom
- A client is fearful or avoidant of activity
- A client is fearful or avoidant of medication and its side effects
- A client needs assistance in changing his or her interpersonal style when interacting with health-care professionals

Table 1 lists a number of examples of behavioral experiments.

When recommending a behavioral experiment, the therapist should assure that the client is prepared for all possible outcomes. Therapists should always be honest with their clients about the possibility that their engagement in an experiment might lead to a confirmation of their fears or concerns, rather than to a disconfirmation. Moreover, whenever engaging in a behavioral experiment that may have medical consequences, a physician should be consulted to make sure there are no contraindications. In addition, the results of a behavioral experiment should be reflected upon in therapy following the actual experiment. Examples of questions that can be used to assist a client in thinking through all aspects of the behavioral experiment are listed in Table 2.

Using Activity Diaries

Activity diaries can be useful to make clients aware of times when their activity patterns are problematic, unsatisfying or otherwise appear to warrant a change. Often the completion of the diary is sufficient to motivate and guide clients to

TABLE 1. Examples of behavioral experiments for individuals with chronic conditions.
- Test the belief that it was my medication that was responsible for my severe diarrhea last night (versus a transient stomach virus or a food contamination) by continuing to take the medication to see if the diarrhea continues.
- Test the belief that I am no longer attractive to my husband by asking him.
- Test the belief that increasing my walking time from 5 to 10 minutes twice per day will limit my energy to do other things I enjoy, by walking for 10 minutes twice a day for the next week.
- Test the belief that refraining from taking naps during the day will improve my overall ability to sleep at night by refraining from naps and logging my sleep patterns for the next week.
- Test the belief that my girlfriend will judge me if I have to stop at a gas station to use the bathroom on our way to the movie by doing so if I need to.
- Test the belief that swimming 5 minutes per day in the warm therapeutic pool will only increase my pain by swimming each day this coming week and logging my pain.
- Test the belief that I will become violently ill after this month's blood transfusion like I did last month, by going through with the transfusion as recommended by my doctor and asking the doctor whether anything can be done to avoid or reduce this side effect.

TABLE 2. Preparatory and processing questions for behavioral experiments.

Preparatory Questions	• How will this experiment test your belief that _____?
	• What would be the best possible outcome of this experiment?
	• What would be the worst possible outcome?
	• What do you predict will actually happen?
	• What will you do if the worst outcome comes true?
Processing Questions	• What happened when you tried _____?
	• Was it consistent with what you predicted would happen?
	• What is the main thing that you learned from this experiment?
	• Can you apply anything you learned from this experiment to other beliefs that you have wanted to test?
	• Would you be willing to use a behavioral experiment in the future for any other beliefs that you may wish to test?

make modifications in their activity patterns. When working with clients with chronic conditions, it is fundamental to obtain a thorough and accurate assessment of the nature, quantity, and attitudes toward activity before supporting a client to make changes or recommending changes in the nature or amount of his or her activity.

This assessment is best accomplished through the use of an activity diary. One example of an activity diary that is frequently used in practice and research is the National Institutes of Health Activity Record (NIH-ACTRE) (Furst et al. 1987; Gerber, and Furst 1992). The NIH-ACTRE is described in more detail in Chapter 13. Using this record, clients

- Record the types and times of their activities during half-hour periods
- Rate each activity in terms of the degree to which it engenders meaning, competence and enjoyment
- Indicate whether the activity is work, self-care, leisure, or rest
- Indicate the difficulty of the activity and whether it caused pain or fatigue
- Indicate whether they stopped to rest during the activity

While it gives a wealth of information, one potential limitation of the NIH-ACTRE is that it is lengthy and time-consuming to complete. A similar but shorter instrument is the Occupational Questionnaire (Smith, Kielhofner, and Watts 1986), which omits such information as that concerning pain, fatigue and rest. (It is available for download at moho.uic.edu).

The way these instruments are rated is consistent with other rating formats recommended in the cognitive behavioral literature. For example, Beck (1995) recommends that clients rate their activities on a scale of 1 to 10, reflecting the degree to which each activity engenders feelings of mastery or accomplishment and the degree to which each activity engenders feelings of pleasure. Rating systems like these are essential when attempting to motivate clients to resume and persist in a given activity following a prolonged relapse or difficult medical treatment. These ratings are also important in assisting clients in determining how to prioritize activities in terms of their available time and energy.

Depending on the needs and treatment goals of the client, activity can also be measured in relationship to physical and cognitive symptoms, beliefs, and mood. Examples of combined measurements that reflect these more complex relationships are provided in later chapters. Therapists may sometimes want to create simpler activity diaries for their clients that target specific needs. An example of a simplified activity diary is provided in Figure 1. In this record the client, Paulette, was asked to describe all activities performed each day and to rate them on a scale of 1 (low) to 10 (high) in terms of the degree to which they are consistent with her values, engender feelings of mastery or competence, and are pleasurable.

Paulette complained in therapy that her pain affected her quality of life negatively since she could not do so many of the things she previously enjoyed. Her psychotherapist recommended that Paulette complete the activity record as a homework assignment before the next session. This simplified activity record was used because Paulette was also reporting she was having difficulty concentrating due to the pain.

A brief look at only a single day in Paulette's activity record can provide information about the activities that she values, enjoys, and feels competent to perform. This was helpful to Paulette and her therapist when they began to make decisions together about prioritizing activities so that she could maximize her quality of life within the constraints imposed by her arthritis.

Daily Activity Record			
Date: July 1			Rating 10=Best 1=Worst
Activities Completed Today	Importance Rating	Competence Rating	Pleasure Rating
Washed and ironed clothes	10	3	3
Took son to school	10	5	5
Went to doctor	10	1	1
Watched son's soccer game	10	5	10
Read a chapter in a novel	3	5	10
Walked	10	5	8

FIGURE 1. Paulette's Daily Activity Record

Supplemental Devices Used to Record Activity

Clients involved in graded exercise programs, overactive clients, and those who are underactive and/or fearful of engaging in too much physical activity may benefit from supplemental devices to assist them in recording the amount of activity in which they are engaging. One of the most common and inexpensive means of recording activity is through the use of a pedometer, or step-counter, which can be obtained at any local sporting goods store. This device is worn on the hip and simply records the vertical stepping motion that occurs when an individual is running or walking. Motion can be recorded in terms of the number of steps taken or in terms of the amount of distance traveled. The total daily or weekly amounts of activity can then be tracked over time to measure a client's progress and setbacks. Actigraphs, which measure multidimensional movement, and other more sophisticated measurement devices can be obtained from a physical therapist or exercise physiologist.

Activity and Exercise Scheduling

Research indicates that individuals can experience consistent health benefits associated with incorporating at least 30 minutes of moderate- to vigorous-intensity physical exercise in their daily routines (United States Department of Health and Human Services, 1996). Engagement in any kind of activity, provided that it is valued, pleasurable, and characterized by feelings of increased competence, can lead to positive health outcomes (Kielhofner 2002, 2003). Yet individuals with chronic conditions who are newly disabled, are recovering from a particularly difficult medical procedure, or are coming out of a relapse will inevitably find it difficult to re-engage in activity or physical exercise for a number of reasons.

Generally, clients that have been forced to change their prior activity patterns dramatically may be vulnerable to patterns of underactivity, overactivity, or imbalances in activity, such as boom-bust patterns that involve periods of high-level activity followed by periods of low to no activity. Each of these three behavioral styles introduces unique challenges into the practice relationship. Scheduling of activity and exercise as part of cognitive behavioral therapy interventions should take into consideration the particular activity pattern the client has previously adopted.

There are a number of approaches that a cognitive behavioral therapist can take to assist a client in reengaging in activity in a positive way. Activity can be prescribed, scheduled, or recommended in the form of a behavioral experiment. Irrespective of the approach taken, the most fundamental rule to keep in mind is that any activity recommendation must be *graded*. Engagement in activity must be graded for a number of reasons.

- Clients that are inactive or have stopped activity due to circumstances involving their condition may experience muscle changes and cardiovascular deconditioning. Initially, activity may lead to increased pain levels, exhaustion, and other symptoms. It may be more difficult for clients with chronic conditions to work through the initial side effects that are often associated with reengagement in activity.

- Individuals that have been forced to stop working or to change their daily routines drastically have lost important roles as well as a sense of structure and routine (Kielhofner 2002). In many cases, they may no longer be able to engage in once-desired activities that were important to them and were characterized by feelings of competency and pleasure. Some clients may be lost or overwhelmed when it comes time to reengage in activity and may react by avoiding activity, by limiting their activity to narrow but essential categories, or by overestimating the amount of activity in which they are able to engage.
- Research indicates that drastic changes in activity levels (both dramatic increases and sudden decreases) alter healthy immune functioning. Clients with chronic conditions will report increased symptoms (and sometimes full-blown relapses) if too much physical activity is initiated too quickly.
- Clients that are not accustomed to regular physical activity as part of their daily routine may feel overwhelmed if too much time is taken up by activity without considering other time commitments within their usual daily routine.
- Clients can become easily discouraged if their expectations for positive outcomes of activity reengagement are too high. Clients should be advised to introduce one new activity at a time. They should be asked for feedback about how they experienced the activity. Feedback about whether the activity was important to the client, whether the client felt competent doing the activity, and whether the activity was pleasurable should serve as the criteria for continued pursuit of that activity.

Underactive Clients

When assessment reveals that a client is underactive, understimulated, and/or deconditioned, reengagement in activity is often recommended. An increase in the range or level of activity might also be recommended for nonsedentary clients with symptoms of depression and anxiety. Anaerobic and aerobic forms of physical exercise represent subtypes of physical activity that are often prescribed by cognitive behavioral therapists because these forms of activity, particularly if performed at an appropriate intensity level (Marcus et al., 2000) can improve endurance, muscle strength, and mood. Therapists prescribing graded exercise schedules for their patients should work collaboratively with physicians, exercise physiologists, and/or physical therapists to ensure that the client is engaging in levels of exercise that are safe, appropriate, and maximally beneficial to the client.

Exercise is not the only appropriate activity to prescribe when designing activity schedules for clients. For some clients with chronic illness, exercise is not well tolerated, and adherence is even more difficult to achieve when clients are not athletically inclined, do not have much prior experience with sports, and do not perceive or experience any significant, tangible benefits of their efforts. Regardless of the type of activity prescribed, any prescribed activity regime should reflect the following considerations (Kielhofner 2002):

- What a client values as important
- What a client feels competent doing
- What a client finds enjoyable or pleasurable.

An example of a graded activity schedule for Alex, when he was recovering from surgery related to Crohn's Disease, is provided in Figure 2. Alex was instructed to list all planned activities during a 24-hour period and to rate each activity on a scale of 1 (low) to 10 (high) in terms if its importance and the degree to which it engendered feelings of competence and pleasure. It was recommended that the number of minutes allocated for each activity correspond to the importance, competence, and pleasure ratings.

Alex's surgery went relatively smoothly. He was up and walking in the halls of the hospital one day later. Given that his general pattern of activity prior to his surgery was that he tended to be sedentary, restricting his activities to computer work, e-mailing friends, sitting in class, online dating, and watching movies, his physician and therapist put together the schedule in Figure 2 to help Alex begin

Week 1: April 15th – April 21st				
Activities Scheduled	**Amount of Time per day**	**Importance**	**Competence**	**Pleasure**
Walking meditation	10 min 3x/day	10	5	5
Watching movies	4 hours	3	3	10
Reading	2 hours	10	10	10
Contact with friends	1 hour	10	5	8
Eating	2.5 hours	10	1	3
Hygiene and wound care	1 hour	10	10	1
Rest/sleep	13 hours/day	10	1	10

FIGURE 2. Alex's Daily Activity Schedule One Week Following Surgery

to establish a daily routine that incorporated physical activity. It is evident from Alex's Week 1 record that he continues to derive most of his pleasure or gratification from more sedentary activities, such as reading, watching movies, and sleeping. Contact with friends was given more time than the walking meditation (Kabat-Zin 1990), which was prescribed by the therapist to give Alex a structured and goal-directed means of engaging in some degree of physical activity while in the hospital and at home recovering. Upon further questioning, the therapist discovered that the walking activity was acceptable to Alex but caused him some pain during his initial stage of recovery. Alex had difficulty training his mind to focus solely on one aspect of his walking. He reported that he discovered that he did not like to meditate while walking but instead preferred to use his walking time to be social with the hospital staff and with other patients. Given this feedback, Alex and his therapist found a way to include a more social form of walking in future activity schedules. Alex made an ad seeking a "walking partner" and placed it in the mailboxes of all of his neighbors. One neighbor, a 65-year-old woman with coronary artery disease, contacted him and they began walking together. However, as Alex increased his physical endurance it became apparent to him that his walking partner could not keep up with him very well. Soon after, Alex met a woman through an online dating service and she became his daily walking partner.

Overactive Clients

Clients with chronic conditions who are overactive can also be challenging to work with. These clients tend to push themselves regardless of how they feel and despite escalations in current symptoms or the emergence of new symptoms. These clients may exercise or perform physical activity with too much intensity or for longer-than-appropriate periods of time. For example, some clients may hold jobs that require engagement in inappropriate levels or types of physical activity. For example, a client with chronic lower back pain and asthma may be exacerbating his symptoms by lifting heavy blocks of cement at his construction job all day, every day, for months. Yet he may be unwilling or unable to change jobs because of union membership and the need to support his children's basic medical and educational needs. Other clients may be overactive and may also work in settings or environments that exacerbate symptoms. For example, a client with fibromyalgia who works as a tour guide for a local museum that has outdoor exhibits may be forced to stand and walk all day on concrete floors in a cold climate. For other clients, overactivity may manifest itself in terms of caring for children or others who are also ill or disabled in the family, or in terms of the number of commitments they make or the number of responsibilities they are forced to take on. Even mental activities that are performed for unusually long periods of time can lead to increased symptoms (e.g., fatigue and headaches) and stress.

Clients with chronic conditions who are overactive can be encouraged to prioritize their activities and then pace themselves according to available energy levels and symptom severity (Pesek, Jason, and Taylor 2000). They can also be encouraged to examine the extent to which they are doing things that they value versus doing things that are required by others around them. This issue is particularly important to examine for clients that are excessively other-oriented and have difficulty with self-care. Interventions for overactive clients can be accomplished with the aid of an activity pacing schedule. This schedule requires a client to list his or her planned activities for each day. Then, for each planned activity, the person uses ascale of 1 (low) to 10 (high) to indicate each activity's:

- Level of intrinsic (important to self) and extrinsic (importance to others) value
- Capacity to produce stress

This schedule can then be used as a means of intervention. Traditionally, over functioning and/or overstressed clients are taught the "50/50 solution," which requires them to eliminate 50 percent of their lower-priority activities in each of the columns (intrinsic and extrinsic) each day to avoid producing fatigue from overexertion.

At the end of each day the client completes the form by

- Indicating whether the planned activities were done or not
- Indicating any other activities done and completing ratings as with the planned activities
- Indicating the overall level of fatigue experienced that day

The final column of this form is designed to allow clients to look at their patterns of activity and fatigue across time and note relationships between fatigue and the level of activity. In this way it serves to teach clients how modulating their activity level can give them some control over their level of fatigue.

The following is an example of using this form and procedure. Nina has been chronically overfunctioning. Her pattern is to engage in too many nonpleasurable or demanding (relative to her capacity) activities. In combination with high stress levels, her activity levels cause her to become extremely fatigued. Following what used to be a normal daily routine consisting of work and household responsibilities, Nina is unable to function for time periods ranging from a day or two to up to a week or longer. Nina agreed to set a goal to practice the "50/50 solution" as a means of reducing her activity, stress, and fatigue levels. Figure 3 shows Nina's unsuccessful attempt to practice this procedure as it was originally intended. To have practiced this technique as intended would have required Nina to have undertaken only half of her planned activities each day (revealing an equal number of "yes" and "no" responses in the "Activity Completed" column. In addition, it would have required her to better prioritize high importance, pleasurable activities and to seek assistance so that she could delegate lower importance, less pleasurable activities to others. However, Nina repeated her pattern of planning and undertaking too much activity, which she did on Friday and Saturday, resulting in a total collapse on Sunday. Chapter 15 contains a second snapshot of Nina's activity pacing schedule after she made significant progress in therapy and learned to successfully apply the "50/50 Solution."

Date Day	Activities planned (numbered in order of priority) Also list unplanned activities that you did at the end of your list	Importance to you	Importance to others	Stress	Activity completed?	Fatigue level for the day
	Remember the 50/50 solution		(low = 1-----------10 = high)		Yes / No	low 1—10 high
June 3 Friday	1. Get ready for work	5	9	2	Yes	8
	2. Drive to work	5	9	9	Yes	
	3. Complete budget spreadsheet	5	10	10	Yes	
	4. Drive home	10	5	8	Yes	
	5. Grocery shopping	5	8	7	Yes	
	6. Take cleaning to cleaners	3	5	5	Yes	
	7. Cook dinner	7	7	7	Yes	
	8. Clean kitchen	7	7	7	Yes	
	9. Call friend	10	8	2	Yes	
	10. Watch TV with partner	10	8	2	Yes	
June 4 Saturday	1. Get ready for the day	5	5	2	Yes	9
	2. Drive daughter to softball practice	5	10	4	Yes	
	3. Take dog to groomer	1	3	7	Yes	
	4. Prepare lunch	3	8	5	Yes	
	5. Do some gardening	10	1	3	No	
	6. Pick up daughter from softball	5	10	4	Yes	
	7. Pick up cleaning	3	3	5	Yes	
	8. Prepare dinner	3	8	8	Yes	
	9. Go to movie with friend	10	9	2	No	
	Had argument with partner	1	1	10	Yes	

June 5 Sunday					10
1. Get ready for the day	1	5	2	No	
2. Prepare lunch	10	1	4	No	
3. Pay bills	8	10	7	No	
4. Do some gardening	5	1	3	No	
5. Spend time with daughter	10	9	3	No	
6. Cook dinner for friends	8	7	9	No	
Too tired to do anything	1	1	10	yes	
watched TV					

FIGURE 3. Nina's Activity Pacing Schedule

The activity pacing schedule can be adapted by clients and their therapists to suit lifestyle preferences and recommended activity levels. Other techniques of energy conservation can be prescribed, including scheduled rest periods and goals that involve arranging for food or grocery delivery, hiring a housekeeper, learning to utilize specialized transportation options, or recruiting assistance with household chores or other mandatory activities from personal care assistants or other hired professionals. Some clients will want to use the form literally and practice the "50/50 solution" religiously, whereas others may wish to gauge their activity levels more subtly depending on weekly symptom patterns and stress tolerance levels.

Unbalanced Clients

Inevitably clients will differ in the extent to which they value balance in their lives. Activity schedules that address imbalance in activity should be pursued only if a client is unhappy with his or her current activities and feels that they are too narrowly focused or limited in the extent to which they are pleasurable and gratifying. A central mistake that therapists make is to assume that balance is a prerequisite for well-being or a positive quality of life.

If clients find that a lack of balance in their lives is leading to feelings of resentment or stress, they can be asked to complete an activity schedule similar to the one presented in Figure 2. Activities can then be examined in terms of their intrinsic importance to an individual and in terms of the degree to which a person finds them pleasurable. A simple pie chart offers an alternative means of examining balance in life activities. Clients can be asked to construct two separate pie charts—one reflecting the actual time spent in daily activities and one reflecting their desired distribution of time (Beck 1995).

Troubleshooting Problems with Activity Scheduling

If activity scheduling is not approached carefully, clients can easily become discouraged. For example, an underactive client might become discouraged if too much of an increase in activity is recommended too quickly. This will inevitably result in the client not being able to complete all of the prescribed activities, in an escalation of symptoms, or both. Prescribed increases in activity should always be graded, and clients should be encouraged to start very slowly. Depending on the client, starting slowly may range from practicing eye blinking (for clients unable to get out of bed) to walking for only two minutes per day.

Despite all of a therapist's careful planning and good intentions, some clients will disregard recommendations to start small and may try to do more than they should. The risk of this occurrence can be reduced by educating clients up front about the potential consequences of increasing activity levels too abruptly. In addition, some clients will want to compare their activity levels to those of others who are not ill, or to their previous activity levels during a time when they were not ill. Clients should be encouraged to compare their current activity levels not to those of others but instead to their activity levels when they were experiencing the worst period during their current illness. Encouraging a client to strive for a realistic "personal best" will prevent comparison against unrealistic standards.

Similarly, a client working on achieving balance in the types of activities he or she engages in might become discouraged if a new type of activity is selected that is too challenging or complex. Because it is new or unfamiliar to the client, the effort involved in mastering it may be overwhelming to him or her. Clients should be encouraged to start with activities that are easy for them and familiar. New hobbies or new vocational activities should be pursued only with sufficient training and supervision. Finally, an overactive client might resent having to cut back on the amount of activities he or she is participating in, particularly if the eliminated activities were pleasurable or if the client does not see any immediate positive results of activity reduction. Any recommendations to reduce or change activity levels should be realistic, should fit with a client's lifestyle, and should render immediate and measurable positive results. Otherwise these changes should not be attempted.

Systematic Desensitization

As a result of the discomfort, pain, or other symptoms that accompany many chronic conditions, some clients with chronic conditions can develop anxiety-based somatic reactions to otherwise neutral stimuli. For example, Curtis repeatedly became nauseous while riding in the car on the way home from a weekly chemotherapy infusion. He began to develop a conditioned nausea whenever he set foot in the car, and sometimes even when he simply thought about riding in a car. For this reason, he had begun to avoid riding in cars whenever it wasn't absolutely required, which was causing him to restrict his social life and some family activities. Moreover, Curtis was embarrassed at having developed this aversion to riding in the car because he felt it made him appear weak. He was highly motivated to change it.

To arrest this process, Curtis was coached to imagine a situation that induces low to moderate levels of anxiety (i.e., to conjure up an image of walking toward the car, then to visualize touching the door handle, and then to visualize sitting in the car) while at the same time practicing relaxation techniques before, during, and after imagining touching, getting in and sitting in the car. As homework, Curtis practiced this procedure multiple times per day until thinking about these things no longer produced anxiety or nausea. This took him nearly two weeks. Then Curtis was guided to take more significant steps toward eventually being able to ride comfortably in a car again. These included sitting (first in a parked car and then in a moving car while his wife or daughter drove) and using the same coping strategies until he longer felt nauseous. By practicing desensitization techniques religiously and gradually (i.e., not proceeding to the next step until he had mastered the first step), Curtis was able to overcome his reaction of anxiety and nausea when riding in a car.

Conclusion

Chapter 6 provided an overview of cognitive behavioral techniques that are commonly utilized in the treatment of individuals with chronic conditions. Chapters 7 and 8 discussed more cognitively oriented techniques, and this chapter discussed techniques that are more behavioral in nature. The cognitive model should serve as a guide and rationale for any technique that is used, and cognitive behavioral approaches should always strive to integrate both cognitive and behavioral techniques. Therapists must use professional judgment in determining which specific techniques are most appropriate for a given client at a particular time. Chapter 10 discusses unique features of cognitive behavioral therapy with persons who have chronic conditions and contains information important for professional judgment when working with this population.

10

Unique Features of Cognitive Behavioral Therapy for Clients with Chronic Conditions

"The most difficult part of this illness is having to cancel out on friends at the last minute . . . . It makes you wonder if they'll be around the next time you can get together. That's certainly happened to me before. I even feel guilty when I have to cancel my therapy appointments at the last minute. It makes you wonder if people think you are selfish or wallowing. Sometimes I think—maybe I'm giving in too much and I could be doing more. But I know this is not true because the pain is very real and it only gets worse when I push myself. Mostly it is very lonely and I don't exactly feel like reaching out only to have to let others down in the end."

With these words, Paulette describes the feelings of isolation, concerns about social stigma, and decreased feelings of control that characterize individuals with chronic conditions. These reflections are closely tied to the reality of living with severe rheumatoid arthritis, particularly during times of flare-up. Although in Paulette's case many of these feelings ultimately stem from her long-standing depression and maladaptive coping patterns, her concerns are nonetheless realistic and might be experienced by anyone with a chronic condition at some point during the course of the illness. None of these feelings and concerns is necessarily a direct reflection of illogical thinking. However, some of these thoughts may reflect negative core beliefs, and others may represent more realistic cognitions that carry low levels of utility.

Clients with chronic conditions can and do differ in clinically significant ways from clients with psychiatric disorders alone (Freeman and Greenwood 1987; Moorey and Greer 2002). Dilemmas and concerns faced by clients with chronic conditions can increase the complexity of the therapeutic process. For example, therapists may not always recognize the extent to which many of a client's cognitions may be related to circumstances surrounding the condition, rather than being the direct result of a psychiatric disorder per se. The degree to which a client's cognition about a given issue reflects reality may be difficult to determine in the case of a chronic condition, since chronic conditions are inherently ambiguous in their nature and course and often produce negative cognitions that are indeed rooted in reality.

Some clients may have energy limitations or other physical or cognitive impairments that will require the therapist to adjust certain structural aspects of the therapy process and/or to utilize assistive technologies when administering cognitive behavioral therapy to clients. Moreover, clients may struggle, initially, in assuming an empowered role as an empirical collaborator within the therapeutic relationship. These and other unique considerations must be incorporated into cognitive behavioral case conceptualizations and when designing treatment plans in collaboration with clients.

Individuals with chronic conditions or disabilities can share a number of unique concerns, many of which may occur independently of any diagnosable forms of psychopathology. Understanding that these concerns are common among individuals with chronic illness and disabilities and not always reflective of enduring psychopathology is vital to developing an accurate case conceptualization in cognitive behavioral therapy. This understanding is also essential to an accurate empathic understanding of a client's cognitions and is vital to establishing a collaborative therapeutic alliance.

A wide range of complexities and challenges can accompany treating a client with a chronic illness or impairment using cognitive behavioral therapy. In this chapter, psychological and social complexities that can be associated with chronic conditions are elaborated. The chapter will cover the following experiences, behaviors and circumstances that can characterize persons with chronic conditions:

- Feelings of isolation, estrangement, and otherness
- Limited patience, limited energy, and high expectations
- Assistance recruiting
- Social judgment, stigma, and discrimination
- Loss of control
- Loss of resources
- Role changes
- Mortality and meaning
- Crisis and suicide
- Contact with health care
- Body image, physical appearance, and sexuality
- Unpredictability and variation in experience

Additionally, this chapter will discuss the kinds of issues that arise when chronic conditions are complicated by Axis I psychiatric overlay and Axis II psychiatric overlay. Finally the chapter will give consideration to disability identity and illness phase and the considerations these two issues can raise in therapy. It will conclude with a discussion of how all the issues addressed in this chapter provide the rationale for an integrative approach to psychotherapy.

Feelings of Isolation, Estrangement, and Otherness

Concerns about, and actual experiences of, isolation, social exclusion, and otherness can be felt by any individual with a chronic condition, particularly when symptoms reach their highest severity, when an individual is undergoing a difficult medical procedure, or when the condition interferes with usual participation in social settings. Some clients, at certain times, may hold a belief in a "just world." As a consequence life may be difficult and even enraging at times for some individuals who question why they have been forced to experience the pain and functional limitations that are often associated with a given chronic condition when others around them have their health.

Beck (1999) has defined two main categories of problems of cognitive distortion involving negative core beliefs:

- Cognitions involving helplessness and
- Cognitions involving unlovability

Some clients will exhibit both categories of negative core beliefs. Clients with chronic conditions who also have significant psychiatric overlay may be particularly vulnerable to demonstrating beliefs associated with helplessness and unlovability. It is important for therapists to keep in mind that these beliefs, in part, may be triggered by real-world traumas and losses that occurred as a result of having a chronic condition.

In addition to these issues, the mere sensations of bodily pain and discomfort associated with many chronic conditions are isolating in that they are often experienced in a unique way and cannot be simultaneously felt or perceived directly by others. People often feel alone in their pain or in their experience of fatigue. Symptoms or medical treatment side effects can be so severe at times that they are highly distracting and can interfere with the ability to even engage comfortably in casual social conversation with someone else. Symptoms and cognitive or physical impairments can limit mobility or make transportation more complicated and cumbersome, decreasing time and opportunities for travel to meet others or to engage in social and recreational activities outside of the home.

Physical attributes of certain illnesses or impairments that are visible to others may lead to cognitions associated with shame or self-consciousness (unlovability), and these feelings and beliefs are likely to be reinforced by real-world experiences of estrangement and judgment. In cases where individuals are most isolated, cognitive distortions may manifest themselves in terms of fears of abandonment, some of which may be reinforced by actual experiences of rejection and abandonment by partners, spouses, family, and friends. In some cases, individuals feeling deep levels of isolation and loss of control may withdraw from others or behave in manipulative or controlling ways that can provoke or invite additional experiences of abandonment.

Limited Patience, Limited Energy, and High Expectations

Many clients with chronic conditions have to make significant sacrifices of time, energy, and resources to attend therapy. Some may risk symptom flare-ups merely as a result of the exertion involved in transportation to and participation in therapy. At any given time, a client may be highly uncomfortable, exhausted, or in pain during a therapy session. These and other symptoms may interfere with attention and concentration in therapy, and they may also limit the extent to which clients are motivated to remain in therapy and able to engage in homework assignments outside of therapy.

At the same time, clients see therapists as health-care professionals and, in some cases, as involved members of a larger health-care team that is immediately involved in care for their physical well-being. As a result, for some clients, and particularly those with more severe conditions or those newer to psychotherapy, patience with more gradual outcomes of the therapy process may be limited, and expectations of the therapist for symptom relief may be high. For these reasons, cognitive behavioral approaches that focus on brevity, on simplicity and on fostering more immediate experiences of efficacy and symptom reduction in clients are very appropriate. Cognitive behavioral therapists must tailor the complexity and length of assessments and therapy activities and the extent of effort required for engagement in therapy.

Many clients face the dilemma of not being able to perform or accomplish as many activities as they could before the condition. With time alone, or in the absence of treatment, some will experience a progressive decline in physical functioning. This will limit their options in terms of occupational and recreational choices, which are often prescribed by cognitive behavioral therapists as part of activity assignments. Until a client and therapist can find an activity that is both possible and gratifying, activity assignments may lead to feelings of demoralization and to noncompliance with therapy.

In addition, some clients may have difficulty attending therapy regularly, or may require shorter sessions because of severe fatigue or symptoms. Adjustments in the therapy schedule can be made. However, within a cognitive behavioral framework, the therapist is encouraged to work with the client to maintain as much consistency and structure within the changed format as possible. For example, if sessions are reduced to 30 minutes, every other week, then this structure should be maintained as consistently as possible. The challenge for cognitive behavioral therapists is to work with the client to identify maladaptive cognitions related to activity performance that may lead to unnecessary levels of social isolation, under-activity, or increased levels of impairment. Activity diaries that incorporate the recording of emotions and automatic thoughts associated with different activities, in addition to preparatory work that explores a client's volition, as discussed in Chapter 13, can assist clients and therapists in this process.

Assistance Recruiting

Even the most independent individuals facing chronic illness or impairments must shift their worldviews and learn to recruit assistance from others to varying degrees. In the absence of psychiatric overlay, recruitment of assistance may, in large part, be mediated by the level of physical or cognitive limitations experienced by an individual at any given time during the course of the condition.

In some cases the progressive course of an illness can cause a person's needs for assistance to escalate irreversibly over time. This can lead to feelings of guilt and powerlessness in the individual with the chronic condition, and can lead to stress, mixed and conflicting feelings of guilt and responsibility, and an increasing sense of burden in the assistant or caregiver.

In conditions characterized by symptoms and impairments that wax and wane in severity, an individual's need to recruit assistance from others can fluctuate according to variations in illness course. This can be confusing, both for the individual requesting help and the caregiver, potentially leading to miscommunication and feelings of resentment on both sides. Because their feelings of personal power, control, and self-efficacy may have been reduced by the illness and or impairment, individuals with chronic conditions may demonstrate significant ambivalence about requesting and accepting assistance and support from others. Others may become habituated to expecting or demanding help in circumstances where they would otherwise be able to manage on their own.

Social Judgment, Stigma, and Discrimination

Apart from the cognitive distortions involving doubts of others' intentions, fears of social exclusion or abandonment, suspicion, mistrust, or concerns about negative judgments or opinions from others, individuals with chronic conditions often face negative evaluations, prejudice, and discrimination from others. These experiences are, indeed, based in reality and they are all too common for individuals with chronic illnesses and impairments. In some clients, particularly in the absence of support, these negative experiences may accumulate over time and may trigger or perpetuate negative cognitions involving self-worth and social acceptability.

Loss of Control

Concerns about loss of control can manifest themselves in terms of preoccupation with loss of control over one's physical body and bodily functions and in terms of worry about loss of emotional control. As an example of loss of physical control, Alex was plagued by concerns about having to rush to the bathroom and possibly remain there for a long period of time during an important exam in school. Given that Alex had Crohn's Disease and was also taking medications that included diarrhea as a side effect, his concern was realistic.

Similarly, an individual with a loss of motor control due to a recent stroke may feel uncomfortable eating in front of others. For many, these concerns are usually based in reality, because the essence of many chronic conditions involves a loss of control over bodily parts or functions. However, some individuals can develop cognitive distortions about loss of control and can become excessively preoccupied or concerned with it. This can interfere with their desire and ability to function well interpersonally.

Having a chronic condition often involves numerous losses and limitations, including recognizing that there is no cure. Any human experience of loss inevitably leads to feelings of frustration, sadness, or anger. Many individuals with chronic conditions struggle with expressing these feelings, because

- They have been taught that it is unacceptable to show negative emotions,
- They are afraid their emotions will scare others or push them away, or
- They fear losing control of their emotions.

Loss of Resources

Inevitably, the circumstance of having a chronic condition is accompanied by losses. Depending on the state of an individual's preexisting resources and ability to acquire new resources, these losses can include:

- Material losses (e.g., money, job, home, car, clothing, food)
- Interpersonal losses (e.g., marriage or partnership, family relationships, friendships, relationships with neighbors or coworkers)
- Intrapersonal losses (e.g., self-esteem, well-being, knowledge, mastery, energy, time).

Within the United States, the cost to individuals of physician visits, hospital stays, medications, and job-related losses resulting from a chronic illness or impairment can be significant. Studies of individuals with chronic health conditions suggest that loss of key resources can have a significant impact on perception of stress and quality of life (Hobfoll 1998; Lane and Hobfoll 1992).

Role Changes

Impairment in physical and cognitive functioning may lead to temporary role changes or permanent role reversals within couples and families. They may also lead to changes in job roles or to changes in other roles within the community, such as those associated with volunteer positions. Though not always negative, these role changes can lead to lowered self-esteem, feelings of guilt, or lowered social status, particularly in the absence of treatment.

For example, as Curtis's prostate cancer progressed, he found himself having to relinquish the more physically demanding aspects of his role as a father. This was particularly disturbing to him since he had always participated in sports and other physically demanding activities with his daughter, since she became old enough to participate. As a result he required assistance with modifying his all-or-nothing thinking associated with his perception of himself as a "worthless father."

A positive circumstance involving a role change can be observed in situations where an individual locates an alternative way to fulfill his or her existing role functioning (e.g., Curtis realizing he can still parent his daughter in psychological and emotional ways, even if he can no longer engage in sports with her). Positive effects of role changes can also be noticed in situations where an individual and his or her larger social context or family system embrace a role change and discover its benefits.

Mortality and Meaning

Chronic conditions can prompt an individual to think about existential issues involving life's overall meaning and significance, his or her personal life meaning and motivations for living, and issues of death and dying. Thoughts of meaning, death, and dying may occur more frequently if an individual is facing a progressive, potentially fatal, or definitely terminal condition.

Cognitive distortions related to death and dying can typically assume one of two forms. That is, clients can

- Deny the severity or terminal nature of the condition or
- Exaggerate the severity of the condition by overestimating or prematurely anticipating that a condition is going to be progressive or terminal (i.e., fearing death).

In the former case many contend that a certain level of denial of the severity or prognosis of a given condition, or even complete denial of an impending death, can lead to positive psychological outcomes. A traditional cognitive behavioral approach to modifying a client's optimistic cognitions surrounding death and dying would not be indicated in this case.

There are some cases in which denial may lead to negative outcomes, both psychologically and physically. For example, if a client's level of denial interferes with his or her willingness to seek a form of treatment that might arrest or delay the progression of the condition, a traditional approach to cognitive behavioral therapy that emphasizes socratic questioning may be warranted. Similarly, if a client's level of denial is inconsistent with his or her partner's or family's ideas about the nature and severity of the condition, a couples' counseling or family-based intervention with cognitive behavioral underpinnings deserves consideration. In the latter instance, where a client overestimates or prematurely anticipates that a condition is going to be progressive or terminal, a more traditional approach to modifying these cognitive distortions would be appropriate.

Clients that fear death and are also undergoing medical treatment may fear that a given treatment could kill them, particularly if the treatment is painful. In this case modification of cognitive distortions, reassurance by the physician, distraction, and relaxation or meditation training may be indicated.

It is important to recognize that in any circumstance where cognitive behavioral therapy might be indicated, the traditional assessment techniques, case conceptualization guidelines, and therapy strategies used by cognitive behavioral therapists may not be sufficient, or they may not always be appropriate in any given therapeutic encounter that involves an individual's personal perception of his or her physical illness experience. This is where behavioral strategies, such as breathing, relaxation, and meditation approaches, commonly used by cognitive behavioral therapists, may be indicated and used independently of other cognitive behavioral techniques.

Though it is a controversial topic (Caro 1998), some cognitive theorists have begun to consider issues of existence and meaning as potential complements to the cognitive behavioral therapy process (Moss 1992). Accordingly, narrative techniques have been recommended as a complementary therapeutic strategy to use in efforts to uncover issues of existence and meaning (Ramsay 1998).

Because changing any client's cognitions about his or her own death may not be possible or, in some cases, may not be ethical, drawing on approaches that aim to increase a client's comfort with uncertainty, or positive psychology approaches that encourage satisfaction with one's past and aim to promote present experiences of pleasure and gratification, may be more appropriate. For those clients in realistic terminal illness situations that are more able to accept and struggle with their impending death, Eastern approaches that aim to facilitate acceptance of death and resolution of existential angst (e.g., Levine and Levine 1982) may also serve as appropriate complements to a more traditional cognitive behavioral approach.

Crisis and Suicide

In addition to concerns about death and mortality, clients with chronic conditions often demonstrate an increased vulnerability to emotional crises, higher rates of suicidal ideation, and an increased risk for actual suicide attempts (White 2001). In some cases, any preexisting psychopathology or subclinical psychological processes may be exacerbated by the resource losses, stressors, physical and cognitive limitations, and pain or discomfort associated with the circumstance of chronic illness.

Any existing psychopathology might also be exacerbated by any effects of disease involvement or medications and treatments on the brain and nervous system. Chronic illness has been cited as one of the most common causes of suicide, and clients with chronic conditions may be more vulnerable to emotional crisis and suicidal ideation for a number of reasons.

Loss of control over physical movements, bodily sensations, and physical and social environments may create an urge to regain control over the timing and nature of one's bodily experience and death, and some individuals may think that this control would be possible through suicide. In other cases, the severe pain and impairments associated with a given condition, particularly if terminal, may lead to long-standing and realistic feelings of hopelessness and to a desire to end life in order to arrest pain and suffering. Other clients may feel they are (or their condition is) a burden to their partners, family, or society. Some may believe that their loved ones would be "better off" without them. Yet other clients may consciously or unconsciously use reports of suicidal ideation as a "cry for help" or as a means of sequestering more of the therapist's attention. In some cases, clients may be motivated by a number of these variables, making their thinking and potential behavior difficult to untangle.

Irrespective of a client's motive to commit suicide and regardless of a therapist's personal feelings about whether these motives are justified, the United States Mental Health Code mandates that mental health professionals thoroughly assess and prevent suicide in any client at risk for suicide. Clinicians must be vigilant to comments and behaviors that may reflect overt or underlying suicidal thoughts, feelings and impulses. It is imperative that cognitive behavioral therapists include suicide assessment in their initial assessments of clients and in their ongoing assessments, when indicated.

Beck, Rush, Shaw, and Emery (1979) conceived of suicide risk in terms of three categories:

- Suicidal ideation and intent,
- Suicide attempt and lethality, and
- Method of completed suicide or attempt.

Later research confirmed that level of suicidal intention is not always linked to the lethality of the attempt, and therefore one must consider all aspects of suicidal ideation and behavior as important in the assessment of risk (Beck, and Kovacs 1975; Weishaar 1996).

Measures that have been utilized in research to identify cognitive risk factors for suicide include:

- The *Beck Depression Inventory*, which must be adapted for use with medical populations due to the risk for overlap in symptoms (Beck, Guth, Steer, and Ball 1997)
- The *Beck Hopelessness Scale* (Beck, Weissman, Lester, and Trexler 1974)
- The *Scale for Suicide Ideation* (Beck, Kovacs, and Weissman 1979)
- The *Dysfunctional Attitude Scale* (Weissman and Beck 1978).

Weishaar (1996) has comprehensively reviewed the extensive body of research in the field of cognitive behavioral therapy that has focused on identifying cognitive risk factors for suicide. Major risk factors include hopelessness, negative self-concept, certain cognitive distortions, cognitive rigidity, dysfunctional assumptions, self-defeating attributions regarding the causes of events, and deficits in problem solving.

Basic suicide assessment strategies that should be common and well-practiced knowledge for therapists include asking the client for more examples of his or her thoughts, and particularly those that pertain to death, asking the client if he or she has ever thought of killing him- or herself, asking the client if he or she has current thoughts of suicide, and asking by what means the client has thought he or she might take his or her own life. Another important line of questioning should focus on the extent to which the client actually intends to harm or kill him- or herself, and the extent to which he or she feels confident that he or she will not make a suicide attempt before the next therapeutic contact. It is also critical that cognitive behavioral therapists notice and respond to automatic thoughts, conditional beliefs, and casual doorknob comments that reflect:

- Existential concerns (e.g., "If I can't have children, then what would be the real point of living?"),
- Feelings of helplessness ("I'm tired of trying and I'm tired of failing... This is something I can't control"),
- Feelings of hopelessness ("It's not like I'll ever get better or be healthy again"), or
- Overt suicidal impulses ("It isn't worth living this way").

If a client is determined to be at risk for suicide, he or she should be escorted to the nearest emergency room for a second assessment. More detailed information about cognitive behavioral approaches to crisis management, suicide assessment and suicide intervention strategies, particularly those used for chronically suicidal clients, can be found in Linehan (1993a).

Contact with Health Care

Individuals with chronic conditions come in contact with a wide range of health-care professionals and health-care settings at a much higher rate than the average person. Rates of client satisfaction with health care within the United States are generally low. Because chronic illnesses and disabilities can be complex and ambiguous, medical professionals can and do provide patients with inaccurate information, only to be contradicted or discounted when new discoveries arise.

In addition, medical professionals do occasionally, though infrequently, make mistakes. Regardless of whether negative sentiments about medical professionals are warranted, patients tend to expect that their providers will be honest and competent in caring for them. At times, even the slightest error or miscommunication can lead to mistrust between a provider and a patient. Given this sentiment, it is inevitable that some clients will report negative experiences with health-care providers, with inpatient settings, and/or with medical treatments and their side effects.

Some clients may have prior negative or traumatic experiences with health care that may further influence their beliefs and behaviors about seeking medical treatment. They may generalize a single negative experience to all future experiences with medical care, or a negative experience may cause some patients to misperceive the intentions of an otherwise earnest physician. Clients may express fears of health care or demonstrate maladaptive behaviors, such as non-compliance with recommended medications or with other medical treatments such as surgery, radiation, or physical therapy.

Other clients may overutilize health care as an attempted means of managing their health-related anxiety, or they may "doctor shop," or travel from provider to provider with the conviction that past providers were not competent or caring enough to provide an adequate assessment or treatment. These behaviors may be observed more frequently in clients with complex, difficult-to-diagnose or difficult-to-treat conditions. Cognitive behavioral methods can be used to assist clients in coping with their interactions with health-care providers and with decision-making regarding treatment options.

Clients with overlapping Axis II disorders may present additional complications in their interactions with providers, and not all medical providers will be aware of or familiar with ways to manage Axis II clients. Therapists working in collaboration with other health-care professionals will inevitably have to navigate issues involving the limits and boundaries of client confidentiality, clients' enlistment of multiple/excessive providers, noncompliance with treatment recommendations, and disagreements regarding treatment approaches. When not managed carefully, these cross-disciplinary dilemmas can result in feelings of divided loyalty and in problems with accuracy in cross-communication of medical and psychological information.

Body Image, Physical Appearance, and Sexuality

Chronic conditions or physical impairments often result in changes in bodily sensations and in changes in the outward appearance of the body. An enhanced level of attention to the body is needed in order to manage the symptoms of a chronic condition. Individuals may need to regulate medication intake, to monitor blood levels for important cellular, glucose, or hormonal fluctuations, to receive periodic radiography to scan for metastasis or monitor the progress of a tumor, and to pace activity or exercise in order to maintain physical fitness, among other self-care needs. The necessity to engage in any number of these health-monitoring activities can result in an increased level of focus on bodily sensations and on bodily appearance, further accentuating any perception of changes that have already occurred or may continue to occur.

In the circumstance of a chronic condition, a client's cognitions about his or her appearance may be well rooted in reality (e.g., "I look emaciated now" or "I have lost the most beautiful part of my body") or they may represent or turn into distortions or exaggerations (e.g., "I am ugly" or "I look like a monster"). In either case, cognitions will need to be evaluated not only in terms of their level of distortion, but also in terms of their overall utility. In either case, cognitions that focus on lost, reduced, or negative aspects of physical appearance will likely be associated with conditional and core beliefs that involve cognitions related to low self-worth, and the pathways of interaction between the cognitions are likely to be mutually reinforcing and bidirectional. These cognitions may, in turn, stimulate interpersonal thoughts or images about how one's physical appearance might be perceived by others.

In addition to the role of cognition, a client's level of concern with body image will, in part, depend upon his or her age, gender, occupation, social context, and prior personal investment in physical appearance and body image. In addition to these issues, a chronic condition may cause real changes in bodily sensations related to sexuality, or in the capacity for physical pleasure. For example, heart disease can cause difficulty with or relative absence of erectile function in men. For some men, these difficulties may be associated with conditional and core beliefs surrounding identification with the male role, one's role as a partner and lover, and one's worth as a man.

In other cases, it may be difficult for both clients and therapists to distinguish between cognitions about sexuality that are associated with real bodily sensations and those that reflect other issues, such as self-image or a long-standing couples issue. In these situations, careful assessment and consultation with the treating physician may help. At times, these distinctions may not be possible, necessary, or useful. Most important is achieving accuracy in these distinctions, or achieving a complex understanding of a multifactorial process. This understanding is often critical to empathy, rapport, and an accurate case conceptualization.

Unpredictability and Variation in Experience

Many chronic conditions are characterized by unpredictability and variation in the nature and severity of symptoms and impairments. This variation may be most frustrating and discouraging to clients that are unable to identify potential triggers involved in symptom changes. With the help of activity and cognition diaries, some of these variations can be linked to changes in cognitions, diet, weather, external stressors, and activity levels. Yet for others unanticipated changes will continue to occur regardless of any hypothesized trigger, and the extent to which triggers are linked to symptom changes will vary depending on the condition and the trigger.

For example, chronic fatigue syndrome is one condition marked by tremendous fluctuations in the type and severity of symptoms. Because chronic fatigue syndrome tends to be a stress-sensitive disorder, in some cases these fluctuations can be linked to specific stressors. However, in other cases new or unexpected symptoms occur for no apparent reason at all. Clients and therapists need to work together so clients ultimately learn to manage as much of this fluctuation as possible through the identification of precipitating and perpetuating contributors.

Axis I Psychiatric Overlay

Moorey and Greer (2002) have found that many clients with chronic conditions such as cancer tend not to demonstrate diagnosable psychopathology. If psychopathology is present, it will tend to be more acute than chronic, it will tend to manifest in terms of one diagnostic category (e.g., anxiety or depression) rather than multiple diagnoses (e.g., Axis I and Axis II pathology), and is likely to be less severe in nature. This said, the stresses and losses associated with chronic conditions may nonetheless increase the likelihood that an individual vulnerable to psychopathology will experience it.

One of the greatest challenges to psychotherapy with individuals with chronic conditions involves accurately distinguishing between symptoms attributable to the condition and symptoms attributable to a psychiatric disorder. Disorders such as depression, anxiety, eating disorders, substance abuse, and somatoform disorders share a number of somatic symptoms that are commonly observed in individuals with chronic conditions. Nonspecific somatic symptoms can also result from increased immune activity as demonstrated in the fatigue, lethargy, and loss of appetite characteristic of acute sickness behavior, and they can emerge as side effects of various medical treatments and pharmacotherapies. These shared, nonspecific symptoms can include fatigue, disturbed sleep, appetite changes, headaches, heart rate changes, difficulty breathing, aches and pains, and gastrointestinal symptoms, among others. Only an experienced clinician, working in tandem with a willing client and the treating physician, can ultimately come to tease apart the causes of these nonspecific symptoms. One measure that has been found to be useful in guiding the process of differentiating medical from psychological symptoms in cognitive-behavioral therapy is the Structured Clinical Interview for the DSM-IV (SCID) (First et al. 1995). Among the Axis I disorders, depressive disorders appear to be the most commonly observed in individuals with chronic conditions, followed by anxiety disorders, and new-onset manic and psychotic episodes that occur in conditions with brain involvement or as side effects of some treatments (American Psychiatric Association, 1994). With reference to depression, its risk of occurrence increases according to the diagnosis, severity, and level of impairment that a given condition causes. In addition, depression may be a characteristic symptom of some chronic conditions with central nervous system involvement. The following is a list of chronic conditions characterized by particularly high rates of depression:

- Heart attack 40–65 percent
- Coronary artery disease without heart attack 18–20 percent
- Parkinson's disease 40 percent
- Multiple sclerosis 40–60 percent
- Stroke 30–50 percent
- Cancer 20–42 percent
- Diabetes 25–33 percent
- Multi-infarct dementia 27–60 percent

Depression that is associated with chronic illness can increase levels of illness-associated impairment and can increase the severity of specific symptoms such as pain and fatigue. It can also increase risk for suicide in some clients, including stroke survivors. Depression is linked with poor adherence to recommended treatments and rehabilitation and can also affect social relationships and increase the risk for social isolation. When it becomes apparent that a client with a chronic condition is depressed, treatment goals must shift, at least temporarily, away from the management of physical symptoms and toward treatment of the depression. In these instances, traditional Beckian cognitive therapy for depression (Beck 1995), in combination with psychotropic medications or modalities, when medically indicated, may offer the most effective means of arresting a depressive episode. Acute anxiety also accompanies a number of chronic conditions at increased rates (American Psychiatric Association, 1994).

In addition to acknowledging that Axis I disorders can emerge as a result of, or become triggered or reactivated by the stressors, lifestyle changes, and resource losses associated with having a chronic illness, cognitive behavioral therapists should also be aware of the significant effects that the conditions themselves can have on brain physiology, behavior, and emotional experience. For example, new manic episodes, new psychotic episodes, and acute confusional states can occur in some chronic conditions, including AIDS-related dementia and advanced cancer (Moorey and Greer 2002). Such episodes may be characterized by restlessness, suspiciousness, increased vocal volume or yelling, other demonstrations of anger or rage, confusion, impaired memory and concentration, and disorientation to place and time (Moorey and Greer 2002).

In addition, manic, psychotic, or other acute confused behavior can be a side effect of some medications in some individuals. Opioid-based pain medications are the most common cause of these symptoms, in addition to some steroidal agents, certain chemotherapy drugs, interferon, vincristine, primary and secondary (i.e., resulting from metastasis) brain tumors, and encephalitis and encephalopathy due to metabolic and immunological diseases (e.g. carcinoid tumors of the gastrointestinal tract, hypercalcaemia and electrolyte imbalance, and neurological paraneoplastic syndromes) (Moorey and Greer 2002). In addition, these symptoms can occur in conjunction with head injury and other organic brain conditions.

Depression can also occur in conjunction with immune dysfunction and with a number of medical treatments, including administration of interferon or other recombinant cytokines for the treatment of conditions such as hepatitis and some cancers. These issues should be considered separately and therapists should be aware of the possibility that an apparent cognitive distortion operant in the client's emotional experience or behavior may be attributable to physiological causes.

In these cases, the practice of cognitive behavioral therapy should be modified, and therapists should work more closely with the treating physicians and psychiatrist, if necessary, to determine indicated psychotropic medications or other medical modalities. In addition, isolated cognitive and behavioral techniques, such as relaxation training, structured activity scheduling, distress tolerance training, or thought-stopping might be utilized, depending on the presenting symptoms. In sum, cognitive behavioral therapy approaches must be tailored and staged appropriately to a given client's symptomatology, and the treatment of psychiatric issues should typically precede the treatment of chronic illness symptoms.

Axis II Psychiatric Overlay

From a cognitive behavioral therapy perspective, Beck and associates (1990) and Beck (1995) have defined the most salient characteristics of a personality disorder as involving inflexible, maladaptive, and compulsive use of otherwise evolutionarily derived patterns of functioning. Beck argued that a wide range of natural strategies used for survival, such as competitiveness, dependence, grandiosity, resistance, avoidance, emotionality, control, aggression, suspiciousness, and isolation, which are typically utilized by psychologically healthy individuals in an ever-changing and flexible manner to adapt to the challenges of existence, are utilized in a dysfunctional manner by individuals with personality disorders. According to Beck (1995), individuals with personality disorders tend to overutilize a small set of these characteristics in rigid and compulsive ways.

Clients with subclinical or preexisting personality disorders prior to the onset of a chronic condition are likely to demonstrate an increase in the manifestation of such disorders with the many stressors associated with managing the condition. Though all personality disorders pose challenges to the treatment process, conditions most likely to complicate the course of cognitive behavioral treatment of a client with a given condition include borderline personality disorder, narcissistic personality disorder, and dependent personality disorder.

For example, clients with borderline pathology may be more likely to enact themes that involve fears of abandonment in therapy, and they will be more likely to vacillate between the idealization and devaluation of the therapist and other health-care professionals involved in their treatment. These clients will be more likely to exhibit episodes of intense rage, and this rage is more likely to be directed interpersonally to significant others and/or treatment providers rather than to the illness itself or to other external circumstances. Splitting is likely to occur. For example, the client may favor one health care provider over another, choose to selectively divulge certain aspects of vital medical or psychological information to one provider over another, or attempt to manipulate one provider into responding more actively and frequently than another. If a provider is not consistently responsive to a client, is not as responsive as the client would wish, or applies limits and boundaries inconsistently or in a manner unacceptable to the client, the client with borderline pathology will inevitably experience underlying feelings of abandonment and engage in maladaptive interpersonal behaviors.

Linehan (1993a, b) has developed a unique and highly effective approach to the cognitive behavioral treatment of individuals with borderline personality disorder. Generally, Linehan's approach, known as Dialectical Behavioral Therapy, involves strategies that range a continuum between problem-solving, irreverent, change-based strategies to validating, reciprocal, acceptance-based strategies. Core concepts that are taught to clients include radical acceptance, distress tolerance, chain analysis, and behavioral skills (Linehan 1993a, b). In radical acceptance clients learn to know and accept themselves in a realistic light, not according to how they would prefer to see themselves. By seeing and accepting themselves as they are, they learn to identify and change dysfunctional beliefs and behaviors (Linehan 1993a). Distress tolerance involves teaching clients to observe their feelings in an objective, nonjudgmental way. As a consequence they are taught and directed to commit themselves to enduring intense negative emotions without acting on them in maladaptive ways. Chain analysis involves constructing a detailed time line of interactions, feelings, and events that lead to maladaptive behaviors with the intention that awareness of these linkages will help clients break the chain that leads to self-destruction. In addition to these strategies, Linehan (1993a, b) employs a number of behavioral techniques, including interpersonal skills training and goal-setting, to assist clients in tolerating and regulating their emotional states. More information about Linehan's theory and treatment approach can be found in Linehan (1993a, b).

Clients with narcissistic disorders are likely to value therapists most when they can serve as idealizable objects and can mirror the client's own sense of grandiosity by providing a unique level of expertise and a high degree of directiveness in therapy. These clients may seek out therapists and health-care providers that are known to be experts in a given area, only to later become disappointed, rageful, or depressed if or when they come to realize any limitations in the provider's capacity to significantly alleviate symptoms or cure their condition. Narcissistic clients may not only expect a lot from their treatment providers, but also demand a lot of their partners, family, and friends, particularly during times of change, stress, or crisis in the course of their illness. Similarly, dependent clients may tend to overutilize health care, make frequent calls to providers, or rely too much on partners, family, and friends to care for them or do things for them that they could otherwise do themselves. Clients with dependency issues will generally oversolicit direction from the therapist and resist goals or other treatment efforts aimed at increasing independence or physical functioning. These clients will more likely adhere to goals that involve symptom reduction and those directed toward improving emotional experience and quality of life. Some clients will present with more than one personality disorder, in which case each disorder must be treated distinctly.

From a cognitive behavioral therapy perspective, Beck and associates (1990) maintain that the treatment of individuals with personality disorders follows a similar structure to that of cognitive behavioral therapy with Axis I disorders such as anxiety and depression. That is, it involves collaborative goal-setting, problem-solving, and the modification of maladaptive thoughts, beliefs, and behavior. Relapse prevention through teaching self-therapy strategies is also a key structural aspect.

However, there are a number of key differences in the more specific and process-oriented aspects of cognitive behavioral therapy with individuals with personality disorders (Beck et al., 1990). Specifically, Beck and associates (1990) emphasize the establishment of a strong therapeutic alliance, a more deliberate focus on modification of core beliefs and assumptions (in addition to automatic thoughts) and a focus on the developmental origins of dysfunctional beliefs.

In addition to Beck and associates (1990) and others (e.g., Safran and McMain), Sperry (1999) has written extensively about cognitive behavioral therapy approaches that have been found to be particularly effective for individuals with a wide range of DSM-IV personality disorders. Sperry (1999) emphasizes the need to borrow techniques from other orientations, to focus more intensively on preparing the client for change, and to deliberately stage treatment in terms of goal phases. From a cognitive behavioral perspective, Sperry (1999) advocates for the conceptualization and assessment of personality disorders according to two dimensions: character (i.e., interpersonal schema change) and temperament (i.e., interpersonal style change). In facilitating character change, schema-focused cognitive behavioral therapy is utilized to assist clients in identifying maladaptive views of themselves and others, to assist them in identifying the goal of treatment, or level at which a change in interpersonal schema is anticipated, and to assist them in developing a strategy to accomplish this change (Sperry 1999).

According to Sperry (1999), temperament change is achieved through modifying the client's interpersonal style using any number of strategies, including anger management, anxiety management training, assertiveness training, cognitive awareness training, distress tolerance training, emotion regulation training, limit-setting, empathy training, impulse control training, interpersonal skills training, problem-solving training, self-management training, sensitivity reduction training, symptom management training, and thought-stopping.

Sperry (1999) endorses a four-phase approach to the treatment of a personality disorder, which includes:

- Engagement (i.e., enlisting the client's trust, respect, and willingness to accept input from the provider—all requirements for true engagement in a collaborative relationship),
- Pattern analysis (i.e., describing a client's specific schemas or characterological features, interpersonal style, triggers to maladaptive interactions, level of functioning, and readiness for change),
- Pattern change (i.e., relinquishing a disordered or maladaptive cognitive, affective, and behavioral interpersonal pattern, adopting a more adaptive pattern, and generalizing and maintaining the new pattern so that it is applied to thoughts, feelings, and behaviors), and
- Pattern maintenance (i.e., prevention of relapse and recurrence).

More information about this approach as it is applied to specific personality disorders can be found in Sperry (1999).

Disability Identity and Illness Phase

Two additional aspects of the inner experience of a chronic condition or impairment that are relevant to cognitive behavioral therapy include disability identity and illness phase. Disability identity has been described as a necessary developmental process of self-definition that involves coming to feel a sense of belonging in a macro-level social context, coming to feel a sense of belonging with disabled peers, integrating similarities and differences with disabled peers, and integrating how one feels with how one presents oneself (Gill 1997). The following quote from Linton (1998, p. 3) describes the sense of pride and integrity that is likely to be felt by an individual that has reclaimed a positive identity as a disabled person and as a member of a larger, positive disability culture: "We have come out not with brown woolen lap robes over our withered legs or dark glasses over our pale eyes, but in shorts and sandals, in overalls and business suits, dressed for play and work—straightforward, unmasked, and unapologetic." Disability identity is likely to be more relevant to persons who experience a permanent and stable impairment than to those who have progressive conditions, conditions that also involve chronic illness, and conditions with less well-defined symptoms, diagnostic criteria, and prognoses.

The concept of illness phase refers to the mapping of a client's psychological adjustment to chronic illness. Fennell (2003) has proposed four-phase model of adjustment. In Phase 1, the "crisis phase," clients physically move from the initial onset of illness to a state of crisis, wherein they respond with uncertainty and emotional distress. In Phase 2, the "stabilization phase," clients continue to experience unpredictability of symptoms and feelings of emotional instability, and are unsure how to respond to the illness in terms of health-related behavior. However, clients do come to recognize some level of stability in symptom patterning and predictability. In Phase 3, the "resolution phase," clients work to accept the chronicity and ambiguities inherent in their illness and begin to search for positive ways of reconstructing their lives. Some may even find new meaning or revelation that has occurred as a result of being forced by chronic illness to view themselves and others differently. In Phase 4, the "integration phase," clients achieve a state of psychological integration in which they are able to reconcile pre- and post-illness self-concepts. They may begin to focus less on the symptoms and circumstances of the chronic illness or disability, and they achieve a positive identity as a disabled person. The Fennell Phase Inventory (Jason et al., 1999) can be utilized by cognitive behavioral therapists to assist in the measurement of illness phase. This measure and its scoring procedures can be accessed on the World Wide Web at *http://condor.depaul.edu/~ljason/cfs/*.

Traditionally, it has not been the focus of cognitive behavioral therapy to directly address issues of disability identity and illness phase with clients. Yet, many contend that a direct discussion and mapping of these issues may be critical to positive self-worth in the context of chronic illness and disability (Gill 1997; Wendell 1996). Cognitive behavioral therapy can play an important role in the process of facilitating positive identity development and integration following chronic illness or disability. Clients can be introduced to the cognitive model as it applies to issues of self-worth, self-efficacy, identity, and to joining or building new social networks.

Automatic thoughts about self and others, and conditional and core beliefs related to illness and disability can be assessed and addressed, when appropriate. Despite the potential contributions that cognitive behavioral therapy can make, many disability studies scholars and activists would argue that cognitive behavioral therapy, or any professionally based treatment modality, for that matter, is not an appropriate avenue by which to attain the requirements for an individual to develop a positive identity as a disabled person.

Though this issue is beyond the subject matter of this book, it is important to consider that psychotherapeutic modalities like cognitive behavioral therapy and many others, no matter how collaborative the client-therapist relationship, necessarily involve a power differential. Unless the psychotherapist has a visible disability or has openly disclosed that he or she has a chronic illness, a second level of diversity introduced into the client-therapist relationship is the fact that a nondisabled therapist may be treating a disabled client. Even if a psychotherapist's disability or illness is apparent, the experience of disability and chronic illness is highly unique to each individual and the therapist's condition may not involve the same characteristics of that of the client.

Though none of these diversity issues precludes a positive therapeutic relationship or positive psychotherapy outcomes, integration of a disability studies perspective would highlight the importance of facilitating exposure to peer disability and advocacy groups that aim to foster positive disability identity and empowerment among peers. Clients unfamiliar with such groups and organizations can be referred to their local center for independent living, or to a self-help organization that has a proactive and empowering mission, when appropriate.

Summary and Rationale for an Integrative Approach

A complex understanding of the unique concerns shared by individuals with chronic conditions is critical to successful outcomes of cognitive behavioral approaches. However, it is equally important that therapists consider the possibility that traditional approaches to cognitive behavioral therapy, alone, may not be adequate in addressing some of the more nuanced challenges involved in conducting psychotherapy with individuals with chronic conditions.

Though there is no other therapy that parallels the empirical evidence for its efficacy with a wide range of client populations (Dobson 2001), other approaches may serve as complementary to cognitive behavioral therapies, and may help to expand the range of clients with chronic conditions for which a cognitive behavioral approach may be appropriate. The next section of this book addresses related knowledge which can complement cognitive behavioral therapy.

Section Two

Related Knowledge

This section argues that a cognitive behavioral approach would be strengthened through an emphasis on three major concepts: empathy, hope, and motivation. An accurate empathic understanding of a client's thoughts, feelings, behaviors, and reactions to the therapist is essential to maintain throughout the therapeutic process. There are a number of reasons to place a high priority on empathy in the conduct of psychotherapy with people with chronic conditions, and these will be discussed in Chapter 11. In addition to empathy, another central issue for many individuals with chronic conditions is hope. In light of significant medical problems and threats to their physical well-being, clients often struggle with how to retain hope for wellness, improvement, or a positive quality of life. Because hope is so critical to therapeutic work with individuals with chronic conditions, cognitive behavioral therapists must assess it on an ongoing basis and target their interventions toward an overarching goal of instilling and preserving it. Hope theory, positive psychology, and their relevance and application to cognitive behavioral therapy will be covered in detail in Chapter 12.

Because fundamental motives to act can be compromised by physical and cognitive changes associated with chronic conditions, assessing and facilitating clients' motivation to engage and act in the world is a third critical aspect of any approach to psychotherapy with individuals with chronic conditions. Chapter 13 argues that volition is the primary source of participation and change for clients participating in cognitive behavioral therapy. Understanding volition will allow therapists and their clients to more accurately select behavioral experiments and other therapy assignments that lead to successful outcomes. It will also allow them to set short- and long-range goals that are more realistic, satisfying, personally significant, and ultimately more likely to be accomplished.

The next three chapters will expand upon the relevance of each of these complementary approaches (empathy, hope and motivation) and how they can be incorporated into the practice of cognitive behavioral therapy with clients with chronic conditions.

11

Believing in Empathy: The Need for a Novel Approach

During her intake interview, Nina told her therapist that the questions were pointless since there was no possible way the therapist could ever understand her or what she was going through. Paulette expressed concern in therapy that her husband was no longer attracted to her since her arthritis had progressed. Curtis, after working hard in therapy with positive results, stopped following through on any homework assignments. He could not explain this new behavior and seemed to accept only empathy and supportive comments from his therapist in therapy. Each of these instances points to potential relevance of using empathy in cognitive behavioral therapy.

Empathy and Chronic Conditions

There are three key reasons to place a high priority on empathy in therapeutic work with people with chronic conditions; that is, empathy

- Is a means by which a therapist can bear witness to a client's past and ongoing experiences of trauma and loss
- Can be helpful to prepare clients to engage in cognitive exploration and change
- Can be used to address "old wounds" that manifest themselves at cognitive and interpersonal levels during the therapy and that are not easily accessed or addressed through standard cognitive behavioral approaches

Each of these three reasons is discussed below.

As discussed in Chapter 10, individuals with chronic conditions can feel isolated and misunderstood, particularly in the presence of others that do not share their illness or disability. At the same time, they often experience physical discomfort and may face discrimination and other barriers to social and occupational participation. Consequently, the initial losses in health-related function that may have occurred as a result of the illness or disability itself may be worsened by the social and environmental context in which a person is living. Because these losses and challenges are significant and painful, clients often have a strong desire to share their experience and have others bear witness to it. In addition, they may experience periods of rage and feelings of demoralization as normal and expected reactions to these many losses. Empathy offers a critical means by which a therapist can bear witness to a client's past and ongoing experiences of trauma and loss throughout the course of the illness or disability.

A new-onset illness or impairment is usually felt and experienced as a significant loss or trauma, particularly for individuals with more Westernized worldviews. The symptoms of physical illness or disability are, in most cases, very real, and clearly unrelated to any errors in thinking or maladaptive belief systems. Most clients with chronic conditions, who do not have a history of chronic or severe psychopathology and are unaccustomed to psychotherapy (Moorey and Greer 2002), may find it difficult to accept psychological definitions of, or solutions to, their problems. Thus, initially, it may be difficult for a client with a chronic condition to adopt the cognitive model or see its relevance in treating a presenting physical symptom or a negative health-care behavior. Yet, some research indicates that acceptance of the cognitive model predicts psychotherapy outcomes (Fennell and Teasdale 1987). Thus, it is crucial that clients are adequately prepared to accept this model as the guiding framework for treatment. In cases where clients may be slow or resistant, empathically based interventions may offer the best means of preparing them to engage in cognitive exploration and change.

It is widely accepted and understood that losses and traumas can trigger or exacerbate feelings of isolation, powerlessness, loss of control, and anger or rage, among other intense reactions. It is likely that any preexisting emotional wounds or aspects of psychological development that may have been arrested earlier in life will inevitably be provoked in situations of new loss or trauma, (Kohut 1984). These reinvoked wounds can threaten an individual's sense of self-cohesion and psychological well being, particularly when the self has not undergone healthy development. In many cases, particularly when these wounds occurred as a result of failures of empathy in prior relationships, an individual is at risk for reenacting disappointments, rejections, and losses that stemmed from old relationships in their current relationships. These "old wounds" are not always concrete, obvious, or easily accessed through standard cognitive behavioral approaches, yet it can be argued that they manifest themselves at cognitive and interpersonal levels during the therapy process.

The Role of Empathy in Psychotherapy Outcomes

Over the past three decades, the significance of empathy to psychotherapy outcomes has been the subject of extensive debate (Morris and Magrath 1983; Turkat and Brantley 1981). This controversy began with comparative psychotherapy studies that suggested that orientations to psychotherapy with opposing causal theories, techniques, and goals, such as psychodynamic and interpersonal approaches, were as effective as cognitive behavioral therapy in the treatment of disorders like depression (Elkin et al., 1989; Rehm, Kaslow, and Rabin 1987; Zeiss, Lewinsohn, and Munoz 1979). It was then hypothesized that these outcomes stemmed from nonspecific positive factors that are common to all approaches to psychotherapy (Bergin and Garfield 1994). Notably, these characteristics include empathy as a key element. Importantly, a major review of 115 studies by Orlinsky and associates (1994) indicated that therapeutic empathy was most strongly and consistently correlated with positive psychotherapy outcomes only when it was measured according to the *client's* perspective and not when it was self-assessed by therapists.

Empathy within Cognitive Behavioral Therapy

The role of empathy within cognitive behavioral therapy is a matter of highly divergent opinion. Ellis (1962) contends that therapeutic empathy is neither a necessary nor a sufficient condition for successful therapy outcomes and may even interfere with progress in psychotherapy. Other critical perspectives assert that empathy may serve to prevent progress or reinforce maladaptive thinking or behaviors in a client (Burns and Auerbach 1996). Some cognitive behavioral therapists argue that a therapist's efforts to display empathy may be more likely to reflect the therapist's unique history, roles, fantasies, and worldviews than the client's *actual* experience (Burns and Auerbach 1996). This critique is supported by research, which indicates that therapists are not usually accurate in their estimations of how their clients perceive them in their attempts to convey empathy and warmth (Free et al., 1985). Accordingly, some cognitive behavioral therapists argue that empathy is useful only to the extent that it is accurately perceived by clients (Beck et al., 1979; Linehan 1995).

In contrast to Rogers (1951), who views empathy as a necessary and sufficient requirement for change, Beck, Rush, Shaw and Emory (1979) refer to empathy as a necessary but *insufficient* condition. According to their perspective, the technical components of cognitive behavioral therapy are highly important for positive therapy outcomes because the underlying theory of psychopathology is based on distorted cognition, rather than on some other hypothesized variable, such as disrupted early relations. From a cognitive behavioral perspective, the technical aspects of cognitive behavioral therapy (i.e., addressing maladaptive cognitions) are not only viewed as important to client change in and of themselves, but they are also viewed as important contributors to the therapeutic relationship in that they convey the therapist's interest in the client and his or her active attempts to support the client in the change process (Keijsers, Schaap and Hoogduin 2000).

Use of Empathy in Cognitive Behavioral Therapy

A growing number of reports and studies indicate that many cognitive behavioral therapists do tend place a high value on empathy and on building and maintaining a positive therapeutic relationship with their clients (Burns and Auerbach 1996; Keijsers, Schaap, and Hoogduin 2000). Although Salvio, Beutler, Wood, and Engle (1992) found no differences in the quality of the therapeutic alliance between cognitive behavioral therapy and other psychotherapy orientations (e.g., gestalt therapy and self-directed supportive therapy), a preponderance of other studies have found that cognitive behavioral therapists tend to engage in a significantly higher proportion of empathic comments (e.g., reassurance, praise, sympathy) as compared with psychoanalytic or gestalt therapists (Brunink and Schroeder 1979). Others have found that cognitive behavioral therapists, in contrast to psychodynamic and psychoanalytic therapists, show more initiative in working to develop a supportive relationship than psychodynamic therapists, are more likely to agree with clients on psychotherapy goals, have a stronger therapeutic alliance, and are rated by their clients as having better interpersonal skills and more accurate empathy (Raue, Castonguay, and Goldfried 1993). Taken together, these findings contradict myths and stereotypes of cognitive behavioral therapists as cold, linear, superficial, unempathic, authoritarian, or more mechanical in their interactions with clients (Keijsers, Shaap and Hoogduin 2000). Instead, they indicate that many cognitive behavioral therapists value the therapeutic relationship and view empathy as having a significant impact upon positive psychotherapy outcomes.

Client Perspectives on Empathy in Cognitive Behavioral Therapy

Some studies suggest that clients of cognitive behavioral therapy may value the relationship they had with their therapist more than the cognitive behavioral techniques that were employed to treat their symptoms (Llewelyn and Hume 1979; Ryan and Gizynski 1971). In addition to these findings, one study found that high helpfulness ratings for relationship variables were associated with more positive therapy outcomes, but high helpfulness ratings for cognitive behavioral techniques were not (Ryan and Gizynski 1971).

Empathy and Client Improvement in Cognitive Behavioral Therapy

A number of more specific findings have been put forth to suggest that empathy is likely to make a significant contribution to clinical improvement in cognitive behavioral therapy (Burns and Nolen-Hoeksema 1992; Keijsers, Shaap and Hoogduin 2000). In one of the earliest studies of this topic, Persons and Burns (1985) measured clients' perceptions of empathy and warmth from therapists after a single session of cognitive behavioral therapy. They found that empathy and warmth were significantly associated with level of improvement following a course of therapy. In a more rigorous study that controlled for the effects of homework compliance and improvement in depression itself, Burns and Nolen-Hoeksema (1992) estimated the effect of therapeutic empathy on clinical improvement using structural equation modeling. The highest levels of clinical improvement were observed in clients of therapists with the highest client-rated empathy scores.

Existing Approaches to Empathy Training in Cognitive Behavioral Therapy

According to the cognitive behavioral therapy perspective, the client is also viewed as an expert on the meanings that he or she has attached to those experiences (Beck, Rush, Shaw, and Emery 1979; Beck 1995). Beck's emphasis on meaning and acknowledgement that each client's manner of ascribing meaning to events is unique and idiosyncratic is critical to the ultimate ability of the therapist to gain an accurate understanding of a client's thinking. It is also critical to a therapist's ability to attain an accurate empathic understanding of other aspects of a client's psyche, including his or her emotional experience and behaviors. From a cognitive behavioral perspective, accurate understanding of a client is also achieved through ongoing assessment and solicitation of feedback about the therapy and the therapist. When problems in the therapeutic relationship arise, a client's concerns are taken seriously, explored, and actively discussed in light of the cognitive model.

Burns and Auerbach (1996) have developed a unique program to train cognitive behavioral therapists to incorporate the use of empathy into the treatment process. The fundamental concept underlying this program is that the effective practice of cognitive behavioral therapy strikes an appropriate balance in shifting between two components: technical interventions and empathic interventions (Burns and Auerbach 1996). Technical interventions comprise the elements of cognitive behavioral therapy that are designed to assist clients with problem-solving and the modification of maladaptive beliefs, emotions, and behaviors.

According to Burns and Auerbach (1996), empathic interventions involve listening and self-expression skills. Listening skills incorporate three approaches. The disarming technique involves finding even the smallest grain of truth in a claim or accusation that a client may be making, even if it seems illogical, distorted, or dysfunctional. Empathy involves paraphrasing a client's words and acknowledging how a client might be feeling. Inquiry involves asking gentle, probing questions in order to better understand what the client is thinking and feeling. Self-expression skills incorporate two approaches. "I feel" statements are used to maintain credibility, convey sincerity, and to avoid blaming the client when attacked. Examples of such statements include "When you say that, I feel that our work together is not important to you." The second self-expression skill, "stroking," is used to convey an attitude of respect and to demonstrate emotional support toward a client, even if a therapist feels that the situation is conflictual or tense. According to Burns and Auerbach (1996), empathic interventions are to be utilized in cognitive behavioral therapy in two circumstances:

- When a client is emotionally upset and needs the therapist to bear witness to his or her feelings, and
- When a client expresses a concern about the therapist or the therapy process.

Shifting between the technical and empathic approaches requires a therapist to possess distinctly different skill sets (Burns and Auerbach 1996).

The Challenge of Empathy within a Cognitive Behavioral Approach

In cognitive behavioral approaches, it is generally assumed that the process of eliciting a client's beliefs and feelings and feedback about therapy on an ongoing basis automatically lends itself to an empathic atmosphere in therapy. The client has the authority to assign meaning to his or her experiences and the power to judge the degree to which he or she is finding the therapy helpful at any given time. Therapists practicing from a cognitive perspective are trained to periodically make summaries of their understanding of what the client has said, particularly following agenda-setting or after an important discovery or intervention has taken place (Beck 1995).

Cognitive behavioral therapists are also trained to solicit and give serious consideration to a client's feedback and to ensure that there is an adequate agreement with the client as to the selected objectives and goals of therapy. Despite this emphasis on summarizing and feedback, therapists practicing from a cognitive behavioral orientation may find it challenging to use more sophisticated approaches to empathy (Burns and Auerbach 1996). Training in cognitive behavioral therapy tends to emphasize the identification and modification of a client's dysfunctional thinking patterns. Therapists newer to this practice may focus too much on assisting the client to identify and modify the negative aspects of dysfunctional thinking. Some therapists may fail to have enough patience to allow the client to recognize dysfunctional patterns on his or her own. This unwitting, implicit conveyance that the client's perceptions are irrational and/or maladaptive may cause some clients to feel belittled, stupid, or judged to be more emotionally impaired than they actually feel, particularly if their main issue is a medical symptom rather than a psychological one. These timing mistakes and other mismatches between therapist and client judgments about the degree to which a given cognition is realistic or useful are more likely to occur during times when there are unrecognized limitations in the therapeutic relationship or when a client is otherwise frustrated, angry, uncomfortable, or in pain.

The required shift into an empathic mode of responding called for in these situations might be more difficult for cognitive behavioral therapists, particularly if they are not adequately trained to assume a more mobile and dialectical approach to treatment (Burns and Auerbach 1996; Linehan 1993a). Such an approach involves moving back and forth between joining with a client to understand his or her worldview and challenge his or her dysfunctional thinking, versus empathizing with his or her more irrational thoughts and feelings or with his or her more difficult experiences of pain, frustration, rage, hopelessness, vulnerability, or feelings of ineptitude.

The capacity to effectively empathize with a client will, in part, depend on a therapist's past life experiences, personal worldview, capacity for vicarious emotional experience, and other characteristics of his or her psychological disposition as they interact with client variables and the given experience being presented. In the absence of a skilled, intentional, and disciplined approach to the use of empathic approaches in therapy, any therapist is vulnerable to reacting to different clients, or even to differing content presented by a single client, in dramatically different ways.

As discussed earlier, Burns and Auerbach (1996) have taken on the challenge of attempting to train therapists to develop an empathy skill set by emphasizing the need to shift between technically based and empathically based intervention strategies. Similarly, Linehan (1993a) emphasizes training therapists to approach the therapeutic relationship from a dialectical point of view (i.e., by striking a balance between change-oriented and acceptance-oriented strategies).

A significant limitation of both of these existing approaches is that they recommend highly technical, cognitive approaches to train therapists in a skill that is arguably neither technical nor cognitively based. There are no definitive rules of timing, perception, and intuition that can guide the use of empathy in real-world therapeutic relationships. If a therapist were to simply rely on the guideline that they are to introduce listening or self-expression skills when a client needs to express emotion or when the client is unhappy with therapy or angry with the therapist, how might we prevent that therapist from choosing the wrong strategy at the wrong time? How can we prevent empathic strategies from appearing affected or insincere?

In the absence of a strong belief in an underlying theoretical framework that can guide their use of empathy throughout the therapeutic process, cognitive behavioral therapists risk coming across as insincere, clumsy, or gimmicky— especially during times of tension or high emotion within the therapeutic relationship. Moreover, therapists are more likely to use empathy in a more mobile and flexible way if they understand its purpose and definition within an underlying theoretical context. That is, cognitive behavioral therapists may be more likely to naturally assimilate the practice of empathy if they come to *believe* in its significance and relevance to their work.

Believing in the Significance of Empathy

For decades, self psychologists practicing according to the theory of Kohut (1971, 1977, 1984) have argued that empathy is the central means by which to access and repair developmental arrests and psychic wounds, which are often played out within the therapeutic relationship. Self psychology is an integrated theory of healthy psychological development, broadly characterized psychopathology, and psychotherapy (Gardner 1991; Kohut 1966, 1971, 1977, 1984; Kohut and Wolf 1978; Wolf 1988). Because it was developed to describe healthy psychological development, it can be used to understand and treat clients facing a wide range of human problems, including acute traumas and losses, difficulties with self-esteem, difficulties with goal attainment, and difficulties with emotion regulation, among others (Gardner, 1991). Because it is not fundamentally pathology based, a self-psychological perspective can be used to understand a number of the losses, psychic injuries, and resulting life dilemmas that can accompany the experience of a chronic condition or new disability.

Kohut's Theory of Self Psychology

In order to understand the significance of empathy to healthy human development, one must understand Kohut's (1966, 1971, 1977, 1984) central theory of self psychology, or the "psychology of the self." Kohut viewed the "self" as the nucleus of the human being and as responsible for all psychological development. His theory holds that the development of a mature and cohesive self is fundamental to healthy psychological functioning. This mature and cohesive self is characterized as possessing psychological structure, or the ability to:

- Self soothe,
- Regulate difficult emotions, and
- Maintain a sense of stability and cohesion.

This healthy and mature self also strives for experiences of mastery, seeks goal attainment, and has basic capabilities and skills (Gardner 1991; Kohut and Wolf 1978).

According to Kohut (1971), the developing self of every young child has three fundamental needs:

- Idealization needs,
- Mirroring needs, and
- Twinship needs.

It is important for these needs to be met in early development so that this need fulfillment can be adequately internalized and adopted by the child's own developing sense of self.

Idealization

Idealization needs refer to a child's need to be close to and accepted by what he or she perceives as a heroic, omnipotent, and ideal caretaker. This "idealized parental imago" conveys to the child that he or she is safe and protected. The idealizable parent or caretaker offers the child a sense of calmness, connection, support, and strength, even in times of high stress or tension. As a result, the child learns healthy ideals and values, is motivated to pursue goals, and develops a sense of respect and admiration for other people. Eventually, the child internalizes a capacity to soothe and comfort him- or herself and regulate emotions under stressful circumstances.

Mirroring

Mirroring needs refer to a child's need to be admired, validated, and bolstered (Kohut 1971). Early in life, children need to feel grandiose in the eyes of their parents or caretakers. Their innate sense of vigor and perfectionism needs to be supported and affirmed. As the child develops, other aspects of the self, even negative affective states, also need to be mirrored and validated. Under circumstances of appropriate mirroring, a child's early grandiosity ultimately matures into a balanced sense of self-esteem, an ability to assert needs appropriately and self-advocate, a desire to be ambitious, an ability to recognize and enjoy success, and an ability to derive pleasure from pursuing interests and activities (Gardner 1991).

Twinship

Twinship needs refer to a child's need to have a sense of belonging and community with like others. As the child develops, experiences of belonging and kinship with others support the self and ultimately lead to the capacity to pursue goals, adopt roles, and utilize one's talents and skills in an optimal way (Gardner 1991).

Development, developmental arrests, and fragmentation of the self

Kohut (1984) maintained that early in development and throughout the life span all individuals need to have interactions with others that provide opportunities for gratification of these three basic needs for idealization, mirroring, and twinship. Kohut (1984) argued that a psychologically healthy individual develops a certain psychological structure, which includes the ability to self-soothe, regulate his or her emotions and inner tensions, and maintain a sense of self-cohesion. According to Kohut, this structure is based on experiences of "optimal frustration," which are minor, nontraumatic, and necessary empathic failures in childhood that are effectively responded to by in-tune parents or caregivers.

   If key others, such as parents, fail to meet a child's needs in one or more of these three areas, arrests to the development of a mature and cohesive self will occur. Later in development, new losses, traumas, threats to self-esteem, or disruptions in relationships will aggravate these areas of unmet need, or developmental arrest, leading to fragmentations of the self. Depending on the individual, this fragmentation might be experienced as rage, despair, anxiety or as other difficulties with self-soothing, emotion regulation, and behavior.

Kohutian Empathy: A Novel Approach in Cognitive Behavioral Therapy

Although Kohut's theory was originally developed as a theory for the treatment of individuals with narcissistic personality disorders, the theory and practice of self psychology have since been broadened to apply to a wide range of human conditions and circumstances (Kohut 1984; Wolf 1980). Today, self psychology theory is considered to be a general theory of human motivation and development (Gardner 1991). Within self psychology, it is now commonly accepted that all human beings require ongoing experiences of need fulfillment in these three areas, and connection to others that can serve to help meet these fundamental needs throughout the life span (Gardner 1991). Conversely, all human relationships will inevitably be characterized by losses, rifts and empathic failures that will need to be repaired. When these occur in therapy, psychotherapists can provide clients with opportunity for resolutions and repair of these woundings through empathic responding within the therapeutic relationship.

The theoretical framework that underlies the Kohutian perspective on psychopathology is distinctly different from the theoretical framework that underlies cognitive behavioral therapy. Nonetheless, there is significant advantage to thinking about empathy from a Kohutian perspective. This can be done largely within the therapists' minds, while they are still practicing according to the structure, principles, and techniques of cognitive behavioral therapy.

The Kohutian perspective emphasizes that therapists must be ever-mindful of the early developmental injuries and arrests that may have led to a client's current behavior. By practicing this mindfulness, an otherwise technically oriented therapist can think beyond the current presenting problems and behaviors. That is, the therapist will also consider the client wholistically, as a once-younger person whose injuries to the self resulted from the failings of more powerful others or from early caretakers in his or her life.

Because self psychology views the resolution of empathic failures and rifts in the therapeutic relationship as central to the reestablishment of a cohesive self, therapists practicing from this perspective are taught to hold sacred the power of making every effort to effectively resolve empathic failures. Therapists are trained to work with clients to resolve these rifts in a way that will preserve the client's self-cohesion and restore any unmet developmental needs in the areas of idealization, mirroring or twinship. In addition, self psychology therapists are trained to convey empathy throughout the therapy process, not only when the client is emoting or frustrated with the therapist.

Kohut (1984) defined empathy primarily as an objective mode of observation in which the therapist comes to understand a client's underlying emotions, needs, longings and motives, while at the same time maintaining an objective viewpoint. Kohut labeled the empathic process of accessing a client's internal world "vicarious introspection" and he consistently emphasized the importance of evaluating each client's experiences and behaviors from the client's unique perspective (Gardner 1991; Kohut 1984).

Practicing Empathy from a Self Psychological Perspective

From a self psychological perspective, the actual practice of empathy is unique and relatively straightforward. It involves speaking back to the client's inner reality and re-conveying an understanding of what a client has said after the client has revealed a significant aspect of his or her experience (Gardner 1991). During this process, a therapist pays particular attention to the client's affect and to his or her reporting of experiences, because one of the central functions of this empathic recounting is not only to aid the therapist in his or her understanding of the client, but also to assist the client in organizing and clarifying the meaning of his or her own feelings and experiences. During this process, the therapist "listens for" the client to express needs, wishes, longings, and motives that likely underlie his or her behaviors (Gardner 1991). According to self psychology, empathy involves the process of recounting accepting, and affirming any perception or experience that a client offers. This process of empathy allows the therapist to gain better access to a client's inner experience and to more fully engage the client in therapy so that a client's communications are more consistent with his or her actual emotional experience.

According to self psychology, an empathic approach to listening and recounting also serves to train clients to identify and focus more inwardly on their thinking and feelings (i.e., become more introspective) (Gardner 1991). This training better prepares clients of cognitive behavioral therapy to listen to periodic summaries of treatment with an open mind, and to provide their therapists with honest feedback about the accuracy of such summaries. In addition, such an empathic approach allows clients to better identify connections between their automatic thoughts and their intermediate and core beliefs. Additionally, it creates an initial atmosphere of safety and acceptance that is facilitative of the client's willingness to share and explore beliefs, feelings and experiences that are otherwise too painful or anxiety-provoking. Thus, empathy is a key means by which to enable many clients dialogue honestly with their therapists and to be willing to even participate in such an active behavioral, problem-solving and change-oriented approach as cognitive behavioral therapy.

In addition to bearing witness to, clarifying, organizing, and assisting the client in assigning meaning to painful and frightening thoughts and experiences, empathy also serves key functions within the therapeutic relationship. Kohut characterized empathy as innately fundamental to all relationships and as a life-sustaining force. A number of self psychologists have suggested that empathy, in and of itself, may have a therapeutic and mutative effect on clients (Kohut 1984; Wolf 1988). Within the self psychological framework, empathy also serves a key function in the resolution of therapeutic impasses, rifts, or other experiences of "optimal frustration" within the therapeutic relationship.

When losses, new traumas, threats to self-esteem, separations, or disruptions in relationships occur, they can trigger a loss of psychic structure, or ability to maintain a sense of self-cohesion. This loss of structure can be acute or chronic, but it is most likely to occur when and if there have been arrests in the client's early development of psychic structure. The loss of structure can lead to feelings of rage, fragmentation, apathy, low self-esteem, and maladaptive behavior. Kohut argued that psychic structure and a sense of self-cohesion can be re-formed, repaired, or rehabilitated through attempts by the therapist to understand and respond to the client's needs, longings, wishes, and motives in an empathic manner. According to Kohut (1984), the most optimal opportunities for the rebuilding of psychic structure arise when the therapist is appropriately and empathically responsive to minor and inevitable rifts within the therapeutic relationship.

The following scenario from Paulette's therapy illustrates how empathic responding can be used as a regular facet of cognitive behavioral therapy to facilitate engagement and a psychologically secure atmosphere.

Paulette: "My husband is getting pretty angry that I can no longer keep the house up like I used to. I'm afraid one day he might just decide I'm not worth it anymore."

Therapist: "You're worried that your difficulties keeping the house clean are driving your husband away." [choosing to make an empathic reflection rather than to probe for more information]

Paulette: "Well it's either that or he's having an affair. He just doesn't seem to care about me anymore. He's like a stone when he gets home from work." [client seems on the verge of tears]

Therapist: "So your real concern is that your husband isn't as available to you, emotionally." [deliberately choosing not to assess, challenge, or plug the client's suspicious, self-blaming, and potentially illogical thinking into the cognitive model prematurely]

Paulette: "I'm no longer the woman he married. I think that he must be sick of me being sick. On the weekends all he wants to do is watch football with his buddies. It just seems like he would do anything just to get away from me and the kids."

Therapist: "In some way you think it's your fault that your husband isn't around as much." [continuing with empathic reflection to facilitate cognitive organization, insight, and personal meaning for this client]

Paulette: "I can't see any other reason he wouldn't want to be with me. I just feel so alone and wish he would help me. Maybe he could help me with the house rather than blaming me for it or running away."

Therapist: "So I just want to summarize my understanding of the problem right now. Your greatest concern is your husband's unavailability and your deepest need is for him to join you in dealing with your illness – like by helping you around the house and things."

Paulette: "Yes, but I can't seem to change him. Nothing seems to work. He just stares at me blankly when I cry and tell him how much it hurts."

Therapist: [now introducing the cognitive model] "I agree with you that we need to figure out an alternative for you. Maybe we can begin by exploring whether there is a specific pattern of thinking, reacting, and interacting going on within your relationship that is leading to your pain and disappointment in him. We clearly know that he is withdrawing. Now we need to figure out how you can survive this, and how you might work with him to change this pattern."

Paulette: "OK."

Similar to what occurs in many real-world therapeutic interactions, in this case example, the therapist was confronted with several choices. It is very possible that an alternative approach to this situation that involved more Socratic questioning, probing, and recording and eventual challenging of the client's maladaptive beliefs may have been effective. However, in this situation the therapist chose to slow the pace of the therapy and build in more opportunities for the client to organize her thinking and derive meaning from her emotional pain and marital experiences.

This empathic process built an atmosphere of greater trust and psychological safety between the client and the therapist, making it more likely that the client would eventually buy into working within the cognitive model to change key aspects of her thinking, her core beliefs regarding lovability, and her behavior within her relationship.

Conclusion

This chapter has argued that the empathic approach of self psychology can be utilized to deliver a more empathically based approach to cognitive behavioral therapy with individuals with chronic conditions. This approach involves the continual striving on the part of the therapist for understanding of a client's experience and the ongoing provision and solicitation of immediate feedback regarding the accuracy of that understanding. Empathy also involves being able to effectively resolve minor but inevitable empathic failures and rifts within the therapeutic relationship.

These fundamental aspects of empathy are particularly relevant to the practice of cognitive behavioral therapy because they can serve to tame the minds of therapists that tend to be over-zealous or premature in their imposition of the more technical aspects of cognitive behavioral therapy with their clients. The incorporation of empathy into cognitive behavioral therapy is also critical in cases where clients may be slow or resistant to accepting the more technical aspects of assessment and intervention and instead require more initial work on gaining understanding and insight into their beliefs and their many potential meanings.

The use of empathy is even more critical in the circumstance of new-onset illness or impairment because individuals with new conditions may be more vulnerable to experiencing episodes of acute emotional crisis and fragmentation. These individuals may have no prior experience or contact with the mental-health-care system and may be less socialized or accustomed to viewing their distressed thought processes as flawed, dysfunctional, or fundamentally irrational. With the increasing emphasis on brief and time-limited approaches to psychotherapy, the use of empathy can create an atmosphere of safety and respect in which people otherwise unwilling to look inward at their dysfunctional patterns of thinking and behaving would be more likely to understand the relevance of the cognitive model to their problem.

12

Instilling Hope in People with Chronic Conditions

It is sometimes observed that models of psychotherapy overemphasize pathology and underemphasize the importance of recognizing, cultivating, and sustaining positive aspects of thinking and experience. In response to this observation, the field of positive psychology was introduced (Seligman and Csikszentmihalyi 2000). Positive psychology involves the study of:

- Positive emotions, such as confidence, hope and trust,
- Positive traits, such as strengths, virtues and abilities, and
- Positive institutions (Seligman 2002).

Positive psychology attempts to understand valued emotions or subjective experiences including well-being, contentment, and satisfaction with the past, hope and optimism for the future, and flow and happiness in the present (Seligman and Csikszentmihalyi 2000). It also studies valued individual traits, including the capacity for love and work, courage, interpersonal aptitude, spirituality, wisdom, high talent, aesthetic sensibility, perseverance, forgiveness, originality, and future-mindedness (Seligman and Csikszentmihalyi 2000).

Positive Psychology and Chronic Conditions

The need for a positive psychological approach to psychotherapy may be more pronounced when treating individuals with chronic conditions. Some clients may perceive cognitive behavioral therapy strategies, such as Socratic questioning, elicitation of automatic thoughts, and frequent summaries of presenting problems, as overly negativistic, pessimistic, frightening, or otherwise threatening. These responses may occur irrespective of whether alternative approaches to thinking and behaving are introduced. Some clients will have a strong need for reassurance and may request a more optimistic approach on the part of their therapists (Moorey and Greer 2002). In these circumstances, positive psychology approaches to cognitive behavioral therapy that emphasize hope and optimism may be useful.

Based on a review of the empirical evidence in this area, Salovey, et al. (2000) contend that positive emotional states can promote physical health through a number of pathways. These include observations that positive emotion may

- Have direct effects on immunity and illness,
- Have a salutatory affect on the experience of and emphasis on symptoms and the tendency to over-rely on help-seeking behavior,
- Be associated with enhanced psychological resources,
- Inspire health-promoting behavior, and
- Lead to social support seeking (Salovey et al., 2000).

Similarly, findings from a study of men with HIV suggest that optimism, personal control, and a sense of meaning may function as health-protective resources in individuals with chronic illness (Taylor et al., 2000).

Hope Theory

This chapter argues that the practice of cognitive behavioral therapy with individuals with chronic conditions would be enhanced by concepts borrowed from hope theory (Snyder, 1989, 2000). Widely embraced by the field of positive psychology, hope theory has been described as a cognitively based metatheory that cuts across many approaches to psychotherapy (Taylor, et al., 2000). Hope theory maintains that hope is rooted in goal-directed thinking and that hopeful people engage in two specific forms of goal-directed thinking:

- Pathway thinking and
- Agency thinking (Snyder 1989).

Snyder defines pathway thinking as an individual's active evaluation of his or her ability to achieve a workable means, or "route," to attaining a goal. Pathway thinking involves planning and the consideration of different options. Agency thinking is defined as the mental energy, determination, and motivation toward goal attainment. According to Snyder (1989) the three central components of hope (goal setting, pathway thinking, and agency thinking) are interrelated and synergistic in nature so that each element of hope builds upon the other as a person takes concrete steps toward attaining both short-term (mainly directed toward symptom relief) and long-term goals in psychotherapy.

When considering application of hope theory or any positive psychology approach in cognitive behavioral therapy, caution should be taken to avoid

- Idealizing positive approaches,
- Using positive psychology as a means of prescribing how people should live, or
- Failing to recognize that there are situations and contexts in which an emphasis on strengths or optimism is not appropriate (Aspinwall and Staudinger, 2003).

Moreover, the suggestion that cognitive behavioral therapy might be enhanced by concepts from positive psychology should not be taken to imply that other positive approaches to psychotherapy, such as Buddist approaches (Levine and Levine 1982), solution-focused therapy (McNeilly 2000) or humanistic approaches (Rogers 1951), are not also worthy of consideration.

Cognitive Behavioral Therapy from a Positive Psychology Perspective

Beck (1996) recognized that "positive modes," or activities aimed at increasing needed resources, should be considered in an overall conceptualization of personality and psychopathology. Seligman (1998, 2002) has applied principles of positive psychology, and more specifically, hope theory, to aspects of the practice of cognitive behavioral therapy. Seligman's (2002) orientation involves

- The promotion of positive emotion and
- The promotion of positive individual traits.

He argues that positive individual traits (e.g., character and other personal strengths) are fundamental to the authentic experience of positive emotion. This argument is valid and important for therapists from any orientation to consider. Because it would be beyond the scope of this chapter to include all aspects of Seligman's approach, readers are referred to Seligman's books *Learned Optimism* (Seligman 1998) and *Authentic Happiness* (Seligman 2002) for more information about the promotion of positive individual traits. In this chapter, the focus will parallel Seligman's approach to positive emotion, with specific emphasis on the promotion of hope and its importance for people with chronic conditions.

Promoting positive emotion is fundamental to effective coping with a chronic condition. Though the primary tradition in cognitive behavioral therapy has been to focus mainly on present circumstances and cognitions (particularly in the initial stages of therapy), Seligman (2002) argues that all time points need to be accounted for in the generation of positive emotional experience. According to Seligman (2002), in order to be hopeful about the future, one must be able to find satisfaction with one's life, which is a historical culmination of past achievements and events, and one must be able to experience pleasure and gratification in the present. Thus, the promotion of positive emotion consists of generating

- Satisfaction about the past,
- Hope about the future, and
- Pleasures and gratifications in the present.

Satisfaction about the Past

Being satisfied with past life experiences, life meanings, and the contributions one has made to others is essential in preventing feelings of existential isolation and angst, particularly in circumstances where chronic conditions are highly impairing or terminal. Beck views meaning from a pragmatic perspective as it is linked to perceived control (Moss 1992). Beck's view is that life meanings are the product of the meanings we attribute to our life situations (Beck, et al., 1979). Seligman (2002) capitalizes on this notion and encourages people to reflect upon issues of meaning and satisfaction with life. People are also encouraged to practice gratitude for other people, situations, gifts, and talents that have been part of their life history. Another aspect of past satisfaction that Seligman (2002) emphasizes is forgiveness. Though it is not always possible or appropriate in some circumstances, practicing forgiveness helps to generate positive emotions such as satisfaction, contentment, fulfillment, pride, and serenity.

The following extraction from a session with Curtis illustrates the difficulties that people with chronic illness can have with finding satisfaction with life and how a therapist practicing cognitive behavioral therapy with a positive emphasis might respond to this issue.

Therapist: [observing a change in affect, therapist probes for negative automatic thought]
  "What was going through your mind just now?"
Curtis: "That, in the end, this life really isn't worth all the effort."
Therapist: "You're feeling deeply disappointed with life right now."
Curtis: "Yeah."
Therapist: "Have you always felt that life has let you down?"
Curtis: "I always thought I'd have more time. Now I'm not sure I have enough time left to do anything really good or important." [Curtis begins to sob.]
Therapist: [bears witness in silence]
Therapist: [probing for an intermediate belief] "Curtis, what do you think would qualify as a good or important life?"
Curtis: "Someone who changed the world, like Martin Luther King or someone like that."
Therapist: [probing further] "What qualities in particular?"
Curtis: "He promoted civil rights and peace and unity and had an influence on human relations everywhere"
Therapist: [probing for underlying core belief] "What does the fact that you admire him say about you?"
Curtis: "I guess that I try to follow his teachings whenever I can."
Therapist: "And how do you do that?"
Curtis: "In my church and at work and stuff – I promote respect, peace and unity when people don't get along."
Therapist: "So it sounds to me like your life hasn't been that meaningless after all."
Curtis: "Guess not in all ways…"
Therapist: "Well, for now let's brainstorm a little longer about peacemaking and other things you've done that you can feel good about."

The experience of chronic illness can prompt thoughts about mortality and meaning in life. The excerpt from Curtis's therapy session illustrates how the therapist's intention to promote life satisfaction can be built into the process of Socratic questioning. The reader may have noticed that the downward arrow technique (working downward from automatic thoughts to intermediate beliefs to core beliefs) was also used in this case. To the therapist's surprise, Curtis's underlying core belief about himself, in this instance, was positive. Instead of making a negative comparison of himself with Martin Luther King and coming up short, Curtis reported that he tries to emulate him. At that point the therapist's main goal was to further capitalize on Curtis's positive core belief about himself as a promoter of dignity, peace and unity and ask questions that would allow Curtis to reflect on his life and his past actions in positive ways.

In addition to supporting positive appraisal of the past within therapy, it can also be useful to provide tasks in therapy or homework assignments that allow clients to explore their satisfaction with their past. Table 1 illustrates three such tasks/assignments. These and other therapy tasks/homework assignments can be used to help clients achieve greater satisfaction with their past.

Some clients with chronic conditions may idealize the past because it seems better to them in light of the losses and limitations they are experiencing in the present. A positive psychology approach to cognitive behavioral therapy would not recommend interfering with this idealized perspective of the past (Taylor et al., 2000a). Other individuals may report that their lives in general, or major aspects of their lives, were not satisfying. They may blame themselves, certain individuals, or life circumstances for negative feelings in the present. Clients having particular difficulty reconciling past experiences and behavior may benefit uniquely from therapy activities and homework assignments that focus on achieving satisfaction with the past.

Instilling Hope

Hope has been found to play a fundamental role in promoting more positive outcomes for individuals with chronic illness (Snyder, Rand, and Sigmon 2002;

TABLE 1. Satisfaction about the past: recommended (therapy or homework) assignments.

Assignment #1 "Life Satisfaction":	Clients complete and score Seligman's (2002) *Satisfaction with Life Scale**. Results are discussed in the next therapy session or following completion of the scale.
Assignment #2 "Cultivating Gratitude":	Clients complete and score the *Gratitude Survey**. Results are discussed in the next therapy session or following completion of the scale.
Assignment #3 "Forgiveness":	Clients are instructed to come up with the name of at least one person they have forgiven and to reflect upon how they feel for having forgiven this person. The purpose of the assignment is to allow clients to see that they are capable of forgiveness.

*Recommended measures for Assignments 1 and 2 can be accessed and scored in Seligman's (2002) book, *Authentic Happiness,* or online at *www.authentichappiness.org.*

Taylor et al., 2000b). Research indicates that hope facilitates better adjustment and coping with the pain, impairment, and other stressors involved in a number of chronic conditions. These include burn injuries, spinal cord injuries, severe arthritis, fibromyalgia, and blindness, among others (Affleck and Tennen, 1996; Snyder, Rand, and Sigmon 2002). Hope has also been shown to affect motivation to engage in self-care and health-promoting behaviors among individuals with chronic conditions (Snyder, Rand, and Sigmon 2002).

Those who incorporate hope theory into therapeutic practice (e.g., Lopez, Floyd, Ulven, and Snyder 2000; Taylor et al., 2000b) recommend that therapists solicit ongoing feedback from clients about both the individual components and overall aspects of hope throughout the therapy process. One means of generating information about the client's degree of hope is the State Hope Scale (Snyder, et al. 1996). It allows therapists and clients to assess hope as it is reflected in goal setting, pathway thinking and agency thinking.

Taylor et al., (2000a) have recommended application of the theoretical and clinical aspects of hope theory to cognitive behavioral therapy. They argue that the generation of hope is a central mediator of clinical improvement in cognitive behavioral therapy (Taylor et al., 2000a). Taylor and colleagues discuss hope as both a cause and a consequence of cognitive behavioral therapy efficacy. They argue that two aspects of cognitive behavioral therapy, in particular, lead to increased hope. The first is a compelling rationale for change provided by the cognitive behavioral therapist in the initial stages of therapy, and the second is the breakdown of long-range clinical goals into more manageable immediate goals. Both serve to catalyze the client's hope and motivate clients to persist in therapy. Taylor and colleagues (2000a) also argue that cognitive behavioral therapy serves to instill hope because therapists from this orientation take special care in using only the specific techniques that have been demonstrated to be effective in promoting goal attainment through clinical research.

Clients that experience more efficacious outcomes of therapy are more likely to maintain a hopeful attitude over time, and their use of pathway and agency thinking is more likely to be reinforced. According to Taylor and colleagues (2000a), many core aspects of the process and practice of cognitive behavioral therapy are directed toward goal attainment, pathway thinking, and/or agency thinking and in those ways serve to generate and retain hope. These include deconstructing long-range goals into smaller subgoals, operationally defining goals, and prioritizing goals (all of these processes leading to more frequent experiences of efficacy). In addition, the cognitive behavioral therapy techniques of presenting a clear rationale and model for therapy, teaching self-monitoring, modification of cognitive distortions, and exposure-based strategies all lead to an increase in motivation, perceived control, and sense of efficacy (Taylor et al., 2000a).

Generating hope is arguably the most fundamental goal of cognitive behavioral therapy for individuals with chronic conditions. Seligman (2002) teaches generation of hope using a number of approaches. Two primary approaches are

- Permanence and pervasiveness
- Disputation of pessimistic beliefs.

Each will be discussed below.

Permanence and pervasiveness.

When interpreting negative events, permanence is defined as a rigid, pessimistic style that defines the timing of events in terms of "always" or "never" (e.g., "My supervisor never gives me the benefit of the doubt)." The converse of a permanent interpretation is the more tentative interpretation of negative events as temporary, or as resulting from ephemeral, situational factors (e.g., "Sometimes my supervisor can be very difficult"). Individuals with a temporary interpretation of negative events consider negative events as occurring "sometimes" and "lately." A positive psychology approach holds that more hopeful people tend to interpret negative events as temporary and positive events as permanent. Similarly, pervasiveness refers to the interpretation of events as either universal or specific. According to this approach, individuals are encouraged to make universal attributions for positive events (e.g., "I am a good worker") and specific attributions for negative events (e.g., "I made a mistake with that client").

The following extraction from a therapy session with Alex illustrates how concepts of permanence and pervasiveness can be used in cognitive behavioral therapy to promote hope.

Alex: "I'm just not smart enough to continue with graduate school"
Therapist: "What evidence do you have that leads you to think that you won't make it?"
Alex: "I don't do well on exams when I don't study enough, and the last time I had a relapse I could only study for about 30 minutes and I ended up with a C."
Therapist: "Well, most people don't do that well on exams when they only have 30 minutes to study. I have a question for you—how does not feeling well enough to study equate with not being smart enough to continue with graduate school?"
Alex: "It doesn't – I just wish I was smarter so I wouldn't have to ask for accommodations all the time."
Therapist: "Alex, do you really think anyone is so smart that they can get an A after studying for only 30 minutes?"
Alex: "No"
Therapist: "Do you remember that section I had you read in Seligman's (2002) book on universal versus specific interpretations of events?"
Alex: "Kind of, but I kind of forgot the specifics."
Therapist: "Well let's define our negative event, here. Would you agree that our negative event is that you received a C the last time you didn't feel well enough to study long?"

Alex: "Yeah, and that my health is heading south again."

Therapist: "OK, well, for now is it OK if we work with the actual event rather than the one you anticipate?"

Alex: (nods)

Therapist: "Would saying that you're not smart enough to continue with grad school be a universal or a specific interpretation of getting that C?"

Alex: "More universal."

Therapist: "Correct. What other evidence do you have that you're not smart enough to continue?"

Alex: "Not much, really"

Therapist: "So do you think a universal statement about your intelligence really applies in this case?"

Alex: "No"

Therapist: "Right, and you remember that universal interpretations of negative events take away our optimism, so we really should try to avoid them. What would be a more specific interpretation of that C grade?"

Alex: "I don't do well when I don't study enough, but that doesn't mean I'm not smart enough to continue."

Therapist: "Do you believe it?"

Alex: "Yeah."

As the excerpt illustrates, it can be helpful for clients to learn about the concepts of permanence and pervasiveness and to practice applying them in their own thinking about events.

Disputation of pessimistic beliefs

Another approach to achieving hope and optimism involves disputing pessimistic beliefs with the ABCDE model. Seligman (2002) explains the malleability of beliefs and how to dispute pessimistic beliefs through what he labels the "ABCDE" model. According to this model:

- A represents adversity or a negative event or circumstance,
- B stands for usual beliefs associated with that event,
- C represents the usual consequences of having that belief,
- D represents one's disputation of the usual belief, and
- E stands for the energy one derives from the successful disputation of a negative belief.

This method is similar to methods used in other orientations to cognitive behavioral therapy, such as identifying and evaluating negative automatic thoughts (Beck 1995) and the disputing of irrational beliefs (ABC method) Ellis (1962). The client uses the ABCDE model as a structured means of disputing a pessimistic belief. For example, Alex was given a homework assignment to use the ABCDE method as a means of responding to what was a particularly disturbing experience for him (i.e., having an urgent need to use the toilet while on a date). Alex's assignment was to use the method mentally while he had to interrupt the date and later to record how it unfolded. Table 2 shows what he recorded.

As illustrated by this example, one advantage of this method is that it can be used as a mental method during stressful events and as a means of later reflecting upon and reinforcing the disputation of pessimistic thoughts.

In addition to the fact that the successful completion of the ABCDE model can function as a means of generating hope and optimism in itself, Seligman's emphasis on energization in the ABCDE model imparts a positive perspective on prior approaches to thought analysis in cognitive behavioral therapy. Training people to focus and reflect upon the positive feelings generated by the effective disputation of a pessimistic belief and on the actual positive outcomes of changing a negative belief serves to reinforce a sense of self-efficacy and positive feelings associated with using this approach.

Summary

This section focused on two primary methods of instilling hope. As illustrated in one case example, homework assignments can be effectively used to generate hope. Table 3 includes three examples of homework assignments designed specifically for this purpose.

TABLE 2. Alex's use of Seligman's (2002) ABCDE model.

Adversity:	Had to stop at the gas station to use the toilet on a first date.
Belief:	I am disgusting.
Consequence:	I'm feeling ugly and inferior and making the situation even worse. I'm feeling depressed and can't have a good time.
Disputation:	It's embarrassing to have to run to a toilet every time I eat, but it does not mean I am disgusting. If Judy doesn't accept my disease, I'll find someone else who does.
Energization:	I'm feeling more empowered and in control with respect to my relationship with Judy. I feel good that I can advocate for myself instead of allowing fears of what others might think to make me feel uncomfortable.

TABLE 3. Hope: recommended therapy activities and homework assignments.

Assignment #1: "How Optimistic are You?"	Clients complete and score the *Optimism Test* (accessed in Seligman's (2002) book, *Authentic Happiness* or online at *www.authentichappieness.org*). Results can be discussed in the next therapy session or following completion of the scale.
Assignment #3: "The ABCDE Approach"	For this assignment, a worksheet consistent with the one presented in the Alex example above can be duplicated or accessed in Seligman's (2002) book or online at *www.authentichappiness.org*.

Here and Now Pleasures and Gratifications

Cognitive behavioral therapy can be used to educate clients about the importance of pleasure and gratification in maintaining positive emotion and in managing pain and discomfort. Seligman (2002) presents a complex and sophisticated analysis of the roles of pleasure and gratification in creating and sustaining positive emotion. According to Seligman (2002), positive emotion in the present is a result of two distinct experiences: pleasures and gratifications. Pleasures are defined as immediate and evanescent delights with clear sensory and strong emotional components. They disappear rapidly, habituate easily, and require little thinking.

Pleasures can be subcategorized in terms of bodily pleasures and higher pleasures. Bodily pleasures come through the senses and are usually momentary. They typically involve sensory experiences related to touch, temperature, taste, smell, motion, sight, and hearing, or combinations thereof. Events such as sitting in a whirlpool, listening to one's favorite music, a taste of one's favorite food, or looking at a picturesque landscape are examples of bodily pleasures. Higher pleasures include rapture, bliss, ecstasy, thrill, hilarity, euphoria, kick, buzz, elation, excitement, ebullience, sparkle, vigor, glee, mirth, gladness, good cheer, enthusiasm, attraction, fun, comfort, harmony, amusement, satiation and relaxation (Seligman 2002). Sharing a good joke with a friend or enjoying all aspects of a ballet performance might be construed as a higher pleasure. Other examples of bodily and higher pleasures and how to create them with limited physical and economic resources can be found in Louden (1992).

Given that they are often fleeting, taken for granted, or can go relatively unnoticed by some, Seligman (2002) recommends three key strategies for enhancing pleasurable experiences:

- Prevention of habituation
- Savoring, and
- Mindfulness

Prevention of habituation

The concept of habituation acknowledges that the human brain is constructed such that repeated indulgence in the same pleasure leads to tolerance, decreased potency of that pleasure, and in some cases, addiction. Habituation can be prevented through plentitude, spacing, surprise, and variation; Seligman (2002) recommends that people aim to experience as many different possible sources of pleasure as are available, that they vary the types of pleasure being experienced, that they spread pleasures out over time, and that they build an element of reciprocal surprise into the experience of pleasure with a friend or lover.

Savoring and mindfulness

Savoring involves deliberate attention to the experience of pleasure. Savoring can be accomplished through sharing the pleasurable experience with others, maintaining mental and physical reminders (e.g., a souvenir), allowing oneself to be proud of one's actions or accomplishments, choosing to focus on the more pleasurable aspects of an experience to the exclusion of other aspects, and allowing oneself to experience pleasure fully and wholly through the senses (Bryant and Veroff 1982 ; Seligman 2002). Mindfulness can involve heightened awareness of pleasure, immersion in pleasure without thinking about it or evaluating it, and shifting perspectives to make an experience new or fresh (Kabat-Zin 1990).

Unlike pleasures, gratifications are comprised of absorbing and enjoyable activities that are not accompanied by a direct sensory or emotional experience. Gratifications are experiences that engage us fully, lead to a loss of self-consciousness, and involve flow (Csikszentmihalyi 2000; Seligman 2002). Gratifications comprise flow situations in which we are challenged, forced to concentrate, pursue clear goals, receive immediate feedback, experience deep involvement without perception of effort, have a sense of control, lack a sense of self, and lose a sense of time (Csikszentmihalyi 2000; Seligman 2002). Examples of gratifications might involve reading a good book, gardening, catching a fish, or teaching a child to ride a bicycle. Chronic conditions can limit the kinds of gratifications and flow experiences that people are able to have. For this reason, knowledge of volition (discussed in Chapter 13) and the generation of new gratifications are essential elements of behavioral experiments, activity scheduling, or other aspects of psychotherapy that involve the facilitation of engagement in activity.

Pleasure assignments have been found to be of particular benefit to clients having difficulty with self-care, mild pain, or discomfort due to a chronic condition. Table 4 illustrates some pleasure and gratification homework assignments. The recommended gratification assignments should be used in conjunction with voli-

TABLE 4. Pleasure and gratification: recommended (homework or therapy) assignments.

Pleasure Assignment #1 "Pleasure Brainstorming":	In preparation for Assignment #2, clients can be instructed to list all possible sources of pleasure (bodily or higher order) that they can imagine, including pleasures they have experienced in the past and ones they have not yet had.
Pleasure Assignment #2 "Pleasures Worksheet":	For this assignment, clients are instructed to utilize the list of experiences that engender pleasure that was constructed in Assignment #1. Clients are instructed to document both the brainstormed pleasures and any newly discovered pleasures that they did not plan or prepare for but that occurred spontaneously or occurred as a result of heightened awareness or a shift in perspective on an old situation. Clients can be instructed to report the situation they were in when they invoked or had the pleasurable experience, the nature of the pleasure that was experienced (brainstormed or newly discovered), and how they were able to enhance the pleasure on any given day.
Gratification Assignment #1:	The client makes a list of gratifying activities. These must be activities that the client enjoys, find challenging, and those in which he or she experiences deep involvement in the absence of time, self-consciousness, or perceived effort. These can then be utilized in activity scheduling and in other behavioral experiments.

tional work (see Chapter 13) and are most useful for individuals that are inactive, feeling bored or functionally constrained by their illness, or lack volition to engage in meaningful activity.

Conclusion

This chapter presented a number of approaches to cognitive behavioral therapy that incorporated concepts and methods of positive psychology, specifically hope theory (Seligman 2002). Undoubtedly, there are additional ways that cognitive behavioral therapy can be modified to incorporate lessons learned from positive psychology. Therapists experienced in the practice of cognitive behavioral therapy are encouraged to view this chapter as a launching pad for additional ideas in this area, and to be creative in the application of positive psychology concepts to cognitive behavioral therapy.

13

Overcoming Motivational Dilemmas in Cognitive Behavioral Therapy

In response to Nina's concern that her fatigue had taken away most of her pleasurable activities, Nina's therapist suggested that she consider the dream she once mentioned of writing a short story. Nina responded that she found that idea overwhelming since she couldn't bear the idea of writing a story that would be rejected for publication. As Curtis' cancer progressed, he saw no point in engaging in any activities, including his old hobby of collecting Word War II memorabilia. He indicated that he felt worthless to his family and, as a result, had just "lost interest" in doing things and that "there [was] no satisfaction in it anymore."

These two clients had difficulty identifying goals for therapy and neither was able to pursue activities that were once important and enjoyable to them and that made them feel competent. Most troublesome is that neither of these clients could entertain ideas about alternative ways of being and acting in their worlds. Given the powerful feelings of demoralization that clients can face, how can cognitive behavioral therapy be used to allow them and others like them to construct new ways of living?

The field of cognitive psychology has made significant advances in its analysis of the role of motivation in human cognition and behavior. For example, in 1986, Albert Bandura put forth his groundbreaking theory of human motivation and action (Bandura 1986). Bandura (2001), whose work is now referred to as social cognitive theory, revised his original theory to emphasize personal agency, or the capacity to exercise control over the nature and quality of one's life experiences, as a fundamental aspect of being human. Bandura (2001) posits that people actively create their own experiences through intentionality, forethought, self-regulation of motivation, affect, action, and self-reflection.

Similarly, Beck (1996) views motivation from a biological-behavioral systems perspective. In his theory of modes, Beck (1996) discusses motivation as a key system participating in a larger mode of synchronous systems that operate together to instruct goal-directed activity. Beck (1996) defines motivation as automatic, outside of conscious control, and as including the biological drives such as hunger, sex, fight-or-flight, and avoidance of danger. Beck (1996) acknowledges that the motivational system can be brought under the control of a conscious control system. This system incorporates an individual's conscious and less automatic goals, values and desires. From a therapeutic perspective, this system can be tapped into for problem-solving, conscious goal-setting, and long-term planning. Beck (1996) explains that it is involved in controlling and limiting the more primal (i.e., motivational and behavioral) systems by allowing for the correction of more primitive, negative states of thinking, such as automatic thoughts, dysfunctional impulses, or unpleasant affect. Thus, from a therapeutic perspective, the conscious control system allows individuals to form conscious intentions and to gain perspective on primitive thinking, affect, and motivation.

Motivation and Cognitive Behavioral Therapy

Despite these and other major theoretical contributions, the theories and practices of cognitive behavioral therapy can be criticized in general for their lack of emphasis on the role of motivation in interpretations of psychopathology and cognitive change (Salkovskis and Freeston 2001). Though there are cognitive behavioral therapists that recognize the importance of the role of motivation in therapeutic change, mention of this topic has, in large part, been limited to the discussion of motivation as a consequence of goal-setting, therapy contracting, or experiences of self-efficacy during therapy. More specifically, techniques geared toward generating motivation have been incorporated into cognitive behavioral therapy interventions that apply conscious control theories of motivation (Bandura 1986; Beck 1996), or into interventions that utilize motivational interviewing or motivational enhancement techniques (MET) (Barrowclough et al., 2001; Diamond et al., 2002; Freidenberg et al., 2002; Haddock et al., 2003). Additionally, motivation has been described as a general byproduct or consequence of cognitive behavioral therapy (Ehlert Wagner and Lupke 1999; Gibbs 2002; Taylor et al., 2000), or more specifically, as a consequence of treatment contracting or goal-setting (Otto et al., 2003) within cognitive behavioral therapy.

The Role of Motivation in Change

Motivation has been implicated as a key variable in clinical trials of cognitive behavioral therapy. Therapy success has typically been associated with motivation for change or "motivational readiness for change" and therapy failure or relapse has been associated with low motivation for change (Halmi et al., 2002; Taft et al., 2004). Many cognitive behavioral therapists make use of the stages of change framework (Prochaska and diClemente 1986) in case formulations in order to understand the perspectives people can have as they are anticipating change. Despite its value as a measurement and formulation tool, this framework was not designed to instruct on how to motivate clients to progress in terms of their readiness for change. Thus, although motivation has been measured in relation to change readiness, and as a means of explaining therapeutic outcomes, cognitive behavioral therapists do not tend to focus on motivation, or more specifically motivation to change, in therapy.

A Volitional Perspective

Prior definitions of motivation as tissue-related, libidinal, or strictly the result of learning or behavioral conditioning were extended by theorists such as Weinberger and McClelland (1990), DeCharms (1992), White (1959), and Smith (1974). These theorists saw motivation as foundational and viewed the pursuit of novel experience, control, mastery and effectiveness as their own drives (DeCharms 1992; McClelland 1985; White 1959). Moreover, theorists (e.g., Higgins and Sorrentino 1990; Weinberger and McClelland 1990) have proposed a reconciliation between the more affective nature of motivation theory and the more intellectual nature of cognitive theories, arguing that the two perspectives can be used in complementary ways in clinical practice.

Based on these revised theories of motivation and other related concepts, Kielhofner (2002) proposed a conceptualization of motivation, which he refers to as volition. The concept has been used and researched in rehabilitation for three decades. Volition is defined as a foundational motive to act that occurs independently of other aspects of motivation, including biological and libidinal drives, and the goal-seeking behaviors they generate (Kielhofner 2002). Volition is viewed as being grounded in the nervous system's need for arousal and in an existential opening provided by having a body and mind with the potential for engagement and doing. While this underlying drive for action is considered universal, the concept of volition recognizes that it is manifest differently in individuals according to each person's innate and acquired tendencies to experience action.

Volition is manifest in the thoughts and feelings an individual has about him- or herself as an actor in the world (Kielhofner 2002). These thoughts and feelings occur as the individual anticipates, chooses, experiences, and evaluates what he or she does (Kielhofner 2004). According to Kielhofner (2002), volitional thoughts and feelings comprise three elements:

- Personal causation,
- Values, and
- Interests.

Personal causation, a concept introduced by DeCharms (1992), involves an individual's ever-evolving thoughts and feelings about his or her capacities and efficacy in performance. Values comprise thoughts and feelings about what is important and meaningful to do. Thoughts and feelings pertaining to interest concern enjoyment and satisfaction in doing. In summary, the thoughts and feelings that comprise volition are involved in a cycle of anticipating, choosing, and evaluating the process of acting in the world (Kielhofner 2002). In this cycle, thought and feeling not only shape choices for action but also are shaped by doing the selected action. Thus the experience of doing plays a major role in shaping feelings and thoughts.

The concept of volition is used as a guide to understanding people's motivation, including their motivational problems. It offers a way of thinking about both choices concerning what one does in everyday life and one's commitment to ongoing and future courses of action (Kielhofner 2002).

The Model of Human Occupation

The concept of volition comes from a conceptual model, the model of human occupation (Kielhofner 2002, 2004). This model is concerned with personal and environmental factors that influence patterns of occupational performance and participation in life in response to chronic illness and disability (Kielhofner 2004). Occupational performance is defined as engaging in a specific sequence of action that is coherent, purposeful, and collectively recognized within a cultural context (Kielhofner 2002). Occupational participation is defined as the larger pattern of engagement in work, play, or activities of daily living that are part of one's sociocultural context and that are desired and/or necessary to one's well-being (Kielhofner 2004).

In brief, the model of human occupation conceptualizes occupational performance and participation as influenced by four factors:

- Volition (personal causation, values, and interests),
- Habituation (acquired patterns of action and ascribed social and occupational roles),
- Performance capacity (underlying physical and cognitive capacities for task performance), and
- Environment (interpersonal and physical opportunities, demands, constraints, and resources) (Kielhofner 2002).

The remainder of this chapter focuses only on the first factor, volition, and the implications of approaches to volition for the practice of cognitive behavioral therapy.

The Role of Volition in Cognitive Behavioral Therapy

Kielhofner views the source of dysfunction in chronic illness as the inability *to do*, and sees volition as foundational to doing (Kielhofner 2004). Thus, evaluating, understanding, and working with volition to remotivate individuals is fundamental to therapy using this approach. Volition is a requirement for authentic engagement in life and, therefore, a vital element of therapy and the change process (Kielhofner 2002). A similar argument can be made that volition is a critical, if not primary, source of participation and change for clients participating in cognitive behavioral therapy. According to Kielhofner (2002), volition is essential to change since change requires decision-making and commitment to enact and sustain courses of action.

Understanding a client's volition will allow therapists and their clients to more accurately select behavioral experiments and other therapy assignments that lead to successful outcomes. It will also allow them to set short- and long-range goals that are more realistic, satisfying, personally significant, and ultimately more likely to be accomplished. A number of symptoms and functional impairments associated with chronic conditions can attenuate or impede motivation. Table 1 provides the example of Nina. It provides a summary of the impact of her fatigue on the three aspects of volition (personal causation, values, and interests).

Kielhofner (2002) recommends using an orientation that recognizes liabilities but emphasizes strengths and motivators. A focus on positive life participation rather than on pathology is used to facilitate authentic involvement in therapy. The following are common empowerment-oriented strategies associated with the concept of volition:

- Actively involving clients in treatment, including sharing the concept of volition as a means for self-understanding
- Rapport-building through careful, narratively oriented interviewing aimed at understanding how the client interprets his/her life and present circumstances coupled with active "checking in" to assure valid understanding
- Use of self-assessments that allow clients to generate insights to their own volition and identify priorities
- Supporting clients to makes choices to engage in volitionally relevant activities and to reflect on the experience of doing them

TABLE 1. Consequences of fatigue on volition.

Aspect of volition	Volitional consequences of Nina's fatigue
Personal Causation	• Lowered sense of capacity and reduced feeling of effectiveness in completing routine tasks • Worry about future including career and family relationships • Difficulty accurately estimating capacity for performance due to fluctuations in available energy • Erosion of confidence in being able to successfully accomplish goals • Gap between pattern of interests and values and what client can do
Values	• Lost sense of meaning associated with occupations that can no longer be done • Inability to attain standards of performance that afford a sense of self-worth • Inability to commit to or see the worth of pursing goals that once were highly motivating
Interests	• Reduced enjoyment in doing familiar and previously enjoyable activities • Decreased anticipatory pleasure in previously engaging work activities and hobbies • Reduced range of satisfying participation • Difficulty forming new interests

Taken together, these strategies can facilitate cognitive organization in clients who are often confused or uncertain about their life circumstances and what the chronic illness means for their present and future lives. They all focus toward engaging the client in activity planning and problem solving, thereby increasing the client's feelings of control over his/her life.

This approach also emphasizes providing opportunities for persons to experiment, reflect, review, and receive feedback on their own capacities and limitations, sense of enjoyment and meaning. This can be accomplished, for instance, through logging activity levels and fatigue and by reviewing recent experience. An important process in the management of chronic illness and impairment is for clients to develop a realistic appraisal of their performance capacity and of the effects of engaging in patterns of activity.

Volitional change can also involve values clarification or reprioritization. With a more restricted capacity for activity, clients with chronic conditions are often forced to choose among those prior activities of most importance. Therapy may involve assisting clients with values change or reprioritization of values by identifying what matters to them most within various occupational domains (e.g., family, work, leisure) or which occupational domains they might wish to relinquish or retain (e.g., relinquishing work to maintain family relationships).

Volitional change can also involve value change. For instance, persons with chronic illness often internalize societal messages that connote illness and disability as essentially "bad." Becoming aware of this internalized oppression can lead persons to focus the parts of self that are essentially valuable. Some persons may need to enlarge the scope of their values to incorporate things for which they are still capable. Clients may need to reformulate how they judge their performance by making reference to their capacities rather than by comparing performance to their past performance and/or to that of others without chronic conditions.

For example, Nina's situation, noted at the outset of this chapter, involves the following volitional components:

- Loss of ability to do activities which were previously enjoyable and satisfying
- Inability to select an activity that is within her present capacity because of too high standards, a component of values (i.e., anything she writes must be publishable)

The concept of volition would suggest the following steps in addressing Nina's situation:

- Underscoring the importance of continuing activities that provide enjoyment and satisfaction
- Acknowledging the reality that some activities and ways of approaching activity (e.g., overfunctioning) that met her needs at one time are no longer possible
- Discussing how values (i.e., unrealistically high standards of performance) are making it difficult to chose an activity that might otherwise bring pleasure
- Identifying why writing was a pleasurable activity in the past and what Nina might enjoy writing about in the present

- Recommending undertaking the activity of writing a brief short story while putting aside worry about whether it is publishable, to see if it is enjoyable (this activity could be assigned as a behavioral experiment and/or for homework)
- Reviewing how the activity was experienced and proceeding accordingly

Measuring and Working with Volition in Cognitive Behavioral Therapy

The essence of volitional work in cognitive behavioral therapy involves ongoing assessment and discovery. Following identification of a volitional problem, the focus of subsequent cognitive and behavioral work should emphasize the choice and performance of activities that create a flow experience and are pleasurable, captivating, meaningful, and gratifying (Seligman and Csikszentmihalyi 2000). The importance of this emphasis on the role of positive psychology in cognitive behavioral therapy is elaborated upon in Chapter 12.

For clients struggling with issues of motivation, values and meaning, and capacity and efficacy, many behaviorally based interventions, activity prescriptions, and behavioral experiments may fail in the absence of a clear understanding of these complex volitional issues. A client's volition may be particularly important to understand during the initial stages of therapy. In addition to the hope of obtaining relief from the emotional pain, negative interpersonal consequences, functional limitations, poor decision-making, or increased physical symptoms associated with faulty thinking, one of the most motivating reasons for a client to pursue cognitive behavioral therapy may involve the rewards and gratifications associated with engaging in activities that are captivating and enriching. When facing a new or escalating condition, many people may have difficulty resuming activities or identifying new activities that matter to them and help to restore a sense of personal competence and fulfillment.

Four assessments derived from the model of human occupation (Kielhofner 2002) can provide critical information about a client's volition and readiness for change and may serve as useful supplements to other measures of cognition and behavior:

- The Occupational Self Assessment (Baron et al., 2002),
- The Modified Interest Checklist (Kielhofner and Neville 1983),
- The NIH Activity Record (Gerber and Furst 1992), and
- The Occupational Performance History Interview – Second Version (Kielhofner et al., 1998).

The Occupational Self Assessment (OSA) (Baron et al., 2002) is a measure of perceived capacity and importance of a variety of activities. In paper-and-pencil format, clients respond to a series of statements about their performance and about characteristics of the environment that affect performance by indicating how well they accomplish each and how important it is. Then, clients select the activities that are priorities for change in order to voice their own perspectives and shape the goals and strategies of therapy. Though it is relatively brief, this assessment can be broken down into shorter steps and can be administered verbally for clients requiring accommodation.

The following example illustrates use of the *Occupational Self Assessment* along with open-ended interview questions to gather more information about Curtis's volition early in his therapy. More information about this measure can be obtained in Kielhofner (2002) and at *www.moho.uic.edu.*

Curtis: "I feel like so many obstacles are in my way right now. Some mornings I can't believe I actually made it to work. My work, my house, myself . . . . everything is like a tornado hit."

Therapist: "What do you think you need most right now?"

Curtis: "I don't know . . . . I'm not sure anything will help. . . . . I just don't feel like I'm of use to anyone anymore. . . . . It seems like I can't do anything right and so nothing matters."

Therapist: "I think it would be a good idea if we systematically looked how well you do everyday things and maybe sort out what really matters to you. How does that sound for a starting point?

Curtis: "I'm not sure it would help. . . . What seems like it mattered doesn't seem to matter anymore. . . and I'm not sure I could do anything about it."

Therapist: "That does seem to be the way things appear to you right now – you're having a hard time seeing what matters in your life right now and you don't feel very competent to do what matters."

Curtis: "I am. That's really the heart of the problem. I feel useless." [Note: Instead of examining this "hot thought," the therapist makes a decision to pursue the client's volitional issues.]

Therapist: "I think that if we explore this together you might get some more clarity on this. How about we start by just taking a look at your daily activities and the obstacles you are facing?"

Curtis: "OK."

Following this exchange, the therapist suggested that Curtis complete the *Occupational Self Assessment*. This tool can be effective in such circumstances because it provides a structured means of reflecting on how well one is performing. It also provides a means of identifying how much different aspects of performance matter. It allows for a structured approach to prioritization of areas for future work in therapy. Figure 1 presents Curtis's responses.

Findings from Curtis's *Occupational Self Assessment* are consistent with those of many individuals facing a significant and new illness. They indicate that Curtis encountered difficulty in a lot of daily life domains, many of which were indeed important to him. Given that he is having difficulty with so many of the average activities of daily living, it makes sense that he would feel

Myself	Priority	Lot of problems	Some difficulty	Well	Extremely well	Not so important	Important	Extremely important
		Competence				Values		
Concentrating on my tasks.			x					x
Physically doing what I need to do.		x					x	
Taking care of the place where I live.		x					x	
Taking care of myself.	1	x						x
Taking care of others for whom I am responsible.		Not Applicable						
Getting where I need to go.				x			x	
Managing my finances.	3	x						x
Managing my basic needs (food, medicine).				x				x
Expressing myself to others.				x			x	
Getting along with others.				x			x	
Identifying and solving problems.					x		x	
Relaxing and enjoying myself.		x				x		
Getting done what I need to do.			x					x
Having a satisfying routine.		x				x		
Handling my responsibilities.	2	x						x
Being involved as a student, worker, volunteer, and/or family member.	4	x						x
Doing activities I like.		x				x		
Working towards my goals.		x					x	
Making decisions based on what I think is important.					x			x
Accomplishing what I set out to do.					x			x
Effectively using my abilities.			x					x

FIGURE 1. Curtis's Responses on the Occupational Self Assessment

demoralized. However, Curtis's results also reveal that he has certain strengths, including his tenacity, decisiveness, problem-solving abilities, and communication and relating skills. Reviewing his ratings of competence reinforced for Curtis that he still managed to maintain some areas of control in things that were important to him.

Often when clients experience so many areas of difficulty, it becomes hard to sort out what should be an area of focus. The Occupational Self Assessment provides a concrete means of doing this. Clients like Curtis can be supported to identify the areas where there are the greatest gaps between the level of performance and how important the activity is. These are shown in Figure 1; they are:

- Taking care of myself
- Managing my finances
- Handling my responsibilities
- Being involved as a student, worker, volunteer, and/or family member

Curtis found the assessment process to be revealing and readily agreed that if he could narrow the gap between how well he was doing in these four areas and the importance of these activities, he would feel better. Using the cognitive model, the therapist also illustrated how addressing these areas would lead to his ultimate goal of improving his sleep (through reducing anxiety and allowing him to practice better sleep hygiene by engaging in activity during the day instead of napping). Consequently, Curtis and his therapist prioritized the four areas of central importance in the numbered order shown in Figure 1. They agreed that improving his performance in these areas would be a useful starting point in therapy. Together they identified the following goals:

- To practice sleep hygiene techniques
- To assume more control in taking his medication, scheduling physician appointments and managing other aspects of his health care that he had defaulted to his wife
- To focus on getting his finances in order, so that his wife and daughter would be taken care of
- To do some of the chores around the house and yard that he had not attended to
- To become reinvolved in his old roles, particularly being a more involved father and husband

After setting these goals, Curtis also identified that if he could take care of these basics he might even feel like dong some of the things he enjoyed in the past. He realized from the discussion that he was feeling so badly about himself that he couldn't allow himself to enjoy anything without feeling guilty.

Clients like Curtis that may become demoralized as a result of changes in their performance capacity will also benefit from cognitive behavioral work that emphasizes remotivation and perspective taking. This can involve the correction of catastrophic or dichotomous thinking, encouragement to focus or meditate on daily goals, tasks, and accomplishments rather than on past experiences or anticipated future outcomes (here and now centering), and the encouragement of self-comparison against current performance, not past performance. Other assessments of volition can aid in this process.

The *Modified Interest Checklist* (Kielhofner and Neville 1983) gives clients an opportunity to indicate what their current interests are, how interests have changed, and whether they participate or wish to participate in an interest in the future. This assessment is helpful in identifying how a chronic illness or impairment has changed interest patterns and participation in interests. It can be completed in sections or administered orally. More information about this measure can be obtained in Kielhofner (2002) and at www.moho.uic.edu.

The *NIH Activity Record* (ACTRE) (Gerber and Furst 1992) is a form on which clients self-report the activities they engaged in during half-hour periods over the course of a weekday and weekend day. It was discussed earlier in Chapter 9. Respondents also indicate whether each activity is work, leisure, a daily living task, or rest. Additionally, the respondents answer questions pertaining to pain, fatigue, difficulty of performance, how enjoyable the activity is, how important it is and how well they do it. Ordinarily the ACTRE is filled out as a log, so that clients can complete it in small sections during the day, but it can be given as an interview.

The ACTRE gives a detailed picture of the daily life routines of the individual, of how symptoms affect both performance and experience (value, competence, interest, difficulty, pain, fatigue) of various daily tasks. It can be useful for identifying troublesome tasks as well as revealing the client's pattern of participation. More information on this instrument can be found in Kielhofner (2002) and at *www.moho.uic.edu.*

In the initial stages of therapy, completing these self-assessments may be overwhelming for some clients who are depressed and still reacting to and learning about the onset of a chronic illness or impairment. In these instances, working with automatic thoughts as they relate to volition is often a good starting point. Table 2 lists some examples of automatic thoughts as they relate to the three aspects of volition.

TABLE 2. Automatic thoughts categorized by volitional domain.

Aspects of Volition	Personal Causation	Values	Interests
Automatic Thoughts	"I'll never be able to paint again."	"Life is meaningless."	"Nothing interests me now."
	"I can't do anything right."	"I don't care about anything."	"I don't like this."
	"Getting to work is impossible."	"Work isn't worth it to me now."	"This is boring."
	"I can no longer make love."	"In the end, people don't care."	"Everything seems the same."
	"I'm losing my mind."	"I feel empty."	"There's not much to choose from."
	"I'm useless."	"Life has lost its flavor."	
	"I have no talents."		

Once clients and their therapists have identified that there are problems with volition they may choose to begin to examine the client's life history, or narrative, as a way of exploring volition over time and locating volitional strengths. Often, but not always, clients can draw from past interests and motivators in the process of creating new work roles and finding new activities that they can engage in. A narrative history approach allows for the identification of motivators and strengths that the client may have drawn upon in the past, rather than strictly focusing on negativistic or dysfunctional thinking by continuing to pursue the identification of intermediate and core beliefs. Ultimately, the choice as to whether to pursue a client's narrative, motivators, and strengths versus pursuing exploration of intermediate and core beliefs will depend on the time available to treat the client, the client's capacity for narrative exploration, and other unique features of the client-therapist relationship.

If a client and therapist choose to pursue this approach to working with volition, a semistructured life history interview, the *Occupational Performance History Interview—Second Version* (OPHI-II) (Kielhofner, et al., 1998) is an effective measure that can guide the process. This measure allows the therapist to collect information about a client's past and present occupational roles, interests, occupational choices, preferred activities, daily routines, values, and the life events and settings that can interact with a client's choices and behaviors. It can be broken down as needed to accommodate a person with energy or concentration difficulties. The OPHI-II can be useful for understanding how a chronic condition has changed a client's life, and it reveals how a client perceives her or his life to be unfolding. More information about this measure can be obtained in Kielhofner (2002) and at www.moho.uic.edu.

These assessments can be utilized on a one-time basis as a starting point for identifying strengths and areas of difficulty, and for the later establishment of therapeutic goals based on item priorities and importance level. Importantly, they also provide information about the client's *perception* of his or her ability to do things as it contrasts with his or her *actual* ability to do things. Thus, the assessment of volition is critical to the process of evaluating distortions or inaccuracies in thinking as they pertain to a client's performance capacity. Distortions or inaccuracies in performance-related cognitions may be particularly salient for clients with new or escalating chronic illnesses or impairments. These assessments may also be used periodically as follow-up measures throughout the course of therapy to inform turning points or to plan termination.

Helping Clients Reclaim Volition

Once clients have identified priorities, capacities, and goals, and have a realistic and accurate perspective on their impairments, activities can be modified so that they are more enjoyable and satisfying to perform. Approaches can range from the use of assistive devices that make performance more comfortable to rescheduling pleasurable activities during available energy periods. Other approaches that can reduce anticipatory anxiety and increase perceived control while engaging in activity include assisting clients in establishing contingency plans that involve escape routes, resting spots, or personal assistants to aiding clients during activity performance.

In cognitive behavioral therapy, there are four commonly utilized means that therapists can use either in combination with assessment or exploration of volitional issues, or after this exploration has taken place and when clients are ready to work on reengaging in functional and meaningful activities. These include: reminder cards, activity assignments, activity scheduling, and behavioral experiments. When planning or recommending that a client engage in a particular activity, therapists should first evaluate the likelihood that the client will enjoy the activity, find it useful or gratifying, and perform it successfully. Table 3 includes a number of variables by which an activity can be evaluated by therapists and their clients in terms of their likely impact on volition before they decide to make it a recommended or prescribed activity.

Behavioral experiments that allow a client to test his or her experience reengaging in a former activity or beginning a new activity may offer the best starting points for clients facing volitional challenges. Behavioral experiments allow the client to have a subjective experience of control in that he or she can participate alongside the therapist in determining whether the activity is worth pursuing. Regardless of which approach to activity a therapist chooses (reminder cards, activity assignments, activity scheduling, or behavioral experiments), clients should begin with activities that are likely going to fulfill at least one of the criteria listed in Table 3 even the very first time the client attempts the activity.

Conclusion

Clients can face challenges to their values, sense of efficacy, and interests at various time points during the course of their illness or impairment. In this chapter

TABLE 3. Suggested volitional criteria for choosing activities.

Personal Causation	• How will this activity sustain/improve the client's self-efficacy?
	• What evidence exists that the client can have success in this activity?
Values	• What is the meaning of this activity in terms of the client's overall worldview? (i.e., how meaningful is this activity)
	• How will this activity help the client accomplish a given goal or realize some kind of meaning?
	• How will this activity relate to the things this client values?
	• Will the client be able to meet his/her own standards of performance?
Interests	• Has this activity been pleasurable to the client in the past? Can those elements that gave pleasure be replicated, or has something changed that may make it no longer enjoyable/satisfying?
	• What will the client's intellectual and sensory experience be during this activity and does it match what he/she finds pleasurable/satisfying?

we have learned that one of the key roles of a therapist can involve enabling clients to recognize and identify these problems of volition so that clients can ultimately reengage in activities that are gratifying, pleasurable, absorbing, and meaningful. This chapter also emphasized how cognitive distortions can be interpreted in terms of their impact upon a client's volition, and it highlighted the importance of considering volitional issues when collaborating with clients to choose and plan activities outside of therapy.

Section Three

Specific Applications of Cognitive Behavioral Therapy to Fatigue, Pain, Sleep Disorders, and Gastrointestinal Dysfunction

Introduction

This second section of the book focuses on the cross-cutting symptoms of fatigue, pain, sleep disorders and gastrointestinal dysfunction. Chapters 14, 16, 18, and 20 cover the epidemiology and role of each of these symptoms in a wide range of chronic conditions. Following each of these chapters, chapters 15, 17, 19, and 21 illustrate specific approaches to assessment of that symptom and review specific therapeutic strategies used in the application of cognitive behavioral therapy to that symptom. In these chapters, case studies of individuals with conditions that involve each of the four cross-cutting symptoms are used to illustrate these applied topics.

14

Fatigue: Subtypes, Prevalence, and Associated Conditions

Fatigue is a highly prevalent and often enduring symptom of a number of chronic conditions. This chapter will define abnormal fatigue and describe its subclassifications. In addition, it will describe the nature and prevalence of fatigue, focusing on conditions for which fatigue is a significant or primary symptom.

This chapter is not intended to provide an exhaustive, systematic, or detailed review of the epidemiology and characteristics of fatigue for each condition covered. A review of this nature would be too lengthy and beyond the scope of this book. However, basic information about a number of fatigue-related conditions is offered to provide therapists with general guidelines and information about the role of fatigue in common chronic conditions. When working with clients with a chronic condition for which fatigue is a primary symptom, therapists will inevitably need to seek out additional information about the role of fatigue in that specific condition from collaborating physicians and research-related resources.

What is Abnormal Fatigue?

Everyone has experienced fatigue as an expected reaction to prolonged physical exertion, mental strain, stress, or lost sleep. However, individuals are only likely to have experienced abnormal fatigue if they have had an underlying medical or psychiatric condition that can explain the fatigue. For example, acute states of abnormal fatigue can accompany severe viral infections (e.g., influenza) or brief periods of depression. Abnormal fatigue can be characterized in any or all of the following ways:

- An ever-present feeling of complete and utter exhaustion that occurs independently of exertion
- Decreased physical endurance to activity
- Muscle weakness
- A feeling of heaviness or resistance to movement (e.g., "swimming through molasses" or "walking uphill")
- Inability to move, talk, or eat

- Inability to tolerate sensory experiences (e.g., intolerance to light, sound, touch, smell)
- Inability to tolerate upright positions, such as sitting or standing
- Feeling faint, dizzy, lightheaded, or as if one is about to faint
- Feeling tired or having a desire to sleep
- Feeling emotionally drained or depressed
- Feeling cognitively or intellectually void or numb (e.g., "mind going blank," "brain dead," or "brain fog")
- Low motivation
- Lack of energy
- Lethargy
- Inability to think, attend, concentrate, or remember recent activities, conversations, or events
- Inability to follow a conversation, movie, or television program
- Disorientation or confusion
- Shortness of breath

While the person with abnormal fatigue will not ordinarily have all the above experiences, it is very common that several are present.

Subtypes of Abnormal Fatigue

Abnormal fatigue can be subclassified in terms of the following dimensions:

- Onset (sudden versus gradual)
- Duration (acute versus chronic)
- Frequency (persistent versus relapsing and remitting)
- Perceived cause (physiological versus psychosocial)
- Perceived severity (mild to severe)
- Functional consequences (mildly disabling to severely disabling)

This section highlights the diversity of fatigue in terms of each of these dimensions.

Onset: Sudden versus Gradual

Asking clients about the circumstances surrounding the onset of their fatigue may, in some cases, provide critical information about the extent to which the fatigue is influenced by psychosocial versus physiological variables. Generally speaking, abnormal fatigue that is described as coming on gradually, as lifelong, or as predating the chronic condition may be unrelated to the physiological features of the chronic condition. Instead, it may be the result of psychosocial or lifestyle influences such as chronic stress, overwork, or an undiagnosed anxiety or depressive disorder.

For some clients, fatigue that is psychosocial in nature and predates a chronic condition may serve to complicate and exacerbate the newer fatigue that is predominantly physiological in nature. There are some exceptions to this guideline.

For example, it is always possible that fatigue that predated a chronic condition was a prodromal symptom of the chronic condition, which developed gradually over a period of months or years. It is important that therapists learn about the role of fatigue in each condition to determine the extent to which it is caused by psychosocial versus physiological variables.

Duration: Acute versus Chronic

Asking clients how long the fatigue has persisted will offer some useful preliminary information regarding the extent of their experience living and coping with the symptom. Prolonged fatigue, which is reported by approximately 25 percent of the population, is defined as abnormal fatigue that persists for at least one month. Chronic fatigue, occurring in between 4 and 18 percent of the general population, is defined as abnormal fatigue that persists for six months or longer (Pawlikowska et al., 1994).

Some individuals with chronic conditions will experience acute episodes of fatigue that are isolated and closely linked to times when they are undergoing a specific treatment, taking a certain medication, or to periods of relapse or symptom escalation. Others will experience fatigue that is chronic in nature and seemingly unrelated to changes in treatments or illness characteristics.

There are some conditions for which this type of chronic fatigue is simply a primary symptom. These include, but are not limited to, chronic fatigue syndrome, multiple sclerosis, fibromyalgia, and lupus. The exact origin of fatigue in these conditions is unknown. Bearing these and other medical exceptions in mind, clients that report that their fatigue is more chronic and insidious may also acknowledge that psychosocial (e.g., depression, anxiety, stress) and lifestyle (e.g., overwork, multiple commitments) variables do play some role in the fatigue.

Frequency: Persistent versus Relapsing and Remitting

Similar to fatigue duration, the frequency with which a client reports fatigue can provide useful information for treatment planning. Clients that report constant fatigue will require a different approach than clients that report that their fatigue waxes and wanes based on illness severity, activity levels, medications, or treatments. Constant fatigue may be present because it is a fundamental aspect of a medical condition, or it may be present because a client is underactive, deconditioned, eating a poor diet, depressed, stressed, overcommitted, or anxious. Alternatively, fatigue that waxes and wanes may manifest as a psychological reaction to the stress involved in undergoing a certain medical treatment or as a result of anxiety about trying a new medication. It may also wax and wane based on activity levels or as a physical side effect of a treatment or medication. Because these differences are difficult to generalize, therapists should elicit information about the frequency with which a client experiences fatigue and compare it against the client's overall psychological, social, lifestyle, and medical history to determine the appropriate approach to addressing the fatigue with cognitive behavioral therapy.

Cause: Physiological versus Psychosocial

For all of the reasons mentioned in the preceding points, determining the primary cause of a client's fatigue is fundamental to planning cognitive behavioral therapy interventions. However, the reality of clinical practice is that fatigue is much more frequently a multidimensional phenomenon with multiple biological, psychological, social, lifestyle, and environmental contributors, rather than a unidimensional phenomenon. Clients with fatigue who experience the most success with cognitive behavioral therapy are those that are able to acknowledge the role of these nonbiological contributors. By the same token, cognitive behavioral therapists that begin their interactions with clients by validating their causal attributions for the fatigue (even if a client feels his or her fatigue is strictly biological in nature) tend to have the greatest success in assisting clients to challenge unrealistic fatigue-related cognitions, should they emerge, later in therapy.

Severity: Mild to Severe

When determining whether to address fatigue as a focal problem for cognitive behavioral therapy therapists should consider the client's perception of the severity of the fatigue. Fatigue severity can also be assessed at key points during the course of therapy. Such assessment can be a means of providing feedback to the therapist and the client about the extent to which the therapy is effective.

Functional Consequences: Mildly Disabling to Severely Disabling

The second issue to consider when assessing the degree to which fatigue poses a problem for a client is the extent to which the fatigue interferes with the client's ability to perform activities of daily living and other occupations. Gathering information on fatigue-related disability as it compares or contrasts with perceived fatigue severity will also shed light on whether a client might be overfunctioning or underfunctioning based on his or her perception of the severity of the fatigue.

Fatigue and Chronic Conditions

Though fatigue is one of the most underrecognized and undertreated symptoms in medical care, it is one of the most debilitating and most commonly reported symptoms of clients with chronic conditions. There have been increasing attempts to bridge this gap in perception of the significance of fatigue in recent years. For instance, there is increasing epidemiological research into the prevalence of fatigue in various chronic conditions. Also, medications have been developed that specifically address some major causes of fatigue.

This section will provide a general overview of the prevalence and nature of fatigue in some of the more common chronic conditions. It should be noted that this review is not intended to be comprehensive. It does not include all of the many chronic conditions that involve or result in fatigue. The conditions that will be covered in this review were selected because they are among the more prevalent conditions that involve fatigue as a primary symptom. They include:

- Anemia
- Asthma and other pulmonary diseases
- Certain cancers and cancer treatments
- Conditions of unknown etiology (chronic fatigue syndrome, multiple chemical sensitivities, irritable bowel syndrome, fibromyalgia and other chronic pain syndromes)
- Diabetes
- Heart and cardiovascular diseases
- Infectious diseases
- Lupus
- Multiple sclerosis
- Myasthenia gravis
- Rheumatoid arthritis
- Spinal cord injury
- Sjogren's syndrome
- Thyroid disorders

Anemia

Anemia is a blood disorder in which an individual does not have enough healthy red blood cells to carry an adequate amount of oxygen to other bodily tissues. This leads to chronic tiredness and fatigue. Numerous types of anemia exist, and each type has a distinct cause. Some of the more common causes of anemia can include an iron or vitamin deficiency, a chronic illness, significant amounts of blood loss, and other genetic or acquired diseases. Anemia is also a common side effect of some medications and medical treatments. It can be acute or chronic, mild or severe. When anemia is life-threatening, it may be treated with blood transfusions.

Within the U.S., anemia is diagnosed in approximately 3.4 million people. Particularly high rates of anemia have been found in individuals with lung (52 percent) and ovarian (51 percent) cancer (Gillespie, 2003). Certain cancer treatments, such as radiation therapy in particular, may cause or exacerbate preexisting anemia in individuals with cancer. For example, of 202 individuals with various types of cancer beginning radiation therapy, rates of anemia increased from 45 percent before therapy to 57 percent by the end of treatment (Gillespie, 2003). Anemia is also common in individuals with chronic heart failure, with prevalence rates ranging from 14 percent to 55 percent.

Asthma and Other Pulmonary Diseases

Asthma is a chronic disease of the airways characterized by airway inflamma-tion, airflow obstruction, and the presence of airway hyperreactivity. Within the U.S., asthma affects approximately 15 million adults. Asthma, bronchitis, emphysema, and chronic obstructive pulmonary disease all represent lung diseases that are characterized by a high prevalence of fatigue. One study found that fatigue is approximately three times more likely to occur in individuals with asthma or emphysema than in the general population (Breslin et al., 1998). Among individuals with chronic obstructive pulmonary disease, 83% reported experiencing fatigue, 47% reported fatigue occurring every day, and 25% reported fatigue as one of their worst symptoms (Theander and Unosson 2004).

Cancer and Cancer Treatments

In general terms, cancer is a neoplastic disease characterized by abnormal cell growth, cell replication, and invasion of bodily tissues or organs. Numerous types of cancer exist. Fatigue has been reported as a common symptom among individuals with cancer and it can be caused by tumor cell byproducts, anemia, prolonged bedrest or inactivity, and various cancer treatments (Witt and Murray-Edwards 2002; Schwartz 1999).

Cancer-related fatigue has been described as relentless, intense, and unrelieved by rest (Schwartz 2000). It has also been characterized as a type of fatigue that is more severe, unpredictable, and overwhelming than any fatigue experienced before cancer (Schwartz, et al. 2001). It involves tiredness, lack of energy, lack of concentration, lack of motivation, weakness, exhaustion, lethargy, depression, and low tolerance for exercise (Mock et al., 2001; Witt and Murray-Edwards 2002).

Studies of individuals with various types of cancer have found that fatigue of any duration occurs at a rate of 52 percent to 58 percent (Goff et al. 2004). In a study of men with testicular cancer, chronic fatigue was reported by 16 percent of the men (Fossa, Dahl, and Loge 2003). Among individuals with cancer that do report fatigue as a major symptom, 90 percent report that their fatigue signifi-cantly interferes with their overall quality of life.

Cancer treatments, including chemotherapy, radiation therapy, surgery, and bone marrow transplantation have also been found to be associated with high rates of reported fatigue. Between 70 and 95 percent of individuals undergo-ing chemotherapy or radiation therapy have been found to report fatigue as a major symptom (Beisecker et al., 1997; Dimeo et al. 1999; Jacobsen et al., 1999; Prince and Jones 2001; Witt and Murray-Edwards 2002). One study of women with breast cancer found that fatigue and low energy persisted for at least six months in 83 percent of women who underwent chemotherapy (Beisecker et al., 1997).

Conditions of Unknown Etiology

Chronic fatigue syndrome, multiple chemical sensitivities, irritable bowel syndrome, fibromyalgia, and other chronic pain conditions are all characterized by high rates of fatigue. Chronic fatigue syndrome is a diagnosis of exclusion made in individuals experiencing six or more months of severe, debilitating fatigue and at least four of eight additional physical and cognitive symptoms that occur in conjunction with the fatigue (Fukuda et al., 1994). These include sore throat, new-type headaches, significant impairment in short-term memory or concentration, unrefreshing sleep, prolonged (>24 hours) malaise following previously usual levels of activity, pain in multiple joints without swelling or redness, muscle pain, and painful lymph nodes (Fukuda et al., 1994). Within the U.S., chronic fatigue syndrome is estimated to occur in approximately 800,000 individuals, and it is more common in women than in men (Jason, Richman, et al., 1999). By definition, fatigue is a primary, debilitating symptom for 100 percent of individuals with chronic fatigue syndrome. Individuals with chronic fatigue syndrome report poor quality of life and significant levels of impairment in physical mobility, cognitive functioning, social functioning, and occupational functioning (Taylor, Friedberg and Jason 2001).

Multiple chemical sensitivity is a chronic condition involving irritation or inflammation of sensory organs, gastrointestinal distress, severe fatigue, and compromised neurological function (Taylor, Friedberg, and Jason 2001). It is a condition in which individuals experience a number of different symptoms in multiple organ systems whenever they come into contact with low-levels of exposure to certain chemical agents (e.g., pesticides, perfumes, petroleum-based products and diesel fuels, automobile exhaust, and detergent residues) (Donnay 1998). Fatigue is a primary symptom of this syndrome, occurring with regularity at a rate of approximately 89 percent (Taylor, Friedberg, and Jason 2001). Other typical symptoms include skin or mucus membrane irritation (e.g., nasal congestion, shortness of breath), muscle and joint pain, fever, irritable mood, dizziness, learning and memory deficits, hypersensitivity to smells, tingling sensations, and sensory discomfort (Davis, Jason, and Banghart 1998). Multiple chemical sensitivities have been reported in approximately 2 percent to 6 percent of the U.S. population and they affect all aspects of daily functioning.

Irritable bowel syndrome is another condition of unknown etiology that is characterized by fatigue. Irritable bowel syndrome involves three or more months of abdominal pain or discomfort, inconsistency in terms of the frequency of defecation, changes in stool consistency, and changes in the way that the stool is passed (Drossman et al., 1994). It also involves passage of mucus and bloating (Drossman et al., 1994). Irritable bowel syndrome occurs in approximately 9 to 22 percent of individuals within the U.S., making it the most common of the functional bowel disorders (Drossman et al. 1982; Drossman et al., 1993; Sandler 1990). Even when it is characterized as being in remission, over 40 percent of individuals with irritable bowel syndrome report fatigue (Minderhoud et al.,

2003). In terms of severity, one study found that the fatigue experienced by individuals with this syndrome is commensurate with that experienced by individuals with cancer (Minderhound et al., 2003).

Fibromyalgia is also a prevalent syndrome characterized by chronic, widespread muscle pain and particular sensitivity to pressure in a minimum of 11 of 18 specific areas of the body (known as "tender points") (Wolfe et al., 1995). Fatigue is a major symptom of figromyalgia, and clinically significant levels of fatigue are reported in 76 to 96 percent of individuals with fibromyalgia (Village 2001; Wolfe et al., 1996). Other symptoms associated with fibromyalgia may include myofascial pain syndrome, recurrent candida infection, headache, disrupted sleep, and chronic gastrointestinal distress. Fibromyalgia is estimated to occur in approximately 2 percent of the population and it is more common in women than in men (Wolfe et al., 1995). The fatigue reported by individuals with fibromyalgia generally occurs in connection with the pain, and it increases as the pain increases. It has also been associated with sleep loss and inactivity. Fatigue is also a primary symptom of other chronic pain conditions. One study of 170 individuals with chronic pain found that 77 percent of participants experienced fatigue during the past one to two weeks, and these individuals also reported becoming fatigued very easily as a result of activity (Iverson and McCracken 1997).

Diabetes

Diabetes is a metabolic disorder characterized by disruption in the way the body processes glucose, one of the central byproducts of food, for growth and energy. Following digestion, glucose is released into the bloodstream for use by cells as a source of energy. Insulin, a hormone produced by the pancreas, must also be present in the bloodstream for glucose to effectively penetrate the cells. For individuals with diabetes, the pancreas fails to produce a sufficient amount of insulin or the cells do not absorb insulin in an effective way. As a result, high amounts of unabsorbed glucose accumulate in the bloodstream and are eventually passed through the urine. This leaves the body lacking in the necessary energy to function. There are three main types of diabetes:

- Type 1 diabetes: an autoimmune disease in which the immune system attacks and destroys the insulin-producing cells in the pancreas.
- Type 2 diabetes: a disease in which the pancreas produces sufficient levels of insulin but the cells fail to absorb and utilize it effectively.
- Gestational diabetes: a form of diabetes that develops only during pregnancy. Women that develop gestational diabetes are at higher risk for developing Type 2 diabetes following pregnancy.

Diabetes is a prevalent condition. It has been estimated to occur in approximately 18 million people within the U.S., or six percent of the population (NIH publication number 04-3873; National Diabetes Information Clearinghouse, April, 2004; *http://diabetes.niddk.nih.gov*). Fatigue is one of the major symptoms of diabetes. It tends to occur most frequently during episodes of hyperglycemia (high blood sugar) and hypoglycemia (low blood sugar). In individuals with diabetes that are under treatment, fatigue is most commonly the result of hypoglycemia, which involves increased levels of insulin in the blood. Excessive insulin levels can be caused by taking too much medication, missing a meal, increased exercise, and increased alcohol intake.

Severe and chronic fatigue also accompanies diabetes-related complications that tend to occur in individuals that have had diabetes for a number of years, such as retinopathy, nephropathy, neuropathy, and cardiovascular disease (Weijman et al. 2003). Fatigue in individuals with diabetes can also result from illness burden and stress associated with the need for ongoing management and treatment of this condition (Weijman et al., 2003).

Heart and Cardiovascular Diseases

Though they are sometimes grouped into the same category, heart diseases and cardiovascular diseases are different kinds of illness that involve different bodily organs. Heart disease includes diseases that involve only the heart and the blood vessels directly within and surrounding the heart. Cardiovascular disease includes diseases of the heart and blood vessels throughout the entire body, including arteries, capillaries, and veins in the brain, legs, and lungs. Generally defined, the main types of heart disease or heart conditions include:

- Coronary heart disease: The most common form of heart disease. It affects the blood vessels (coronary arteries) in and surrounding the heart. It is characterized by chest pain and heart attacks.
- Heart failure: Occurs when the heart is not able to pump blood through the body as efficiently as expected. Systolic heart failure occurs when the heart has difficulty contracting, or pumping blood. Diastolic heart failure occurs when the heart malfunctions in terms of its ability to release or relax. Over time, heart failure results in major impairments in activities of daily living, such as bathing, dressing, and walking.
- Angina: Crushing, pressing, or squeezing pain or discomfort in the chest and sometimes in the shoulders, arms, neck, back, or jaw. Angina usually occurs when the heart does not receive a sufficient amount of blood supply.

The main types of cardiovascular disease include:

- Atherosclerosis: Thickening, narrowing, and hardening of the arteries, leading to blood clots, blockages in blood flow, and ultimately, to heart attack or stroke.
- Stroke (cerebrovascular accident): Disruption of blood flow to the brain resulting in damage to the brain and subsequent impairment in movement (e.g., hemipeligia) and/or cognition. Stroke is caused by clotting of the blood in the brain or excessive bleeding within the brain from a ruptured blood vessel.
- High blood pressure (hypertension): Occurs when the force of blood pumped from the heart into the walls of the blood vessels is too great, resulting in readings that are consistently over 140/90. High blood pressure is associated with heart failure, stroke, kidney failure, and other health problems.

Heart disease is the first leading cause of death among chronic conditions within the U.S., and stroke is the third leading cause. Severe and chronic fatigue are prevalent symptoms of all types of heart and cardiovascular diseases. In women, unusual fatigue is the most prevalent of all the early symptoms of heart attack, occurring in 70 percent of women within one month prior to the attack. Fatigue in individuals with cardiovascular and heart disease is a byproduct of the condition itself, a side effect of certain medications, and a byproduct of psychological and social factors, such as depression, anxiety, stress, and overexertion.

Infectious Diseases

Infectious diseases, such as acute infectious mononucleosis, hepatitis C, and HIV/AIDS are all associated with significant levels of acute and chronic fatigue. The primary symptom of mono is severe and unrelenting fatigue. Other symptoms include, but are not limited to, severe sore throat, swollen lymph nodes, fever, and enlarged spleen or liver. It is typically a self-limiting infection that resolves within one to two months of onset. However, in approximately 10 percent of cases, a syndrome characterized by chronic, disabling fatigue has been found to occur six or more months following the initial diagnosis of mono (Buchwald et al., 2000, White et al., 2001). This syndrome is often referred to as "post-infectious fatigue syndrome."

Hepatitis C is one of many viruses that can cause inflammation of the liver. Approximately four million individuals living within the U.S. have been infected with the hepatitis C virus, but only about half of them are aware of the infection. In 75 percent of individuals with Hepatitis C, the inflammation is no longer reversible and has become chronic. Most (80 percent) of people infected with the virus do not have any symptoms. In the 20 percent of individuals that do develop symptoms, most do not report symptoms until 10–20 years after the initial infection. Few individuals have symptoms during the early acute phase of the infection, which typically occurs 5–12 weeks following the initial infection.

Fatigue is a primary symptom of Hepatitis C in both the acute and chronic phases. Approximately 67 percent of symptomatic individuals with Hepatitis C report fatigue, and 49 percent report fatigue as their worst symptom (Hassoun et al. 2002). In a study of 92 individuals with Hepatitis C, 25 percent reported that their fatigue was present every day and 12 percent reported that it was present for more than 12 hours per day (Hassoun et al., 2002). Other symptoms of Hepatitis C include nausea, vomiting, diarrhea, loss of appetite, abdominal pain, jaundice, urine dark in color, and stools pale in color. Fatigue is also a major symptom of cirrhosis, which is a complication of Hepatitis C. Cirrhosis eventually causes liver failure, requiring individuals to have a liver transplant.

HIV (human immunodeficiency virus) is the virus that causes AIDS (acquired immune dysfunction syndrome). HIV progressively kills and damages cells within the body's immune system and it eventually destroys the body's immunity against certain infections and cancers. Opportunistic infections that do not typically affect the general population, are common among individuals with AIDS.

AIDS is a highly prevalent infectious disease that has been reported in more than 830,000 people within the U.S. With few exceptions, it is considered to be fatal, but recently developed medications have been found to prolong the life span significantly for many individuals. Many individuals do not become ill when they are first infected with HIV, but those that do become ill report a brief flu-like illness characterized by fatigue, fever, headache, and swollen lymph nodes.

As HIV continues to affect the immune system, fatigue continues to be a primary symptom that interferes with major life activities, such as employment and the ability to drive an automobile (Darko et al., 1992). Fatigue occurs in approximately 37–57 percent of individuals with HIV infection (Sullivan and Dworkin 2002; Wolfe 1999). Fatigue can result from immune dysfunction, nutritional deficits, antiviral medications, anemia, and psychosocial variables (e.g., stress, depression, and sleep disturbance). Other symptoms of HIV infection include weight loss, fevers and sweats, chronic candida infection, skin problems, short-term memory loss, and, in women, pelvic inflammatory disease that does not resolve with treatment. Severe, debilitating fatigue is also one of the most prevalent symptoms of many opportunistic infections and cancers that occur in individuals that develop AIDS.

Lupus

Lupus (systemic lupus erythematosus) is a chronic autoimmune disease characterized by immune dysfunction, severe joint pain and arthritis, muscle pain, persistent fever, weight loss, vascular lesions, and skin rash. It is estimated to occur in between 500,000 and 2,000,000 individuals within the U.S. and can be fatal. Symptoms and severity can relapse and remit without apparent cause. Between 50 and 90 percent of individuals with lupus experience disabling fatigue (Bruce et al., 1999; Giles and Isenberg 2000). Lupus is a systemic disease, which means it can affect multiple organs within the body. Some have described fatigue as a byproduct of the primary pathological processes of the disease, and others have found no correlation between fatigue and disease activity or organ damage in lupus (Bruce, Mak, Hallett, Gladman and Urowitz 1999). Thus, the role of psychosocial variables in fatigue is unclear.

Multiple Sclerosis

Multiple sclerosis is a chronic autoimmune disease that affects nerve fibers in the brain and spinal cord. It is characterized by intermittent damage to myelin, which is the fatty substance that surrounds and insulates nerve fibers and allows for the transmission of nerve impulses. Damage to the nerve fibers usually occurs within the brain, spinal cord, and optic nerves. This can result in weakness, numbness, pain, and loss of vision. Multiple sclerosis affects different nerve fiber systems within the body at different times. As a result, the disease is often characterized by relapses and remissions of different symptom clusters. However, some subtypes of the disease are characterized by progressive degeneration with few periods of remission. Multiple sclerosis is estimated to occur in approximately 500,000 individuals within the U.S. and is more common in women than in men.

Fatigue has been reported by 75–90 percent of individuals diagnosed with multiple sclerosis (Ward and Winters 2003). Fatigue in multiple sclerosis has been thought to be associated with impaired nerve conduction, axonal loss, immune dysfunction, physical deconditioning, and psychosocial variables, though not much empirical evidence supports any of these hypotheses (Ward and Winters 2003). In one study, fatigue was described as lasting for up to six hours and becoming more severe as the day progressed (Ward and Winters 2003). It was described as an overwhelming sense of physical exhaustion and as being associated with the exacerbation of other symptoms of multiple sclerosis, including increased visual disturbances, decreased mobility, cognitive functioning, and anxiety and depression (Ward and Winters 2003).

Myasthenia Gravis

Myasthenia Gravis is an autoimmune disorder that involves progressive skeletal muscle weakness. It results in rapid fatigue (fatigability) and loss of muscle strength upon exertion. In its early stages this disease primarily affects the muscles of the eyes, face, and jaw, and those that control swallowing. As the disease progresses and in the absence of treatment, it affects respiratory muscles and eventually causes respiratory failure. Myasthenia gravis is reported in approximately 2 of every 100,000 people. Between 82 and 89 percent of people with this disease report experiencing physical fatigue as an ongoing symptom (Paul et al., 2000). In myasthenia gravis, fatigue worsens with activity and improves with rest, but it reoccurs as soon as activity is reinitiated (Howard 1998). Fatigue in this disease is associated with moderate impairment in cognitive, physical, and social functioning (Paul et al., 2000).

Rheumatoid Arthritis

Rheumatoid arthritis is a chronic, progressive autoimmune disease characterized by inflammation of the lining (synovium) of the joints. It generally progresses in three stages:

- Stage 1: Stage 1 involves swelling of the joint lining. Stage 1 symptoms are pain, warmth, stiffness, redness and swelling around the joint.
- Stage 2: Stage 2 involves rapid division and growth of cells, which causes the joint lining to thicken.
- Stage 3: In Stage 3, the inflamed cells release enzymes that cause destruction of bone and cartilage, causing the joint to loose its shape and alignment. This results in more severe, chronic pain, loss of mobility, and decreased ability to work and perform activities of daily living.

Rheumatoid arthritis is frequently characterized by flare-ups, or periods of increased severity. It is a systemic disease, which means it can affect other organs within the body. However, new drugs, exercise, joint-protection techniques, and self-management techniques all help in controlling the disease. Rheumatoid arthritis is estimated to occur in approximately 2.1 million individuals within the U.S.

Fatigue is reported by 80 to 93 percent of individuals with this disease, regardless of stage and severity (Huyser et al., 1998). In one study, 57 percent reported that fatigue was the most problematic aspect of rheumatoid arthritis, and 32 percent reported that they were too tired to work more than four hours without rest (Huyser et al., 1998). Fatigue in rheumatoid arthritis has been described as being associated with the disease activity itself, pain, sleep disturbance, decreased activity levels, greater functional limitation, more comorbidities, depressed mood, stress, medications, and environmental variables (Huyser et al., 1998; Wolfe, Hawley, and Wilson 1996).

Spinal Cord Injury

Spinal cord injury is the result of a trauma that damages cells within the spinal cord or severs the nerve tracts that transmit information up and down the spinal cord and to the rest of the body. Spinal cord injury can be caused in a number of ways, but the most common causes include lacerations of nerve fibers from wounds (e.g., gunshot wounds), compression wounds (pressure on the spinal cord), contusion wounds (bruising of the spinal cord), and central cord syndrome (damage to the corticospinal tracts of the cervical spinal cord). Spinal cord injuries that are severe result in paralysis, which is defined as a loss of control over the movement of muscles. The extent and location of the paralysis depends on the location of the damage to the spinal cord. Spinal cord injuries also result in loss of sensation and reflex function below the point of injury. This includes the loss of autonomic nervous system activity (e.g., breathing, bowel, and urinary control). Depending upon the location of the injury along the spinal cord, loss of reflex function and autonomic activity may result in loss of bowel and bladder control and, if the injury is high enough, impairment in independent breathing.

Estimates of the prevalence of spinal cord injury vary, but they generally range between 183,000 and 230,000 individuals living within the U.S. (DeVivo et al., 1980; Harvey et al., 1990; Lasfarques, Custis et al., 1995). Associated symptoms of spinal cord injury, including pain, unusual sensitivity to stimuli, muscle spasms, and sexual dysfunction typically develop over time. Individuals with spinal cord injury are also at risk for development of a range of secondary, recurring conditions, such as pressure sores, pulmonary infections, and bladder infections.

Fatigue in spinal cord injury tends to develop gradually over time. One study of approximately 300 individuals that had been living with spinal cord injury for over 23 years found that more than half of those interviewed reported experiencing ongoing exhaustion and other fatigue-related symptoms (Craig Hospital, 2004). In this study, fatigue was associated with depression, decreased quality of life, lack of mobility, decreased social contact, reduced mental activity, and reduced motivation (Craig Hospital, 2004).

Sjogren's Syndrome

Sjogren's syndrome is a chronic autoimmune disease characterized by inflammation of the glands of the body (mainly the salivary and tear glands). This leads to chronic dryness of the eyes and mouth. Chronic inflammation of the tear glands can progressively lead to irritation of the eyes, decreased tear production, a "gritty" sensation in the eyes, eye infections, and significant corneal abrasions. Chronic inflammation of the salivary glands can result in difficulty swallowing, mouth sores, tooth decay, gum disease, mouth swelling, and stones or infections of the salivary glands. Additional glands that become inflamed as a result of Sjogren's syndrome include those that line breathing passages (resulting in lung infections) and vagina (resulting in pain during intercourse). The prevalence of Sjogren's syndrome has been estimated at 500,000. There are two categories of Sjogren's syndrome:

- Primary: The syndrome is localized to inflammation of the salivary and tear glands and does not involve connective tissue disease.
- Secondary: The syndrome not only involves gland inflammation but is it also associated with connective tissue diseases, such as rheumatoid arthritis, lupus, or scleroderma.

Other autoimmune diseases associated with Sjogren's syndrome include autoimmune thyroiditis (Hashimoto's disease) and gastroesophageal reflux disease. Raynaud's phenomenon, sleep disturbance, lymph node swelling, kidney, nerve, and muscle disease can also accompany Sjogren's syndrome.

Because both the primary and secondary types of Sjogren's syndrome are systemic, the syndrome inevitably affects other organs within the body. As a result, the more predominant symptoms of the disease include fatigue, joint pain, and widespread muscle pain. Because fatigue and pain are often experienced by individuals as the most problematic symptoms, individuals often forget to report symptoms of dry eyes and mouth to their doctors, making the actual diagnosis of this condition infrequent.

Extreme debilitating fatigue occurs in between 50 percent and 68 percent of individuals with primary Sjogren's syndrome, and rates increase in individuals with secondary Sjogren's syndrome (Giles and Isenberg 2000; Kassan and Moutsopoulos 2004). For many individuals, fatigue is the most troublesome and disabling symptom of the syndrome (Giles and Isenberg 2000; Kassan and Moutsopoulos 2004). Participants reported spending several extra hours in bed trying to rest or sleep without feeling refreshed or energized as a result of this extra time spent (Kassan and Moutsopoulos 2004).

Thyroid Disorders

Thyroid disorders affect the thyroid gland. The thyroid gland is a small endocrine gland in the neck that produces thyroid hormones (i.e., T4 thyroxine and T3 triiodothyronine) that regulate metabolism (the rate at which the body uses and stores energy from food) and control the rate at which every other part of the body functions. Generally, disorders of the thyroid affect body weight, energy levels, skin health, menstruation, muscle strength, cholesterol levels, heart rate, and memory. Thyroid disorders are highly prevalent within the U.S. More than 20 million individuals have been estimated to be receiving treatment for a thyroid disorder (*http://cpmcnet.columbia.edu*).

There are two primary ways in which thyroid disorders can affect thyroid functioning:

- **Hypothyroidism**: This occurs when the thyroid is underactive and it is not producing enough (or any) thyroid hormone. When there is not enough thyroid hormone in the bloodstream, metabolism and the rate at which other bodily organs function slow down. The symptoms of hypothyroidism develop gradually. Some of the most common symptoms include: fatigue, muscle weakness, weight gain, decreased appetite, change in menstruation, loss of sex drive, feeling cold when others do not, hair loss, constipation, puffiness around the eye area, brittle nails, and muscle aches.
- **Hyperthyroidism**: This occurs when the thyroid is overactive in its production of thyroid hormone. This causes the metabolism and rate at which other bodily organs function to accelerate. Some of the more common symptoms include: fatigue, weight loss, nervousness, heat intolerance, heart palpitations, increased sweating, changes in menstruation, more frequent bowel movements, and tremors.

Hypothyroidism and hyperthyroidism occur as primary components of specific thyroid conditions. The most common thyroid disorders include:

- Autoimmune hypothyroidism (Hashimoto's Disease), which is the most common cause of hypothyroidism. In Hashimoto's disease, the immune system perceives the cells of the thyroid as foreign and begins to attack the thyroid gland. This causes the gland to become swollen, irritated, and less able to produce thyroid hormone.
- Subacute (viral) thyroiditis, defined as an inflammation of the thyroid gland, which is thought to be the result of a self-limiting infectious process within the body. The thyroid can become swollen, enlarged, and painful. The inflammation may temporarily result in an overproduction of thyroid hormone, particularly when in the initial stages of infection. Associated symptoms include symptoms of hyperthyroidism, fatigue, fever, and muscle and joint pain. This condition usually resolves within a six-month period with no lasting damage to the thyroid.
- Postpartum thyroiditis, in which the thyroid becomes swollen or inflamed after child birth. This causes changes in the levels of thyroid hormone within the body, and these changes can involve periods of both hypothyroidism and

hyperthyroidism. This condition usually disappears within six months after pregnancy with no permanent damage to the thyroid. However, some women do develop chronic thyroid conditions (primarily hypothyroidism) following pregnancy.

- Thyroid nodules, which are lumps in the thyroid gland that occur when tissues of the thyroid grow. Roughly 5 percent of the worldwide population has benign thyroid enlargement or nodules. Most thyroid nodules are asymptomatic and harmless, but some can lead to hyperthyroidism and others may be cancerous.
- Thyroid cancer, which occurs when growth of the thyroid tissues is caused by cancer cells. Though various types of thyroid cancer exist, the most common types can be fully removed with surgery and are associated with five-year survival rates that exceed 90 percent. For most individuals with thyroid cancer, the prognosis is excellent.
- Goiter, which is a diffused enlargement of the thyroid gland.
- Grave's Disease, which is the most common cause of hyperthyroidism. In Grave's disease, the immune system produces antibodies that falsely stimulate the thyroid gland to produce unnecessary amounts of thyroid hormone. This causes enlargement, inflammation, and chronic overactivation of the thyroid gland.

Fatigue is one of the most prevalent symptoms of thyroid disorders. It occurs as a primary symptom of both hypothyroidism and hyperthyroidism and severe fatigue is present in up to 84 percent of individuals with thyroid disorders (Trivalle et al. 1996).

Conclusion

This chapter provided an overview of the prevalence of abnormal fatigue within the general population and described common ways in which fatigue is subclassified and experienced. In addition, basic information about a number of conditions for which fatigue is a primary symptom was provided, and the role of fatigue in each condition was described. The next chapter next chapter will discuss Nina, a woman with chronic fatigue syndrome. That chapter will illustrate unique considerations of assessment and intervention with a person whose primary chronic condition is characterized by debilitating fatigue.

15

Cognitive Behavioral Assessment and Treatment Outcomes for Chronic Fatigue: The Case of Nina

Chapter 14 described the variegated features of fatigue as a major symptom category. It reviewed the prevalence and causes of fatigue within the general population. In addition, it provided an overview of common chronic conditions that involve fatigue as a primary symptom. This chapter will illustrate the application of cognitive behavioral therapy to Nina, a woman with chronic fatigue syndrome. Nina was introduced in Chapter 1 and periodically discussed throughout the text.

This chapter aims to synthesize earlier examples of Nina and present her case, including the outcomes of her therapy, in its entirety. Moreover, this chapter will illustrate unique assessment and intervention approaches that can be incorporated into cognitive behavioral interventions that focus on fatigue. In this regard, the chapter will illustrate the application of clinical assessments that, in the author's experience, are useful for the client with fatigue. Copies of the assessments developed by the author are reproduced in the Appendix of this chapter. It should also be noted that this chapter will illustrate cognitive behavioral strategies that are specific to the treatment of persons with fatigue. The chapter will close with an overview of the unique considerations in treating individuals with fatigue.

As described in Chapter 1, Nina is a 35-year-old woman with chronic fatigue syndrome (CFS). Nina was referred for cognitive behavioral therapy by her physician because he was concerned that psychological variables were having a negative impact upon Nina's health status and overall compliance with treatment recommendations. Although she initially rejected the referral, Nina was eventually willing to see a psychotherapist when she was told that the therapist would focus on teaching her alternative ways to manage her fatigue.

Initial Orientation, Approach to Assessment and Assessment Findings

For Nina, the initial orientation and assessment period was protracted, taking place over a period of five sessions. Medical records and verbal information from all of Nina's health-care providers was collected and ultimately the following assessments were completed:

- Semistructured clinical interview
- Problem list
- Activity pacing schedule
- Occupational self-assessment

These assessments were administered in the order listed. They were gradually selected over time as the therapist gathered increasing knowledge about Nina's interpersonal style, primary goal for therapy, and preferred approach to therapy.

Orientation and Rapport-Building

Rapport-building is a fundamental aspect of cognitive behavioral therapy. Because Nina demonstrated an unusual level of ambivalence about therapy during her initial phone conversation with the therapist, the therapist spent the entire first session orienting Nina to cognitive behavioral therapy and working to strengthen the therapeutic relationship. Continuing to build upon the initial telephone conversation with Nina, the therapist spent additional time describing the basic structure and steps of cognitive behavioral therapy, and getting to know Nina in terms of her basic competencies, perceived strengths, primary concerns, and goals and expectations for therapy. The therapist made it a point to mention examples of studies that have demonstrated empirical support for the use of cognitive behavioral therapy with individuals with chronic fatigue syndrome. She also spent a significant amount of time answering the numerous questions that Nina had about the process and expected outcomes of therapy in terms of improving her fatigue and functioning.

During this exchange, Nina informed the therapist that her primary goal was to reach a complete recovery from chronic fatigue syndrome, and her expectation was that this would occur after only attending two or three sessions. This required the therapist to have a longer conversation with Nina about her expectations for therapy and about the variability in each individual's pace and response to cognitive behavioral therapy. As the first session was drawing to an end, it became clear to the therapist that they would not be able to complete all nine steps of the initial orientation and assessment phase during the first session. Because it is important to maintain and teach clients as much of the basic structure of cognitive behavioral therapy as possible, the therapist decided to ask Nina to complete a problem list (described in Chapter 4) as her first homework assignment.

During the initial summary and feedback, Nina mentioned that she was unsure about whether this process would really be helpful, but that she agreed to come for a second session because she had promised her doctor she would give it a try. The therapist thanked Nina for her honesty and informed Nina that this is exactly the kind of feedback needed for cognitive therapy. At that time the therapist also informed Nina that feelings of doubt about the process are very common at the beginning, and she made a plan with Nina for how to manage any challenges or negative feelings that could potentially arise during therapy and/or within the therapeutic relationship. The plan involved Nina providing immediate feedback whenever she felt doubtful, invalidated or misunderstood.

Nina failed to complete the problem list as the initial homework assignment. The therapist decided to complete the problem list with Nina during the second session as part of a semistructured clinical interview. This interview was used to elicit information about Nina's physical health history, present symptoms and impairments, psychosocial history, and family background (reviewed in Chapter 1). Nina was asked to describe her experience with CFS in general, including circumstances surrounding CFS onset, reactions of health care providers and individuals in her social network, illness-related losses, what she considers her most troublesome symptoms, and issues involving self-concept and adaptation to illness.

A semistructured interview format was selected over more structured interviews or formal self-report measures because of Nina's

- Initial ambivalence about entering therapy,
- Failure to complete her first written assessment (the problem list) independently, and
- Initial doubts about the therapeutic process.

The therapist's rationale was that Nina would feel more comfortable with self-disclosure about negative automatic thoughts and emotions during the treatment process if she felt that the therapist

- Took her illness seriously,
- Understood that it was not a psychiatric disorder,
- Validated her experience, and
- Normalized her reactions to it.

In addition, the therapist was hopeful that this approach would increase the likelihood that Nina would actively participate in a collaborative relationship.

Problem List

Because initially Nina had difficulty reporting any problems outside of her concerns about having chronic fatigue syndrome, the therapist introduced the problem list during the clinical interview. After two sessions, Nina completed a problem list that consisted of the following three presenting problems:

- Extreme fatigue and too many other symptoms
- Not working or functioning to my full capacity because of my fatigue
- Feeling overwhelmed by my fatigue

Activity Pacing Schedule

Because Nina wanted to focus on reducing the functional consequences of chronic fatigue syndrome, the therapist introduced a more behaviorally based and volition-oriented assessment (the activity pacing schedule) to gather information that was directly relevant to her presenting problems. Nina's first few entries on the activity record were completed retrospectively during the third session with guidance from the therapist. Results from Nina's initial entries (which were originally presented in Chapter 9) are shown in Figure 1.

Date Day	Activities planned (numbered in order of priority) Also list unplanned activities that you did at the end of your list Remember the 50/50 solution	Importance to you (low = 1 ------10 = high)	Importance to others	Stress (1 ------10 = high)	Activity completed? Yes / No	Fatigue level for the day low 1—10 high
June 3 Friday	1. Get ready for work	5	9	2	Yes	8
	2. Drive to work	5	9	9	Yes	
	3. Complete budget spreadsheet	5	10	10	Yes	
	4. Drive home	10	5	8	Yes	
	5. Grocery shopping	5	8	7	Yes	
	6. Take cleaning to cleaners	3	5	5	Yes	
	7. Cook dinner	7	7	7	Yes	
	8. Clean kitchen	7	7	7	Yes	
	9. Call friend	10	8	2	Yes	
	10. Watch TV with partner	10	8	2	Yes	
June 4 Saturday	1. Get ready for the day	5	5	2	Yes	9
	2. Drive daughter to softball practice	5	10	4	Yes	
	3. Take dog to groomer	1	3	7	Yes	
	4. Prepare lunch	3	8	5	Yes	
	5. Do some gardening	10	1	3	No	
	6. Pick up daughter from softball	5	10	4	Yes	
	7. Pick up cleaning	3	3	5	Yes	
	8. Prepare dinner	3	8	8	Yes	
	9. Go to movie with friend	10	9	2	No	
	Had argument with partner	1	1	10	Yes	

June 5 Sunday						10
1. Get ready for the day	1	5	2	No		
2. Prepare lunch	10	1	4	No		
3. Pay bills	8	10	7	No		
4. Do some gardening	5	1	3	No		
5. Spend time with daughter	10	9	3	No		
6. Cook dinner for friends	8	7	9	No		
Too tired to do anything – watched TV	1	1	10	yes		

FIGURE 1. Nina's Initial Activity Pacing Schedule

Results of this assessment indicate that Nina initially had difficulty limiting the number of high-stress activities she performed. In addition, she engaged in more high-stress activities than low-stress activities. She did not prioritize and reduce her activity levels in response to her fatigue levels until she reached a point when her symptoms forced her to remain in bed all day. Overall, Nina appears to be leading a lifestyle oriented around doing activities that are, at times, significantly more important to others than to her. With the exception of gardening, cooking, and driving her car to run errands and meet with people, Nina is sedentary and does not exercise. Findings from a snapshot of the activity pacing schedule obtained after Nina completed her first 20 sessions of cognitive behavioral therapy are presented in Figure 4 of this chapter and discussed in the outcomes section.

Fatigue Cognitions Scale

The therapist chose to administer the Fatigue Cognitions Scale (shown in Figure 2 and in the Appendix) in order to obtain a clear idea of the nature and extent of Nina's cognitions concerning her fatigue. The scale is a clinical measure developed by the author for use in practice. It can be used to assess the presence and types of a client's dysfunctional cognitions that are related to fatigue. Because it is

Fatigue Cognitions Scale	
Please answer "true" or "false" to the following statements.	
1. I cannot predict when my fatigue will occur.	T
2. No one cares about my fatigue.	T
3. My doctor does not know how to treat my fatigue.	T
4. My fatigue makes me less attractive to others.	T
5. My fatigue never goes away.	T
6. No one understands my fatigue.	T
7. I cannot keep my mind off my fatigue.	T
8. My fatigue will never improve.	F
9. My doctor does not care about my fatigue.	F
10. My fatigue renders me useless at work.	F
11. My fatigue causes social/interpersonal difficulties.	T
12. I can no longer live with my fatigue.	F
13. People think my fatigue is "all in my head".	T
14. My fatigue has made me an ineffective parent.	T
15. People think I exaggerate my fatigue.	T
16. I cannot control my fatigue.	T
17. I am looking for a complete cure for my fatigue.	T
18. My fatigue has changed my personality.	T
19. I feel I have failed in life because of my fatigue.	T
20. I cannot do anything without feeling fatigued.	T
21. At times my fatigue makes me want to die.	T
22. I cannot cope with my fatigue.	T
23. My fatigue has changed who I am as a person.	F

FIGURE 2. Nina's Responses to the Fatigue Cognitions Scale

brief and offers an easy "true" or "false" response format, it can be administered rapidly during a session or assigned for homework. A second strength of this scale is that it allows therapists and their clients (when appropriate) to use clinical judgment and contextual information about the client's illness and life circumstances to determine which of the statements endorsed as "true" reflect cognitive distortions (as opposed to realistic cognitions of low utility).

For example, it may be realistic for some clients to report "my doctor does not know how to treat my fatigue" if indeed the doctor has indicated this to the client. Similarly, some clients who are severely ill or experiencing a relapse may be realistic in their endorsement of the statement, "I cannot do anything without feeling fatigued." The number and nature of statements that a client endorses as "true" can also aid a clinician in making more global clinical judgments regarding the degree to which a given client's cognitions about fatigue are, in general, dysfunctional. A similar scale (which will be presented in Chapter 17) has been developed by the author to assess pain-related cognitions.

Occupational Self Assessment

Because one of Nina's central concerns involved improving her work performance and everyday functioning, the therapist included volition-oriented questions within the clinical interview. The therapist used selected items in the occupational self assessment (introduced in Chapter 13) as a guide for questioning. Using this assessment, the therapist asked about Nina's ability to perform certain tasks and their meaning/importance to her. This allowed the therapist to get a general idea about the nature of Nina's occupational and volitional strengths and difficulties without asking her to complete an entire assessment.

What became apparent from this part of the interview was that Nina had lost the ability to participate in many activities that she once found gratifying, including sports. Despite the fact that she was functioning well beyond her available energy levels and pushing herself until she was unable to get out of bed in the morning, Nina was no longer able to work at the pace that she once did before she became ill. Fluctuations in her energy level were leading her to believe she was improving one day, only to realize that she was relapsing the following day. This led to difficulties estimating her current performance capacity. Because of her high expectations for her own performance, Nina was unable to find much gratification or meaning in any activity and was concerned about the future. A summary of these findings, which were discussed in Chapter 13, is presented in Table 1.

DSM-IV Diagnostic Profile

Following the assessment process the therapist arrived at the following DSM-IV diagnoses.
Axis I: Depressive disorder, not otherwise specified
Axis II: Obsessive-Compulsive personality disorder

TABLE 1. Consequences of fatigue on Nina's volition.

Aspect of volition	Volitional consequences of Nina's fatigue
Personal Causation	– Lowered sense of capacity and reduced feeling of effectiveness in completing routine tasks
	– Worry about future, including career and family relationships
	– Difficulty accurately estimating capacity for performance due to fluctuations in available energy
	– Erosion of confidence in being able to successfully accomplish goals
	– Gap between pattern of interests and values and what client can do
Values	– Lost sense of meaning associated with occupations that can no longer be done
	– Inability to attain standards of performance that afford a sense of self-worth
	– Inability to commit to or see the worth of pursing goals that once were highly motivating
Interests	– Reduced enjoyment in doing familiar and previously enjoyable activities
	– Decreased anticipatory pleasure in previously engaging work activities and hobbies
	– Reduced range of satisfying participation
	– Difficulty forming new interests

Axis III: Chronic fatigue syndrome, herpes simplex virus -II

Axis IV: Psychosocial issues: occupational problems, problems with primary support group

Axis V: Global assessment of functioning = 61

Treatment Goals

In the third session, as noted above, Nina and her therapist identified two treatment goals. They agreed that Goal 1, reducing fatigue, was the priority. The therapist recommended corresponding objectives, or steps that Nina would need to take to accomplish that goal. The therapist reminded Nina that they would focus only on Goal 1 for a period of 20 sessions and then review progress on that goal during the 20th session. At that time they could decide whether to move on to Goal 2 or to continue working on Goal 1. When Goal 1 was initially established, Nina rated her confidence level for attaining the goal by the 20th session as an "8" on a scale of 1–10. Table 2 shows this first goal and three objectives that Nina and the therapist agreed upon.

Nina's second goal for the future was to improve work functioning. The objectives for this goal were to decide upon an appropriate structure within which Nina could set limits on the number of work activities she engaged in, to plan ahead for anticipated workloads, and to increase her willingness to delegate tasks to the company secretaries, while at the same time increasing her overall productivity through greater consistency. This goal was placed on hold until 11/3/02.

TABLE 2. Nina's first goal and objectives.

Goal Form			
Date: _____			
Goal(s)	Confidence rating (1–10)	Objectives (realistic steps I can take to achieve goal)	Target date
Goal 1: Reduce fatigue and CFS symptoms	8	a) Explore and test beliefs about the relationship between stress, types of activities performed, and fatigue. b) Practice 50/50 solution with an aim toward prioritizing low-stress activities and reducing high-stress activities. c) Gradually increase the amount of low-stress activities performed over time, with an emphasis on increasing activities that both are enjoyable and involve physical activity.	20th session on 11/3/02)

Cognitive Behavioral Case Conceptualization

By the fourth session, the therapist was ready to develop a cognitive behavioral case conceptualization that would guide the subsequent sessions of therapy. For the fourth and fifth sessions, Nina and the therapist reviewed the basic aspects of the cognitive model. This included a review of the relationships between health event triggers, automatic thoughts, and emotional, behavioral, and physiological outcomes. They also reviewed the three levels of beliefs and their role in the cognitive model.

When it was initially presented to her, Nina questioned the cognitive model repeatedly. She asked how the cognitive model would be incorporated into her treatment and how it would help her address her central goal, which was to reduce her fatigue and symptoms. The therapist explained that chronic fatigue syndrome is a stress-sensitive condition in which symptoms vary not only in relationship to activity levels, sleep, nutrition and other self-care activities, but also in relationship to stress. The therapist explained that there are now decades of research in the field of psychoneuroimmunology that demonstrates that the immune system is highly responsive and highly sensitive to human emotion and behavior.

Nina initially rejected this explanation as overemphasizing the role of stress, and complained of difficulties concentrating, which she said prevented her from understanding the cognitive model. The therapist reassured Nina that the therapist's belief is that chronic fatigue syndrome is a legitimate systemic condition. Like all chronic conditions, it needs to be managed not only with medications but also by cognitive behavioral strategies, which include stress reduction and behavioral modification. The therapist then recommended that together they try to apply examples from Nina's life to the cognitive model.

Together and over the course of two sessions, the therapist and Nina worked on the case conceptualization worksheet (introduced in Chapter 4) to come up with a "real world" case conceptualization for Nina that would accurately reflect the basic aspects of the cognitive model. First, the therapist made some suggestions for how to fill in the blanks to form an initial case conceptualization. Together, Nina and her therapist worked on revising the case conceptualization diagram until Nina not only understood it, but also felt that it accurately represented how her beliefs played a role in her emotional, behavioral, and physiological reactions to triggering events. The final version of Nina's case conceptualization is presented in Figure 3.

As the case conceptualization illustrates, the core belief that underlies Nina's feelings of anxiety and depression is that she is worthless as a wife, parent, and coworker. When Nina experiences an increase in fatigue and symptoms, she typically concludes that she is headed for a prolonged relapse, and her conditional belief is that she must rush to take care of all of her responsibilities before the relapse occurs (otherwise, she is worthless). The consequences of her beliefs are that she feels anxious and sad, pushes herself to work harder, becomes hostile toward her husband and daughter, and eventually develops additional physical complications (e.g., an outbreak of genital herpes). Nina's understanding of her case conceptualization was her first significant achievement in therapy.

Summary of the Orientation and Assessment Phase

In Nina's case, six central objectives were important in socializing her into cognitive behavioral therapy. These included:

- Validating her belief that chronic fatigue syndrome is a legitimate physiological illness
- Establishing an empathic understanding of her illness experience
- Planning with Nina for negative feelings that could arise within the therapeutic relationship and agreeing on an approach to manage them together
- Outlining the structure, process, and other essential elements of cognitive behavioral therapy.
- Defining problems, setting a goal, and setting a provisional target date for completion
- Teaching the cognitive model as it applied to Nina's situation

By the end of the initial assessment and orientation period, the therapist was more confident that Nina understood the basic structure and process of cognitive

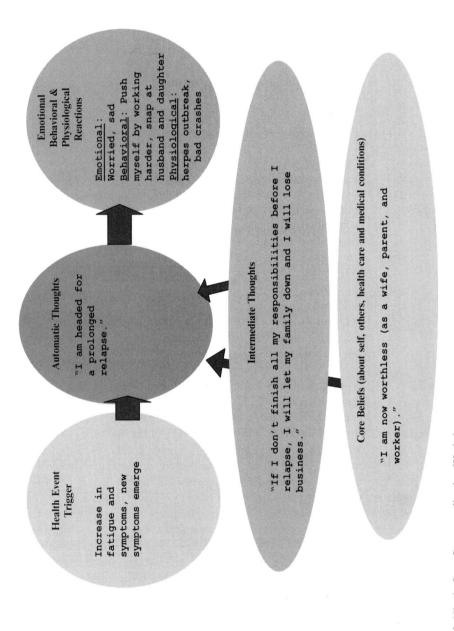

FIGURE 3. Nina's Case Conceptualization Worksheet

behavioral therapy. Nina appeared motivated to work toward the primary goal she had identified, which was to reduce her fatigue and symptoms. As anticipated, Nina did not find the initial assessments that the therapist selected to be threatening— possibly because they did not appear to emphasize emotional or psychological issues. In addition, they allowed her to describe her symptoms and experiences in her own words with little external structure or implied interpretation.

Subsequent Sessions: Course of Treatment

Nina received a total of 40 sessions of cognitive behavioral therapy over a one-year period. Her first course of therapy, which lasted 20 sessions, aimed to address Goal 1 (to reduce her fatigue and CFS symptoms). By the 20th session, Nina had made significant progress on Goal 1, but she agreed with the therapist that she had not yet mastered objective (c), which was to gradually increase activities that are enjoyable and also involve physical activity. During the remaining 20 sessions, Nina continued to work on Goal 1 (with a focus on objective (c)) and also began to work on her second goal, which was to improve her ability to function in her work role through increased planning, delegation, and limit-setting.

Main Emphasis of the Socratic Questioning

Socratic questioning was used carefully and strategically throughout the course of treatment to facilitate examination of Nina's beliefs about responsibility-taking and her role as a wife, parent, and worker. During the first course of 20 sessions, Nina occasionally provided the therapist with feedback that she found some of the Socratic questions to be "obvious," "inappropriately rhetorical," and "almost a gamey treatment of my disease." The therapist acknowledged and validated her reactions, and explored them further. Nina reported that CFS does not always escalate predictably in reaction to stress or activity, and that questions that asked her to examine the consequences of her choices to engage in certain responsibilities were "pointless." The therapist took Nina's reactions seriously and instead began to draw more heavily upon achieving an empathic understanding of Nina's experience with CFS.

In addition, the therapist became more vigilant about using only the kinds of Socratic questions that Nina would consider to be worthy of contemplation. For example, Nina appeared to view questions that probed evidence, assumptions, and viewpoint as nonthreatening types of Socratic questions. During the second course of 20 sessions, Nina had become more comfortable with the therapist and more trusting in the therapy process. At that time, Socratic questioning was used with greater frequency to address core issues of self-worth and guilt as they pertained to maintaining the 50/50 solution, setting limits and delegating at work, and being willing to pursue leisure activities that she enjoyed.

In-Session Cognitive and Behavioral Activities

Using the case conceptualization worksheet (introduced in Chapter 4 and presented in Figure 3) Nina's case conceptualization was reviewed periodically during the course of treatment. Thought records (presented in Chapters 7 and 8) were used liberally as an in-session activity during the treatment process. Nina initially became defensive whenever any of her more entrenched core beliefs about herself or her illness were directly questioned. Because many of Nina's negative beliefs could be considered realistic, the therapist decided to utilize a thought record that was adapted for use with both realistic and unrealistic cognitions (i.e., the reversal record, presented in Chapter 8) during the initial course of therapy (i.e., first 20 sessions). The reversal record allowed Nina to decide at her own pace which of her cognitions were realistic versus unrealistic and to choose how to respond to them. Over time during sessions 21–40, Nina became more comfortable with the idea that not all of her thoughts about her illness were necessarily accurate or realistic at all times, and she began to utilize the response record (presented in Chapter 7) to consider alternatives to her more maladaptive beliefs.

In addition to thought records, the activity pacing schedule was introduced during one of the initial sessions but was typically completed as homework. To facilitate the likelihood that Nina would be able to successfully practice the 50/50 solution using this schedule, Nina's husband and daughter were brought into one therapy session in order to explain how use of the schedule and the 50/50 solution were essential for goal attainment.

In addition, Nina was provided with self-advocacy training toward the end of the therapy process as a means of preparing her to set more limits at work, to plan ahead for her workload, and to delegate more of her lower-level work responsibilities to the company secretaries. Ultimately, Nina used her self-advocacy training at home to better communicate her needs to her husband. One of the outcomes of this process was that the family hired a housekeeper to come twice per week to relieve Nina and Nina's daughter of some of the daily chores, such as cooking, housecleaning, loading and retrieving dishes from the dishwasher, and laundry. Finally, thought-stopping was introduced as an alternative means by which Nina could respond to negative automatic thoughts about her condition that were unhelpful and low in utility value.

Homework Prescribed

Nina did not respond favorably to the idea of homework assignments. Initially, she reported that her limitations of time, energy and concentration would make it very hard for her to complete homework assignments, and she stated that she only wanted to do them if they would be of "direct benefit" to her. For this reason, the therapist relied upon a single format for homework throughout the course therapy—the activity pacing schedule. Using this schedule, Nina was assigned to complete various activities over time. First she was assigned to record her daily activities and their importance value, stress level, and fatigue levels.

As she became more comfortable with the idea of practicing the 50/50 solution, Nina began to utilize the schedule to better prioritize her activities in terms of their personal importance value, and was increasingly able to eliminate lower-priority activities, particularly at times when her fatigue levels became high. The notion that reducing stressful activities would lead to a decrease in fatigue and symptoms was treated as a possibility rather than a fact (i.e., a "hypothesis"), and Nina was encouraged to test this possibility by reducing or eliminating stressful activities for homework each week (i.e., behavioral experiments). By the fifteenth session Nina commented that she simply needed someone to "keep her honest" in her efforts to "avoid stress."

During the second course of therapy (sessions 20–40), Nina continued to use the activity schedule to maintain consistency in her practice of the 50/50 solution. At the same time, Nina was encouraged to identify "possibilities" for physical activities that she found enjoyable. By the 30th session and after trying numerous activities ranging from a graded walking schedule to anaerobic yoga, Nina had identified swimming as a physical activity that she not only found enjoyable but also found to be most effective in improving her energy levels and overall symptoms.

At this time, Nina also explored "possibilities" related to Goal 2 for homework. She used principles of self-advocacy that she wrote on flash cards to support her in setting limits on the amount of work she took on and in delegating more of the secretarial aspects of her job to the company secretaries. She recorded these attempts and their outcomes on her activity pacing schedule as if they were normal parts of her daily routine.

Difficulties Encountered

In addition to difficulties concentrating during therapy, Nina's Axis II disorder presented a number of challenges to the therapy process. Initially, she became consumed in the details of any educational content or Socratic questioning that the therapist used. She typically dwelled on issues of word usage and missed the overall objective of the therapist's communication. For example, Nina did not respond well to word "hypothesis" and to the therapist's reference to the therapeutic relationship as "collaborative empiricism" because she thought that the notion of testing out ideas and behaviors through experimentation was "manipulative and gamey." It was clear to the therapist that Nina would not be open to exploring any cognitions or core beliefs that led to this interpretation, so the therapist simply changed her word usage when discussing issues pertaining to hypothesis testing or experimentation. This was an effective strategy and Nina eventually let go of her suspicions about the process.

In addition, it was important for Nina to maintain a high level of control over the therapy process and the content of the therapy, despite the fact that she was not always able to do this very effectively because of her cognitive symptoms and fatigue. When the therapist assumed a more directive stance in reaction to her difficulties, Nina became mistrustful and often provided the therapist with negative feedback. As a result, the pace of therapy was slowed and the therapist relied heavily upon empathy. This helped to smooth the therapeutic relationship, facilitate compliance with in-session activities and homework assignments, and maintain Nina's active collaboration in the therapy process.

Use of Related Knowledge as a Supplemental Approach

As mentioned, the therapist drew heavily upon related knowledge of volition and empathy in introducing and developing a cognitive behavioral treatment plan for Nina. The therapist informally assessed Nina's volition during clinical interviews and encouraged her to define new activities (e.g., swimming) to replace former activities that she was no longer able to perform (e.g., snowmobiling). This approach allowed her to achieve a renewed sense of satisfaction with an aspect of life and a new motivation to continue to engage activities to support her health and functioning. Swimming also allowed her to build muscle strength, endurance, and ultimately support her immune functioning. During therapy, Nina also identified a new sedentary activity that she wanted to pursue, which was writing a short story. Without this emphasis on volition, the therapist's use of a cognitive behavioral approach might have been less effective with Nina because it was difficult for her to rely strictly upon her case conceptualization as the only guiding principle for treatment.

In addition to the therapist's emphasis on volition, the therapist utilized empathy frequently and liberally. Nina had several past negative interactions with health-care providers and did not trust the therapist or the therapy process, initially. For these reasons, ongoing emphasis was placed on achieving an empathic understanding of Nina's illness experience and everyday work and family interactions through the continual use of summary statements. In addition, the therapist made sure to respond to Nina's negative feedback and resistances during the therapy process by validating her responses, by seeking to understand them from an empathic perspective, and by providing corrective emotional experiences through responding more effectively to Nina's needs and preferences in future therapeutic interactions and activities. Without the use of these strategies, it is very likely that Nina would have discontinued therapy prematurely.

Treatment Outcome: Termination and Relapse Prevention

Nina's termination date was initially set for the 20th session, but because Nina felt that she needed to continue work on Goal 1 and also wanted to initiate work on Goal 2, her final termination date was set and retained as the 40th session. Though the 50/50 solution was somewhat effective in reducing fatigue and symptom levels following the first course of 20 sessions, Nina did not notice a significant change in her symptoms until she began to swim on a regular basis and reduce her work responsibilities during the later half of therapy. She reported that at this time she also noticed a significant change in her mood and in her emotional reactions to her CFS symptoms. Nina also reported that she received feedback from both her husband and her daughter that she was "easier to live with" after having attended therapy. Figure 4 is an example of one of Nina's final activity pacing schedules.

As evident from her entries, Nina learned how to reduce higher-stress, lower-priority activities by 50 percent on days when her fatigue levels were high (e.g., Friday). This typically resulted in a lower fatigue level the following day. In addition, Nina learned to delegate more of her household responsibilities to her housekeeper, relieving her husband and daughter of some of the burden and allowing Nina to pursue swimming at the local health club (e.g., Saturday and Sunday).

In order to maintain a temporal structure to the therapy process, the therapist suggested that they periodically rate Nina's level of goal attainment every 10 sessions. By the 40th session, Nina reported that she felt she had accomplished both of her goals. Though she continued to experience significant levels of physical and cognitive impairment resulting from chronic fatigue syndrome, she reported that she had a new sense of control over the severity of her fatigue and symptoms, felt she could prevent severe relapses more than half of the time, and thought she was becoming stronger physically. Nina also reported that she had not had a herpes virus outbreak since the beginning of therapy.

At the 30th session, one of the in-session activities included constructing a plan for relapse prevention. This involved keeping a supply of activity pacing schedules at hand and utilizing them whenever her fatigue and symptoms increased, and continuing to swim and find other nonstressful activities, such as writing, that she found enjoyable. Nina was also invited to return to therapy should she ever need a booster session or another course of treatment.

Learning from Nina: Unique Features of Individuals with Fatigue

Like many individuals with invisible chronic illnesses involving severe fatigue, Nina had a history of negative interactions with health care providers characterized by invalidation, rejection, and misunderstanding. In many cases, her fatigue was not taken seriously or was attributed to psychological variables. In addition, she struggled with energy limitations and difficulties concentrating, and these symptoms influenced the pacing of the therapy process. Finally, Nina and her therapist struggled to determine the degree to which her beliefs about her illness were realistic and the degree to which she was able to control and manage her symptoms. The unpredictability and variability in her fatigue levels over time was confusing to both Nina and her therapist, and this added a unique level of complexity to the treatment process. In summary, there are three unique considerations to bear in mind when conducting cognitive behavioral therapy with individuals with fatigue:

Date Day	Activities Planned (numbered in order of priority) Also list unplanned activities that you did at the end of your list	Importance to you	Importance to others	Stress	Activity completed?	Fatigue level for the day
	Remember the 50/50 solution	(low = 1----------10 = high)			Yes / No	low 1---10 high
May 10 Friday	1. Get ready for work	5	9	2	Yes	9
	2. Drive to see client	10	10	8	Yes	
	3. Lunch with client	10	10	5	Yes	
	4. Drive home	10	5	7	Yes	
	5. Prepare dinner	4	10	5	No	
	6. Eat dinner with family	10	10	1	Yes	
	7. Watch movie at home	5	5	1	No	
	8. Purchase housewarming gift online	2	8	4	No	
	9. Pay bills	2	10	10	No	
	Husband prepared dinner					
May 11 Saturday	1. Get ready for the day	5	1	2	Yes	6
	2. Purchase housewarming gift online	2	8	4	Yes	
	3. Grocery shopping	3	5	5	Yes	
	4. Drive daughter to slumber party	2	10	8	Yes	
	5. Prepare dinner	4	10	5	No	
	6. Eat dinner with partner	10	10	1	Yes	
	7. Work on short story	10	1	4	No	
	Housekeeper came	10	5	1	Yes	
	Husband prepared dinner	10	5	1	Yes	
	Went swimming at club	10	1	1	Yes	

FIGURE 4. Nina's Final Activity Pacing Schedule

May 12, Sunday					5
1. Get ready for the day	1	5	2	Yes	
2. Furniture shopping	10	8	4	Yes	
3. Get lunch while shopping	5	5	1	Yes	
4. Pay bills	10	1	10	Yes	
5. Order pizza for delivery	10	10	1	Yes	
6. Help daughter with homework					
Went swimming at club	10	10	8	No	
Husband's turn to help daughter with homework	10	1	1	Yes	

FIGURE 4. *Continued*

- Individuals with fatigue will have energy limitations that affect their physical and cognitive functioning. These limitations will inevitably affect their ability to participate in certain therapy activities and will slow the overall pace of the therapy process.
- Individuals with fatigue and their therapists will be confused and frustrated by the unpredictability and wide variability of the severity of a fatigue at any given time.
- Because fatigue is an invisible condition that has not been given much credibility with the medical profession, individuals may feel embarrassed by or ashamed of their fatigue. If they have a history of interactions with health-care providers that have been characterized by misunderstanding and invalidation, the internalization of this public stigma may be particularly intense.

Appendix

Fatigue assessments developed by the author.

Fatigue cognitions scale

Please answer "true" or "false" to the following statements.

1. I cannot predict when my fatigue will occur.
2. No one cares about my fatigue.
3. My doctor does not know how to treat my fatigue.
4. My fatigue makes me less attractive to others.
5. My fatigue never goes away.
6. No one understands my fatigue.
7. I cannot keep my mind off my fatigue.
8. My fatigue will never improve.
9. My doctor does not care about my fatigue.
10. My fatigue renders me useless at work.
11. My fatigue causes social/interpersonal difficulties.
12. I can no longer live with my fatigue.
13. People think my fatigue is "all in my head".
14. My fatigue has made me an ineffective parent.
15. People think I exaggerate my fatigue.
16. I cannot control my fatigue.
17. I am looking for a complete cure for my fatigue.
18. My fatigue has changed my personality.
19. I feel I have failed in life because of my fatigue.
20. I cannot do anything without feeling fatigued.
21. At times my fatigue makes me want to die.
22. I cannot cope with my fatigue.
23. My fatigue has changed who I am as a person.

Activity Record

Date Day	Activities planned (numbered in order of priority) Also list unplanned activities that you did at the end of your list Remember the 50/50 solution	Importance to you	Importance to others	Stress (low = 1——10 = high)	Activity completed? Yes/No	Fatigue level for the day (low 1—10 high)
Day 1						
Day 2						
Day 3						
Day 4						
Day 5						
Day 6						
Day 7						

16

Pain: Subtypes, Prevalence, and Associated Conditions

Pain is a pervasive and usually negative human experience that has been defined and described in numerous ways throughout history. Within the U.S., pain is the most common reason for seeking medical care and the leading cause of decreased productivity among workers (Hadjistavropoulos and Craig 2004; Stucky, Gold and Zhang 2001). Chronic pain, or pain that continues beyond the expected time-frame or long after an injury has healed, is a highly prevalent and often enduring symptom of a number of chronic conditions. It has been reported by approximately 75 to 80 million people within the U.S. (Tollison 1993), and it has been estimated that approximately 45 percent of people will experience chronic pain at some point during their lives.

Despite its significance as a medical complaint and its enduring impact on quality of life and functioning, unrelieved pain has been a relatively neglected area within medical care. In 2003, the National Pain Care Policy Act was introduced in Congress to address the need to prioritize pain care treatment, education, and research within federally funded health-care programs and facilities. If passed, this bill would facilitate increased patient access to important pain care services throughout the United States.

This chapter will define pain, describe the various types and subclassifications of pain, and provide a basic overview of existing theories of pain. In addition, it will describe the nature and prevalence of pain in common chronic conditions that involve pain. It should be noted that this chapter is not intended to provide an exhaustive, systematic, or detailed review of the epidemiology and characteristics of pain for each condition covered. Rather, basic information about a number of pain-related conditions and general guidelines and information about the role of pain in each of these conditions is provided. When working with clients with conditions that involve chronic pain and/or acute pain resulting from medical procedures, therapists will need to seek out additional information about the role of pain in that specific condition or medical procedure from collaborating physicians and research-related resources.

What Is Pain?

The most basic definition of pain is a sensation that can range from mild discomfort that is limited to a specific area to more generalized and severe sensations of distress and agony. Pain comprises both physical and psychological components. The physical aspect of pain results from the stimulation of specialized nerve endings. When pain results from nerve stimulation, it can signal actual or potential harm to the body. However, pain as a psychological phenomenon can exist even in the absence of actual harm or threat of actual harm to the body.

Recent advances in the understanding of pain as a biopsychosocial phenomenon are consistent with definitions that emphasize the complex interactions between the psychological and sociocultural aspects of pain as well as the sensory, physiological, and anatomical aspects (Asmundson and Wright 2004). The psychological aspects of this conceptualization are often most pertinent in psychotherapeutic interventions. Research in cognitive psychology has examined the role of pain as it relates to cognition. For example, Turk, Michenbaum, and Genest (1993) describe pain as a subjective experience involving one's senses, emotions, beliefs, and behaviors. Melzack and Casey (1968) define pain as a predominantly perceptual phenomenon that involves conscious awareness, ascribed meaning, cognitive appraisal, selective abstraction, and learning. These definitions are particularly relevant to the interpretation of pain from the standpoint of cognitive behavioral therapy. Cognitive behavioral therapy places value not only on clients' subjective reports of their experience but also on their beliefs and interpretations of that experience and the resulting behavioral and emotional consequences.

Common Descriptions of Pain

Though common pathophysiological features of certain conditions tend produce similar experiences and descriptions of pain across clients, each individual's experience of pain is nonetheless unique to some extent. When using cognitive behavioral therapy with individuals with pain-related conditions, it is important to ask clients to describe their pain in detail. In doing so, some therapists may wish to use certain structured assessments, visual analog scales, and pain diaries, such as those presented in Chapter 17.

Asking patients to describe their pain facilitates understanding, situates clients and their therapists to develop more appropriate cognitive behavioral interventions, and may facilitate an increased sense of control among clients. Pain has been described in multiple ways. The following are common adjectives often used to describe pain:

- Aching
- Biting (gnawing)

- Boring (drilling, lancinating, penetrating, pricking, stabbing, or piercing)
- Burning (also described as hot, searing, or scalding)
- Cold (also described as cool or freezing)
- Cramping
- Crushing, pressing/pressure, or squeezing
- Dull
- Nagging
- Numb (also described as "pins and needles," itching, scratching, or tingling)
- Pinching
- Pulling (tugging or wrenching)
- Radiating (spreading)
- Sharp (cutting, lacerating, tearing, splitting)
- Shooting (also described as darting, fulgurant, jumping, flashing, or lightning)
- Sore
- Stinging
- Tender
- Throbbing (pulsing, beating, pounding, quivering, flickering)
- Tight
- Wandering (traveling)

Individual and Cross-Cultural Differences

Pain is a highly individualized experience and also exists within a sociocultural context. It is experienced and expressed differently depending upon one's sex, age, and ethnocultural identification (Rollman 2004). These differences are also a function of the condition under study and its course and progression across the life span. For example, musculoskeletal pain is more commonly reported by women than men and tends to increase with age (LeReshe 1999). Abdominal pain is more prevalent in women than in men but does not increase with age (LeReshe 1999). Headaches are also more common in women than in men. Chronic back pain, which tends to occur more frequently in men, is the only extensively documented exception to this trend (Hadjistavropoulos and Craig 2004).

Lipton and Marbach (1984) introduced a model that summarized ethnocultural differences in pain according to three dimensions:

- The way physical experience is communicated to others (intensity, quality, location, and duration);
- The behavioral reaction to pain (cognitive interpretation, or the way pain is perceived and evaluated, emotional response of fear, anxiety, depression, or anger, including whether pain is expressed openly or covertly, and function, or how the pain effects social interaction and daily activities); and
- Response to medical intervention, or the extent to which an individual is compliant and trusting versus challenging and uncooperative.

Because the cross-cultural research on reactions of specific ethnic and cultural groups to pain is contradictory and limited by methodological flaws, it is now considered premature to make any broad statements about how a member of one cultural group might respond to pain as compared to another (Rollman 2004). It is also important for clinicians and researchers not to place value-judgments on one individual's reaction to pain (e.g., expressive and combative) as compared to another's (e.g., stoical and cooperative).

Classifying Pain

Pain can be subclassified in terms of the following dimensions:

- Duration (acute versus chronic)
- Frequency (transient, intermittent, or constant)
- Hypothesized cause (nociceptive, neuropathic, combined-type, idiopathic, or psychogenic)
- Phantom limb pain: pain or other sensations felt as if they are occurring in a limb that has been amputated.
- Perceived severity (mild to severe)
- Functional consequences (mildly disabling to severely disabling)

The following section outlines the heterogeneous aspects of pain in terms of each of these dimensions.

Duration: Acute versus Chronic

Acute pain is generally defined as pain that lasts less than three-to-six months and is directly related to injury or nerve stimulation resulting from some other pathology or damage to the body. Chronic pain is defined as pain that continues well after an injury has healed or beyond the time frame in which an individual would otherwise expect pain to occur. Characteristically, chronic pain is often the result of a wide range of converging variables. It may be caused by a single injury or by a series of injuries. Certain invasive medical procedures may also lead to chronic pain. Coexisting chronic illness or other sources of physiological pathology that can make the body and brain vulnerable to pain can also play significant roles in the experience of chronic pain. Stress and other psychological problems can have a marked impact on a client's experience of pain.

Individuals with chronic pain are more likely to demonstrate coexisting psychological problems, such as depression, anxiety, somatization, posttraumatic stress disorder, and anger (Banks and Kerns 1996; Gaskin, et al. 1992; Miller, 1993). Estimates of Axis I psychiatric comorbidity among individuals with chronic pain range from 30 to 100 percent (Turk, Rudy, and Steig 1987). In addition, the prevalence of personality disorders among individuals with chronic pain is also high. One study found that between 31 percent and 51 percent of clients with chronic pain were diagnosed with at least one personality disorder (Weisberg and Keefe 1999).

Frequency: Transient, Intermittent, or Constant:

Pain can be described as transient or brief—lasting only seconds or minutes. It can also occur intermittently with or without a specific trigger, rhythm, or pattern. Pain that is continuous never relents and may or may not vary in terms of severity. The frequency with which a client experiences pain and the degree to which this frequency varies will play a significant role in planning an appropriate cognitive behavioral therapy intervention.

Hypothesized Cause

The causes of pain are multifactorial and complex. They include nociceptive, neuropathic, mixed, psychogenic, or unknown causes. A number of theories have been developed to explain pain. The most frequently cited models include the gate control theory of pain (Melzack and Wall 1965), neuromatrix theory (Melzack 1999; Melzack and Katz 2004), the operant model (Fordyce 1976), the Glasgow model (Waddell 1987, 1991, 1992), the biobehavioral model (Turk and Flor 1999; Turk 2002), fear-avoidance models (Asmundson et al., 1999; Vlaeyen and Linton 2000) and diathesis-stress models (Asmundson and Wright 2004).

To varying degrees, all of these models emphasize the roles of cognitive, emotional, and/or behavioral contributors to pain. Because a full review of each of these models is beyond the scope of this book, the hypothesized causes of pain will be discussed in terms of the broad categories of nociceptive, neuropathic, mixed, psychogenic, or unexplained causes of pain. Each of these will be summarized below.

Nociceptive pain

Nociceptive pain involves nerve stimulation, or activation of specialized pain receptors in the spinal cord and brain (nociceptors) that signal the brain that an injury has occurred (Hadjistavropoulos and Craig 2004). Nociceptive pain most commonly results from an injury or pathology within the musculoskeletal system. Some examples of nociceptive pain include arthritis pain, bone breaks, burns, dislocations, injury to an internal organ, pulled muscles, torn ligaments, or wounds. Nociceptive pain, in itself, does not involve nerve damage or permanent changes in the central nervous system. As such, it usually ceases to exist once the injury has healed (Winterowd, Beck, and Gruener 2003).

Neuropathic pain

Neuropathic pain is defined as pain that results from actual damage to the nerves or other nerve dysfunction. Neuropathic pain often involves changes within the peripheral (nerves leading to the spinal cord) and central (brain and spinal cord) nervous systems that become permanent over time. Damage to the central nervous system is often referred to as "central pain." In its advanced stages, neuropathic pain can involve significant sensory changes, such as allodynia (pain produced by light touch, the feel of the wind, clothing against the skin, or some other trigger that would not produce pain in most people), hyperalgesia (increased sensitivity to a painful stimulus), and hyperpathia (an abnormally painful reaction to a painful stimulus and a lowered pain threshold). Neuropathic pain is difficult to diagnose and often missed because it is not typically detectible using standard diagnostic approaches, such as X ray or magnetic resonance imaging (MRI). Examples of neuropathic pain include: AIDS-related neuropathy, diabetic neuropathy, complex regional pain syndrome (a chronic pain condition resulting from an injury to the bone or soft tissue), and postherpetic neuralgia (a chronic pain condition resulting from shingles) (Winterowd, Beck, and Gruener 2003).

Mixed pain

Mixed pain involves a combination of nociceptive and neuropathic pain (Winterowd, Beck, and Gruener, 2003). It typically involves an injury to the musculoskeletal system that also results in irreversible nerve damage.

Psychogenic pain

Psychogenic pain is pain that occurs in the absence of evidence of injury or other pathology and results solely from psychological variables. Though psychological variables play a role in pain regardless of its cause, purely psychogenic pain is rare (Winterowd, Beck, and Gruener 2003). When it does occur, it often manifests itself in terms of a conversion disorder.

Unexplained pain

Unexplained pain is not linked to any tangible musculoskeletal or nerve damage and is not purely attributable to psychological causes. Some individuals with unexplained pain may have undiagnosed neuropathic pain (Winterowd, Beck, and Gruener 2003).

Although the most widely accepted modern theories of pain emphasize its biopsychosocial nature, clients will nonetheless differ widely within that biopsychosocial framework in terms of the degree to which their pain is linked to an identifiable source of injury or pathology. For this reason, it is imperative that therapists gather as much information as possible about the client's particular illness or impairment and the extent to which psychological variables are expected to play a role in the experience of pain within that condition. Knowledge of the degree to which a client is able to link his or her experience of pain to specific physical, cognitive, emotional, or behavioral triggers can provide useful information about the timing and approach required when introducing the cognitive model as the basis for cognitive behavioral therapy. Clients that are not able to link their experiences of pain to a specific trigger, cognition, or behavioral and emotional consequence will require greater reliance on the supplemental approaches to cognitive behavioral therapy introduced in this book. These include a greater degree of empathic understanding and summary statements, a greater emphasis on directing the cognitive behavioral therapy toward identifying strengths and instilling hope, and a more concerted effort to understand the client's volition from a practical, occupational perspective. Only after the client and therapist have established sufficient trust and rapport will the client be able to approach his or her experience of pain with understanding of the roles of cognition, behavior, and emotion.

Severity: Mild to Severe

When determining whether to address pain as a focal problem for cognitive behavioral therapy, a central issue to consider is the client's perception of the severity of the pain. If pain is identified as a focal problem, pain severity can then be assessed at key points during the course of therapy as a means of providing feedback to the therapist and the client about the extent to which the therapy is effective in reducing the pain.

Functional Consequences: Mildly Disabling to Severely Disabling

A second important issue to consider when assessing the degree to which pain presents a problem for a client is the extent to which the pain interferes with the client's ability to perform activities of daily living and other occupations. Gathering information on the extent of impairment resulting from pain as it compares or contrasts with a client's perception and report of the severity of the pain will also shed light on whether a client might be overfunctioning or underfunctioning.

Pain and Chronic Conditions

This section will provide a general overview of the prevalence and nature of pain in some of the more common chronic illnesses and impairments. It should be noted that many other chronic illnesses and impairments involve or result in pain. The conditions that will be covered in this review were selected because they are among the more prevalent conditions that involve pain as a primary symptom. They include:

- Arthritis (rheumatoid, osteoarthritis)
- Cancer and cancer treatments
- Central pain syndrome
- Crohn's disease
- Complex regional pain syndrome (reflex sympathetic dystrophy)
- Cystic fibrosis
- Diabetes
- Endometriosis/pelvic pain
- Fibromyalgia

- HIV/AIDS
- Lower back pain
- Lupus
- Head injury
- Multiple sclerosis
- Peripheral neuropathy
- Phantom pain
- Renal (kidney) disease
- Sjogren's syndrome
- Spinal cord injury
- Stroke

Arthritis (Rheumatoid, Osteoarthritis)

Various forms of arthritis exist. The two most common forms of arthritis are osteoarthritis and rheumatoid arthritis. A basic description of rheumatoid arthritis was provided in Chapter 14. Rheumatoid arthritis activates the inflammatory immune response in joints and leads to joint tissue damage. Nearly 70 percent of adults with rheumatoid arthritis experience pain on a daily basis. Pain is characterized by general soreness, stiffness, and aching. Joint pain and swelling often occurs in multiple joints, and joints are typically affected bilaterally. Early in the disease, pain is first experienced in the hands and feet.

Osteoarthritis is a degenerative joint disease characterized by pain and loss of mobility, particularly in the weight-bearing joints of the body, such as the vertebrae, knees and hips. It can also occur in the hands and feet. Pain and swelling is often felt in the joints and is accompanied by stiffness and loss of mobility. Pain is usually worsened with exercise and alleviated with rest. Pain arises from a change in the health of the joint tissue (e.g., breakdown of cartilage and deterioration of joint fluid). The change may be idiopathic or may arise as a result of secondary causes, including genetic vulnerabilities, joint overuse, or trauma. Among the subtypes of osteoarthritis, rapidly destructive osteoarthritis typically affects the shoulders, hips, and knees. Osteoarthritis is the most common joint disease and the leading cause of pain and impairment among the aging population, with more than 80 percent of individuals over the age of 70 demonstrating musculoskeletal changes indicative of osteoarthritis.

Cancer and Cancer Treatments

A basic overview of cancer and some of its treatments was provided in Chapter 14. Pain is a common symptom of various forms of cancer. In a sample of individuals newly diagnosed with cancer in Taiwan, with no history of recent surgery or cancer treatments, 38 percent reported having cancer-related pain

(Ger et al., 1998). Similar studies of inpatients and outpatients with cancer estimate pain to occur in between 57 percent and 80 percent of individuals (Beck and Falkson 2001; Chang et al., 2000; Wells 2000). One study of inpatients with cancer in South Africa found that 57 percent of individuals reported pain seven days a week and 24 percent reported pain 24 hours per day (Beck and Falkson, 2001). The most common causes of pain in cancer are tumor growth, bone metastasis, postsurgical pain, pain resulting from radiation treatment, and postchemotherapy neuropathy.

Tumor growth

Tumor growth can lead to pressure on pain receptors in different parts throughout the body, including the periosteum of the bone or the capsule around the liver, for example. Tumors can also interrupt blood flow, infiltrate or put pressure on the nerves, and block hollow organs of the body (e.g., intestines), causing pain. Tumor pain varies according to the location of the tumor and the types of pain receptors that are involved. Tumors closest to neural structures tend to cause the most severe pain.

Bone metastasis

The most common form of cancer-related pain results from the metastasis of tumors to the bone. As they grow, bone tumors compress healthy bone tissue, deposit abnormal bone tissue, and cause pathological fractures. Pain occurs when tumors push on bone tissue, nerves, or other organs (Diel, Solomayer, and Bastert 2000). Symptoms of bone pain include swelling, bruising, tenderness, joint pain, stiffness, decreased joint mobility, and aching or sharp pain that can be constant or intermittent. Approximately 60 to 80 percent of individuals with bone metastasis experience severe pain.

Postsurgical pain

Pain is expected to follow any surgery due to the tissue damage surgery causes. However, in some instances chronic pain can result from complications of surgery aimed at removing cancerous tissue. Depending on the site of the surgery and the extent of nerve damage, some individuals may develop a complex regional pain syndrome as a complication. Post-mastectomy pain syndrome is one example of a postsurgical chronic pain syndrome that involves neuropathic pain (Blunt and Schmiedel 2004). Postmastectomy pain is often described as long-lasting, continuous pain in the axilla, medial upper arm, and lateral chest wall starting shortly after surgery. The pain is often described as piercing pain against a background of burning, aching, and tightening sensations. This type of chronic arm pain has been reported by 65 percent of women in the year following surgery (Maunsell, Brisson, and Deschenes 1993) and by 31 percent of women for up to five years following surgery (Tengrup et al. 2000).

Postradiation therapy pain

Because radiation therapy is a local treatment, irritation and pain resulting from radiation therapy is usually limited to the skin and the area being treated. Effects can begin within a few days of treatment and can last for several weeks after treatment. General effects can include skin redness, irritation, and a sunburned sensation. Radiation to the head, neck, or chest can cause difficulty or soreness when swallowing, irritation in the mouth, dry mouth, changes in taste, and nausea. Radiation to the pelvic region can cause localized pain and digestive symptoms.

Chemotherapy-induced neuropathy

This condition occurs because the mechanism of action of most chemotherapy treatments causes the peripheral nerves to be vulnerable to chronic nerve compression (Dellon et al., 2004). Over 60 percent of individuals that receive chemotherapy for breast, lung, and colon cancer report symptoms of neuropathic pain (Rinat Neuroscience 2004). Peripheral pain and paresthesia may be accompanied by sensory changes and losses in motor functioning.

Central Pain Syndrome

Central pain syndrome occurs as a result of injury or damage to the central nervous system. This damage can be caused by stroke, multiple sclerosis, tumors, epilepsy, brain injury, spinal cord injury, or Parkinson's disease. Central pain is experienced by up to 8 percent of stroke survivors and by up to 30 percent of individuals with spinal cord injury (Schwartzman et al., 2001). Central pain can affect a large portion of the body or a discrete area. The pain may be constant and can worsen with touch, movement, emotions, and temperature changes. It is most commonly felt as a burning pain but it can also be experienced as sensations of "pins and needles," pressing, sharp, or aching pain.

Crohn's Disease

Crohn's disease is discussed more fully in Chapter 20. Pain can be attributable to a number of causes in Crohn's disease, but the most common causes of pain are intestinal obstruction and inflammation. Abdominal pain is generally localized and most likely to occur in the right lower quadrant of the abdomen. In a sample of 105 individuals with Crohn's disease, 91 percent presented with pain in the right lower quadrant of the abdomen upon admission to the hospital (Ozdil et al., 2003). In addition, ulcers that tunnel through tissues surrounding the intestines (fistulas) can develop, become infected, and cause pain.

In addition to abdominal pain, a number of other painful extra-intestinal complications from Crohn's disease can occur. These can involve the skin, eyes, joints, and kidneys. Painful raised spots, referred to as erythema nodosum, can develop on a client's legs, and an ulcerating skin condition (pyoderma gangrenosum) may occur near the ankles. An individual's eyes may be affected by uveitis or episcleritis (pain due to inflammation of tissues within the eye). Lower back pain and pain in various joints may result from arthritis (e.g., sacroiliac joint arthritis) or from a degenerative spinal condition referred to as ankylosing spondylitis (Marks and Kam 2002). One study found that 52 percent of individuals with Crohn's disease reported lower back pain, and 45 percent of those had evidence of sacroiliac joint arthritis (Steer et al., 2003). Kidney stones may also be more likely to develop in individuals with Crohn's disease. In addition to these potential complications, side effects of some medications used to treat Crohn's disease may be painful and include heartburn and headache.

Complex Regional Pain Syndrome (Reflex Sympathetic Dystrophy)

There are two subtypes of complex regional pain syndrome (CRPS). CRPS type 1 (or Reflex Sympathetic Dystrophy) is a chronic pain state with onset due to soft tissue injury or bone injury. CRPS type 2 is a chronic pain state with onset due to nerve injury. CRPS type 1 has been estimated to occur in 21 people per 100,000 and CRPS type 2 has been estimated to occur in 4 people per 100,000 (Sandroni et al., 2003). In addition to chronic pain, which is experienced by individuals with both subtypes of CRPS, CRPS type 2 pain is also associated with autonomic changes such as sweating, trophic changes (e.g., skin atrophy), hair loss, and joint contractures. Injury in both subtypes can result from a surgery, car accident, or other injury to the body.

Cystic Fibrosis

Cystic fibrosis is an inherited disease of the exocrine glands that causes secretion of abnormal mucus in the lungs and problems with breathing, pancreatic function, and food absorption. Due to recent advances in medical treatments, the life expectancy for individuals with cystic fibrosis is increasing. Chronic pain is a major symptom of cystic fibrosis and is expected to increase with age. One study of a pediatric sample reported the following rates of pain: headache (55 percent), chest pain (65 percent), back pain (94 percent), abdominal pain (19 percent), and joint/limb pain (16 percent) (Parasa and Maffulli 1999; Ravilly et al., 1996). Chronic abdominal pain in cystic fibrosis can be caused by a range of sources, including periappendiceal abscess, pancreatitis, and gastroesophageal reflux. These gastrointestinal symptoms can all occur as a result of involvement of the exocrine glands in the disease. Joint pain, which is another common symptom of cystic fibrosis, may be attributable to decreased bone mineral content and bone density.

Diabetic Neuropathy

A general description of diabetes was provided in Chapter 14. Up to 25 percent of individuals with diabetes report chronic pain. The most common reason for this pain involves damage to the peripheral nerves, which can cause various forms of diabetic neuropathy (Loftus 2004). Diabetic neuropathy is often experienced as a pattern of ascending nerve damage. In diabetic neuropathy and polyneuropathy, pain is typically first experienced in the feet and can travel up the legs. Diabetic amyotrophy involves pain in the upper leg and back. This usually occurs in individuals whose diabetes has been poorly controlled. Diabetic thoracic neuralgia involves chest or abdominal pain that is due to damage to a peripheral nerve from the thoracic spine.

Endometriosis

Endometriosis is defined as an abnormal growth of endometrial cells, which typically form within the uterus and are shed with menstruation. In endometriosis, endometrial cells grow outside of the uterus and attach themselves to other tissues and organs such as the ovaries, other surfaces on the uterus, the intestines, the fallopian tubes, and the surface lining of the pelvic cavity. The attached tissue is typically referred to as an endometrial implant. Endometriosis affects approximately 3 percent to 18 percent of women within the U.S. and is the leading cause of pelvic pain, laparoscopic surgery, and hysterectomy. Approximately 85 percent of women with endometriosis experience pain in the pelvic region. Pelvic pain typically begins before or during menstruation and decreases following menstruation. Pain intensity can vary from month to month. Some women with endometriosis experience pain and cramping during intercourse, pain with bowel movements, and pain with urination. Pain can depend, in part, on the extent to which endometrial tissue has attached itself to certain organs and the proximity of this endometrial tissue to nerve tissues. Endometrial implants can also produce substances that circulate in the bloodstream and cause pain. Pain can also result from scarring that occurs as a result of endometrial implants.

Fibromyalgia

An overview of fibromyalgia was provided in Chapter 14. Chronic, unexplained, widespread pain is the defining symptom of fibromyalgia. It occurs in 100 percent of individuals with this condition. To receive a diagnosis of fibromyalgia, the pain must occur in all four quadrants of the body for at least three months (American College of Rheumatology 2003). Fibromyalgia pain is characterized by widespread aching in the muscles and soft tissues, pain when pressure is put on specific tender points, and pain that is usually felt in the neck, shoulders, upper back, elbows, lower back, and hip girdle (American College of Rheumatology 2003).

Head injury

The most commonly described type of pain associated with traumatic brain injury is headache (Rees 2003). Depending on the severity of the head injury, headaches can vary in terms of frequency and severity. One study found that 23 percent of individuals with chronic daily headaches had a history of head trauma (Bekkelund and Salvesen 2002). Another potential complication of head injury is rigid body posture that can lead to painful contractures.

HIV/AIDS

HIV/AIDS was already described in Chapter 14. Pain is a common symptom of HIV and AIDS. The prevalence of pain during infection with HIV or AIDS has been estimated to range from 30 percent to 80 percent (Larue, Fontaine, and Colleau 1997). Larue and colleagues (1997) found that pain related to HIV/AIDS was consistently underestimated and undertreated by providers. Pain in HIV/AIDS can result from opportunistic infections, cancer, and anti-HIV medications that can all cause peripheral neuropathy (O'Neill and Sherrard 1993). Peripheral neuropathy (described in more detail in this section) is a common cause of debilitating pain in HIV/AIDS. More than one-third of individuals with HIV/AIDS have peripheral neuropathy, which first involves burning pain, tingling, or numbness in the feet and hands that results from nerve damage. As it progresses and in the absence of treatment, peripheral neuropathy can involve sharp, shooting pains or severe, continuous burning pain.

Lower Back Pain

Chronic lower back pain is diagnosed when pain persists beyond 12 weeks. There are many potential causes of chronic lower back pain, the most common being disc protrusion and disk herniation. In cases where the extent of protrusion and herniation do not correlate with clinical symptoms and when diagnostic workup yields no structural cause, psychological and social variables are more likely to be considered (Wheeler, Stubbart, and Hicks, 2004). Chronic lower back pain may also result from complications resulting from back surgery, including nerve damage. Before initiating cognitive behavioral therapy, all potential causes of the pain should be ruled out and clarified so that both the client and the therapist are aware of the extent to which psychological and behavioral variables should be emphasized.

Chronic lower back pain can be sudden and sharp or may be experienced as a dull ache. It may be localized or may radiate or cover a broad area (Gallagher et al., 2003). Pain is usually experienced while standing or sitting for prolonged periods of time, or when performing activities with arms extended away from the body (e.g., vacuuming) (Wheeler, Stubbart, and Hicks, 2004). Chronic lower back pain is reported by 56 percent of people that experience pain (Education Development Center, 2000). Of those who report chronic lower back pain, 11.7 million are impaired by it and for 2.6 million this impairment is permanent (Education Development Center 2000).

Lupus

An overview of systemic lupus erythematosus (lupus) was provided in Chapter 14. Over 90 percent of individuals with lupus report joint and/or muscle pain at some time during the course of their illness. Joint pain, which occurs in more than half of individuals with lupus, is often the most frequent presenting symptom at the time of illness onset (Quismorio 2001). Joint pain in lupus is primarily caused by inflammation of the joints (arthritis). This pain is experienced with swelling, tenderness, and a feeling of warmth and fluid collection around the joints (Quismorio 2001).

Multiple Sclerosis

Basic aspects of multiple sclerosis were described in Chapter 14. Pain occurs in an estimated 29 percent to 86 percent of individuals with multiple sclerosis (Solaro et al., 2004). Pain in multiple sclerosis is caused by the demyelination of and damage to nerve fibers. A multicenter cross-sectional study found the following causes and rates of pain in individuals with multiple sclerosis (Solaro et al., 2004):

- Trigeminal neuralgia (2 percent): Trigeminal neuralgia is described as stabbing pain in the face that feels similar to dental pain. Excruciating pain is felt in the distribution area of the trigeminal nerve, usually near the eyes, lips, nose, or ears. Pain is described as piercing or lancinating and it occurs in bouts of a few seconds to two minutes. Pain results from compression of the trigeminal nerve root and may be triggered by a sensory trigger, such as brushing the teeth. In multiple sclerosis, trigeminal neuralgia is ultimately caused by damage to the myelin sheath.
- Lhermitte's sign (9 percent): Lhermitte's sign is described as a sudden or brief, stabbing, electric-shock-like sensation that runs from the back of the head down the spine. It is felt when flexing the neck forward and is caused by demyelination.
- Dysesthetic pain (18.1 percent): Dysesthetic pain is described as spontaneous burning, aching, and lancinating pain that is sometimes described as "girdling" around the body. It is neurological in origin.
- Musculoskeletal pain (16.4 percent): There are many potential causes for this pain, including spasticity and pressure due to lack of mobility, muscular weakness, and imbalance. Musculoskeletal pain is most often felt in the back, arms, hips, and legs. Back pain can be exacerbated with improper seating or incorrect posture while walking.
- Painful tonic spasms (11 percent) Spasticity in multiple sclerosis can lead to muscle spasms and cramps as well as aching joints. Leg spasms often occur during sleep.

Peripheral Neuropathy

More than 100 types of peripheral neuropathy have been identified. Peripheral neuropathy describes a wide range of pain syndromes that can result from damage to the large network of nerves outside of the brain and spinal cord that send communications from all other parts of the body into the brain and spinal cord.

Neuropathy that involves damage to only one nerve is referred to as "mononeuropathy" and neuropathy that affects multiple nerves in multiple locations within the body is referred to as "polyneuropathy." When two or more isolated nerves are affected in separate areas of the body, the condition is referred to as "mononeuritis multiplex."

Peripheral neuropathy has numerous potential causes. Some of these explanations include:

- Physical injury and repetitive stress
- Systemic diseases
- Infections
- Tumors (benign and malignant)
- Genetically inherited nerve disease

Physical injury can result in direct damage to nerves. Auto accidents, falls, penetrating wounds, contusions, and bone fractures and dislocations can sever, crush, compress, or stretch nerves. Repetitive stress injuries, superficial nerve pressure (e.g., use of crutches), or remaining in one position for too long can lead to compression and entrapment neuropathies. One example of an entrapment neuropathy is carpal tunnel syndrome.

Systemic diseases that affect multiple organs within the body can cause damage to nerve tissue. These include metabolic and endocrine diseases, such as diabetes, kidney disease, thyroid disease, alcohol-related vitamin deficiencies, vascular and blood diseases, connective tissue disorders and chronic inflammation. In these diseases, nerve damage can result from impairment in the body's ability to metabolize key nutrients, process wastes, or generate healthy tissues. Autoimmune diseases, including lupus, multiple sclerosis, and rheumatoid arthritis can also cause peripheral neuropathies. In these conditions cells within the immune system can attack the myelin sheath or axons of nerves. In addition, chronic inflammation that occurs within a wide range of autoimmune disorders can cause damage to sensory and motor nerves.

Viral and bacterial agents can directly attack nerve tissues and, in some cases, can attack nerves within both the peripheral and central nervous systems. Some of the viruses known to attack nerve tissues include: Epstein-Barr virus (one member of the human herpesvirus family responsible for mononucleosis), cytomegalovirus (another member of the human herpesvirus family that can cause mononucleosis), herpes varicella-zoster (the virus responsible for shingles), and herpes simplex viruses. These viruses can cause damage to sensory nerves, leading to sharp and shooting pains. Postherpetic neuralgia is a common pain syndrome that results from peripheral nerve damage caused by shingles (herpes zoster). Shingles affects 800,000 individuals in the United States annually. Posttherpetic pain three months following onset of the shingles rash affects 25 percent to 50 percent of those with shingles over the age of 50. The HIV virus can directly attack nerves within the central and peripheral nervous systems. Certain bacterial agents, such as Lyme disease, diphtheria, and leprosy can cause extensive damage to peripheral nerves.

Inflammation related to these infections can also serve as an indirect cause of nerve damage.

As discussed earlier in this section, benign and malignant tumors can infiltrate, damage, or compress nerves. Peripheral neuropathy can also be inherited in the form of nerve diseases that affect the myelin sheath. Because each peripheral nerve in the body serves a unique function within a particular region of the body, sensations and pain associated with peripheral neuropathy can take on many forms and can range in terms of severity and functional impact. Sensations can include numbness, tingling and pricking sensations, sensitivity to touch, and muscle weakness. In its advanced stages, sensations can include burning pain (particularly at night), paralysis and muscle wasting, and organ and gland dysfunction. Sexual dysfunction occurs, and individuals may become unable to digest food easily, maintain normal blood pressure, and sweat normally. In the most severe cases, organ failure and breathing difficulties may occur.

Phantom Pain

Phantom limb pain is the most common form of phantom pain. It is generally felt as pain in an absent part of the body—typically in the place where an amputated limb once existed. As many as 51 percent of people with upper limb amputations report phantom pain, and 64 percent report that this pain is moderate to severe (Kooijman et al., 2000).

Renal (Kidney) Disease

A wide range of kidney diseases exist. Pain is a significant problem in most kidney diseases. It occurs in more than 50 percent of dialysis patients and often stems from multiple causes (Davison 2003). One study found that almost 20 percent of patients receiving dialysis had more than one cause for their pain. Musculoskeletal pain is the most common type of pain experienced, followed by severe dialysis-related headache (attributable to electrolyte changes) (Davison 2003; Goksan et al., 2004).

Kidney stones are another source of pain. Kidney stone pain can be experienced anywhere along the urinary tract and can be severe. One kidney disease commonly referenced in the literature is autosomal dominant polycystic kidney disease (which progresses to end-stage renal disease) and often involves kidney stones. In autosomal dominant polycystic kidney disease, severe and debilitating flank, back, and abdominal pain has been reported in as many as 60 percent of individuals (Badani, Hemal, and Menon 2004). In this condition, pain is caused by cyst enlargement, cyst rupture, and cyst infection. Kidney stones are another frequent cause of pain in individuals with autosomal dominant polycystic kidney disease (Bajwa et al., 2001). Individuals with end-stage renal disease often require dialysis, and as a result, individuals with autosomal dominant polycystic kidney disease also experience severe dialysis-related headaches and musculoskeletal pain.

Sjogren's Syndrome

A basic description of Sjogren's syndrome is provided in Chapter 14. In this syndrome, underlying autoimmune dysfunction causes an inflammatory response that leads to muscle pain and joint pain. Up to 44 percent of individuals with Sjogren's syndrome report muscle pain on an ongoing basis (Lindvall et al., 2002).

Spinal Cord Injury

Spinal cord injury has been described in Chapter 14. Over 65 percent of people with spinal cord injury report pain, and one-third of those rate their pain as severe (NINDS 2003). Spinal cord injury can involve mixed pain (both neurogenic and nociceptive). Neurogenic pain results from damage to nerves in the spinal cord. The nerves may become hyperexcitable and this may lead to spinal cord pain syndromes. In addition, secondary damage to the spinal cord may be responsible for such syndromes. Pain at the level of injury is hypothesized to result from damage to gray and white matter just above the injury site, whereas pain below the injury results from the interruption of axon pathways and the formation of abnormal connections within the spinal cord near the site of injury (NINDS 2003). These various forms of neurogenic pain may be felt as an intense burning or stinging sensation. In many cases, the pain is unremitting due to hypersensitivity in some parts of the body (NINDS, 2003). Musculoskeletal pain, such as shoulder pain, may be due to overuse from pushing a wheelchair and using one's arms to transfer in and out of bed and in and out of chairs (NINDS, 2003).

Stroke

A basic description of stroke is provided in Chapter 14. The most common type of pain following stroke is shoulder pain. Within two weeks after a stroke, approximately 25 percent of non-hemiplegic patients will experience shoulder pain (Gamble et al., 2000). If hemiplegia (paralysis) is involved, then shoulder pain is reported by approximately 65 percent of patients (Aras et al., 2004; Wanklyn, Forster, and Young 1996). It is hypothesized that this kind of musculoskeletal pain is caused by lack of mobility during recovery from the stroke, which can lead to limitations in joint mobility (e.g., "frozen shoulder"). Lack of mobility occurs due to the nature of the damage in the brain, rendering an individual unable to move the joint voluntarily. Frozen shoulder pain is felt when the joint is moved or while the person is lying on the shoulder.

Between 5 percent and 8 percent of individuals that have had a stroke develop central neurogenic pain that is referred to as central poststroke pain (Pain Relief Foundation 2003a). Damage to brain matter disrupts normal nerve function and causes individuals to perceive pain in the absence of painful stimuli. Central poststroke pain is often described as burning, throbbing, shooting, or stabbing. The pain is usually felt in a part of the body that has been affected by the stroke. In this area other disruptions to normal sensation are likely to occur.

Conclusion

This chapter provided an overview of the prevalence and nature of pain within the general population. It also presented common ways in which pain is subclassified and described. Information about the role of pain in a number of conditions for which pain is a prominent symptom was provided. The next chapter will present a case example of Paulette, a woman with rheumatoid arthritis. This chapter will illustrate some unique considerations of assessment and therapy with a person who has a primary symptom of pain.

17

Cognitive Behavioral Assessment and Treatment Outcomes for Chronic Pain: The Case of Paulette

Chapter 16 presented chronic pain as a major symptom category, noting its prevalence and some of its causes, and overviewed common chronic conditions that involve pain. The chapter also discussed the variegated nature of pain and how it is experienced by different people. This chapter will illustrate the application of cognitive behavioral therapy to Paulette, who was introduced in Chapter 1 and periodically discussed throughout the text.

The aim of this case presentation is twofold. First, it will synthesize the earlier examples of Paulette, discussing the case as a whole and illustrating her outcomes. Second, this chapter will illustrate unique assessment and intervention approaches that can be incorporated into cognitive behavioral therapy with people who have chronic pain. In this regard, the chapter will illustrate pain-related assessments that in the author's experience are useful for the client with chronic pain. Information on the published assessments is found in the Appendix of this chapter and copies of the assessments developed by the author are reproduced in the Appendix. It should also be noted that this chapter will illustrate cognitive behavioral strategies that are specific to the treatment of people with chronic pain. The chapter will close with an overview of the unique considerations in treating individuals with chronic pain.

As described in Chapter 1, Paulette is a 42-year-old woman with rheumatoid arthritis (RA). Paulette referred herself for cognitive behavioral therapy after reading an article about its potential utility for pain management in a magazine published by an RA self-help organization.

Initial Orientation, Approach to Assessment and Assessment Findings

Because she had prior experience in psychotherapy, Paulette was somewhat familiar with the basic process of therapy, and her expectations for therapy outcomes were realistic. She wanted to learn how to better manage her pain. Although she was unfamiliar with the specifics of cognitive behavioral therapy, she responded well to the imposed structure of therapy. Paulette was able to complete all of the steps involved in the initial orientation and assessment within the first two sessions.

The clinical interview and problem list were conducted during the first session and Paulette completed other assessments as homework that was due for the second session. With written authorization, medical records were collected from all of her health-care providers. In addition, the therapist contacted Paulette's rheumatologist by telephone, at which time she learned more about Paulette's noncompliance in taking the prescribed antirheumatic medication and the rheumatologist's threat to discontinue her corticosteroid injections if she did not take the medication.

By the end of the second session, the following assessments were completed:

- Semistructured clinical interview
- Problem list
- McGill pain questionnaire
- Pain cognitions scale
- Suicide assessment and prevention plan

In the sections that follow, the rationale behind each assessment is covered.

Orientation and Rapport-Building

In addition to her concerns about her pain, Paulette was very open in describing a long history of interpersonal difficulties and losses. Most recently, these difficulties centered on her relationship with her husband and around her dealings with her rheumatologist. In developing rapport, the therapist took Paulette's interpersonal history into consideration. The therapist paid particular attention to Paulette's body language, facial expressions, and verbal reactions when orienting her to the structure and process of cognitive behavioral therapy. In addition, the therapist periodically paused to check in with Paulette about her reactions and relied upon the frequent use of empathic summary statements to create as much of a nonjudgmental and emotionally safe atmosphere as possible. Because Paulette reported that her past experiences with psychotherapy had ranged from being neutral to negative, the therapist paid particular attention to educating Paulette about the importance of providing honest feedback to the therapist regarding what aspects of therapy were more and less helpful at the end of each session.

Paulette volunteered that it is not always easy for her to provide direct, face-to-face feedback to people when things are ot going well. She predicted she might have difficulty with this aspect of cognitive behavioral therapy, even if the source of her discontent was relatively minor. After further exploration, Paulette reported that she is not always able to verbalize her discontent with something or someone at the time it occurs. Instead, her discontent and anger usually build over time after an interaction has already taken place and she has "had time to think about it." Although the therapist could have suggested that Paulette work on achieving an ability to provide immediate feedback in therapy as one of her goals in cognitive behavioral therapy, instead she suggested that Paulette consider writing her feedback down as part of her assigned homework each week for review during the following session. Paulette reported that she felt more comfortable with this approach and agreed to try it.

Semistructured Clinical Interview

The therapist first decided to conduct a semistructured interview to elicit information about Paulette's physical health history, present symptoms and impairments, psychosocial history, and family background (preliminary findings from this interview are presented in Chapter 1). Paulette was asked to describe her experience with RA in her own words, including the circumstances surrounding her diagnosis, reactions of health-care providers and individuals in her social network, illness-related losses, what she considers her most troublesome symptoms, the types of treatments and medications she has tried, and issues involving self-concept and adaptation to illness.

Additional questions that focused specifically on the nature and circumstances of her pain were included in this interview. The questions were considered critical in achieving an initial understanding of Paulette's pain-related cognitions and behavioral reactions; some of these questions and the responses they elicited are presented in Table 1. Importantly, these questions revealed some of her underlying beliefs about health-care professionals, herself, and others in her social network.

Based on this and other information gathered from the clinical interview, the therapist generated some initial hypotheses about Paulette's pain-related cognitions. Namely, she hypothesized that Paulette viewed her pain as being a very powerful influence within her life. Paulette saw the pain as uncontrollable, unpredictable, and, in her words, "imprisoning." In addition to these beliefs about her pain, Paulette's core beliefs about herself appeared to reflect themes of unlovability and worthlessness.

Other important information that the therapist gathered from this interview was that Paulette was well aware of the consequences of not taking the recommended antirheumatic medications in terms of her overall health, pain levels, and functioning. At this point in the process, the therapist decided to ask Paulette to complete a problem list to obtain a more focused idea of what Paulette considered to be her priorities for therapy.

Problem List

Paulette and the therapist completed the problem list during the first session. Paulette identified the following three problems as priorities:

- Severe Pain
- Fatigue
- Problems with partner

TABLE 1. Extractions from the semistructured clinical interview.

Therapist:	". . . What does is mean to you now to have RA? What thoughts pass through your mind when you think about it?"
Paulette:	"That I am a prisoner . . . . I feel like I am going through a series of torture exercises. I resent the fact that I have it. It has limited me a lot, especially during the past few years. I feel like it has taken my life away, the few friendships I had, and it is damaging my marriage. The pain is just unbearable at times."
Therapist:	". . . Would you tell me more about the ways RA has affected your life in these past few years?"
Paulette:	"I no longer go out unless I have to and I am about to lose my job. I feel so alone and I'm worried that my husband is unhappy with me."
Therapist:	"It has affected your life significantly . . . . May I ask, how has RA affected the way you feel about yourself?"
Paulette:	"It has made me feel more unattractive, lazy, and pretty much of a drag on other people. Like a chronic complainer . . . . I just want to scream – don't you understand that the pain is so bad! – I try really, really hard to do things for others – to meet their needs when I can – but I think I always come up short because I just can't seem to be helpful enough to anyone anymore. That's why I'd just as soon stay alone most of the time. I feel better not bothering people."
Therapist:	". . . OK, just so I am clear I understand. You started to experience more intense pain and limitations, and you started to lose the ability to participate in more and more activities. You stopped seeing people that were important to you. Do you remember whether anything happened to trigger this kind of cascade of symptoms and losses?"
Paulette:	"No. It just came on – the illness just suddenly took a turn for the worse and it dragged my life with it."
Therapist:	"At this point what do you know about RA? What kind of factual information do you have about what causes it, how it works, and how it is treated?"
Paulette:	"Well I didn't know much about it until recently when I started reading the magazines . . . . I know it's like an autoimmune disease in which the body's own immune system kind of turns against itself and destroys the joints. I guess it eventually destroys the joints altogether and then you have to have joint replacements. Obviously this is why my doctor wants me to take the antirheumatic drugs now."
Therapist:	". . . Another important job for us is to decide on a plan for you to begin to manage your pain on your own. Have you done anything so far to try to manage your pain on your own?"
Paulette:	"When it first started to get bad a few years ago, I tried tai chi, yoga, acupuncture, and massage therapy. I just felt worse after each one. Nothing really seemed to work."
Therapist:	"Are there any symptoms that you think you can control just by virtue of what you do in your daily life?"
Paulette:	"No, there is no rhyme or reason to this illness. The only thing I know is that the pain gets worse when I do too much."
Therapist:	"Is there anything else that you do or experience that you know makes your symptoms worse?"
Paulette:	"Do you mean stress or things like that?"
Therapist:	"Yes, stress, certain interactions with people, and certain activities that tend to increase the pain?"
Paulette:	"Yes, work and feeling pressured at work brings it on, arguing with my husband, and doing too much around the house. That's why I've stopped doing so much . . . . I just decided to surrender to it."

In reviewing the problem list, Paulette and the therapist agreed that they would consider her severe pain as the initial focus of therapy. During the second session and after having collected more information from the rheumatologist, the therapist asked Paulette whether she was aware of the possibility that there might be some discrepancies between her problem list and the one that her rheumatologist had come up with. Specifically, the rheumatologist identified anxiety, noncompliance with treatment recommendations, and activity avoidance as the central concerns.

Chapter 4 highlighted the importance of the therapist's decision to support Paulette in pursuing her concerns in therapy as opposed to those of her rheumatologist. However, it is important to recognize that the therapist's decision to support Paulette's perspective did not occur in the absence of a direct and explicit conversation about the discrepancies between Paulette's perspective on her problems versus that of her rheumatologist. Paulette reported that she suspected that her rheumatologist had a different agenda for her care. Paulette reported that she did not want to face this dilemma initially, and that what she really needed right now was pain relief. The therapist agreed to follow Paulette's wishes and together they agreed to revisit this issue whenever Paulette felt she was ready to address it.

McGill Pain Questionnaire – Short Form

The Short-Form McGill Pain Questionnaire (Melzack 1987) was used to measure Paulette's perception of the nature and intensity of her pain. This questionnaire was administered as homework as a baseline measure at the beginning of therapy, as a measure of progress at key points during the course of therapy, and as a measure of outcomes at the end of therapy. Information about how to obtain a copy of this questionnaire without charge is provided in the Appendix.

This questionnaire has three components. Part I (the pain rating index) lists 15 adjectives that describe pain. These adjectives are subclassified in terms of sensory (items 1–11) and affective (items 12–15) qualities of pain. Paulette was asked to rate the level of pain she experienced for each word on the scale, where 0 = none, 1 = mild, 2 = moderate, and 3 = severe. She was instructed to leave the column blank if the word did not apply to her. Her responses to the first part of the questionnaire are presented in Table 2.

For the second aspect of this questionnaire (Part II, overall pain intensity), Paulette was asked to rate the overall intensity of her pain on an average day on a visual-analogue scale. The scale ranged from "no pain" to "worst possible pain." Figure 1 presents her responses on the visual-analogue scale.

The third aspect of the questionnaire (Part III, present pain intensity) required Paulette to make an evaluative rating of the intensity of her pain in the present moment by choosing an appropriate word on a 0 to 5 scale. Table 3 presents Paulette's rating of her present pain intensity at baseline.

Paulette's scores on the short form of the McGill Pain Questionnaire were converted into percentage scores, as illustrated in Table 4.

TABLE 2. Paulette's baseline responses to the first part of the McGill pain question-naire – short form (reproduced with permission*).

	None 0	Mild 1	Moderate 2	Severe 3
1. Throbbing	×			
2. Shooting	×			
3. Stabbing				×
4. Sharp	×			
5. Cramping	×			
6. Gnawing				×
7. Hot—Burning		×		
8. Aching				×
9. Heavy	×			
10. Tender		×		
11. Splitting		×		
12. Tiring—Exhausting				×
13. Sickening				×
14. Fearful			×	
15. Cruel—Punishing				×

* The McGill Pain Questionnaire-Short Form was reprinted from PAIN, V30, Melzack, R. The short -form of the McGill Pain Questionnaire, pp. 191–197, (© 1987), with permission from International Association for the Study of Pain.

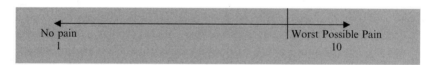

FIGURE 1. Paulette's Baseline Rating of Pain Intensity on the Visual Analogue Scale of the McGill Pain Questionnaire – Short Form (Reproduced with Permission*)
*The McGill Pain Questionnaire-Short Form was reprinted from PAIN, V30, Melzack, R. The short -form of the McGill Pain Questionnaire, pp. 191–197, (© 1987), with permission from International Association for the Study of Pain.

TABLE 3. Paulette's baseline rating of present pain intensity on the McGill pain questionnaire – short form (reproduced with permission*).

Present Pain Intensity		
0	No Pain	
1	Mild	
2	Discomforting	
3	Distressing	
4	Horrible	×
5	Excruciating	

* The McGill Pain Questionnaire-Short Form was reprinted from PAIN, V30, Melzack, R. The short -form of the McGill Pain Questionnaire, pp. 191–197, (© 1987), with permission from International Association for the Study of Pain.

TABLE 4. Paulette's baseline scores on the McGill pain questionnaire – short form.

Part I (items 1–11)	Sensory Pain Rating Index	12/33 = 36%
Part I (items 12–15)	Affective Pain Rating Index	11/12 = 92%
Part I (items 1–15)	Total Pain Rating Index	23/45 = 51%
Part II	Overall Pain Rating – Visual Analog Scale	8/10 = 80%
Part III	Evaluative Rating of Present Pain Intensity from 0 -5	4/5 = Horrible = 80%

As observed in Tables 2–4 and Figure 1, Paulette reports experiencing a great deal of pain and her affective pain ratings are particularly high. This suggests that Paulette's experience of pain is being influenced rather strongly by emotional and psychological variables, making her a good candidate for cognitive behavioral therapy.

Pain Cognitions Scale

The therapist assigned the pain cognitions scale to Paulette as part of her home-work assignment in order to elicit Paulette's beliefs about her pain and to deter-mine the extent of dysfunction involving her beliefs. The pain cognitions scale is a 23-item clinical measure developed by the author for use in clinical practice. It can be used to assess the presence and types of a client's dysfunctional cogni-tions that are related to pain.

Because it is brief and offers a simple "true" or "false" response format, it can be administered rapidly during a session or assigned for homework. Similar to the fatigue cognitions scale, the pain cognitions scale should be evaluated from a qual-itative perspective; it requires consideration of the nature of the client's chronic ill-ness and other aspects of his or her life situation in determining whether some of the statements that are endorsed as true reflect cognitive distortions (as opposed to realistic cognitions with low utility). Paulette's responses to the pain cognitions scale are presented in Table 5.

Paulette endorsed 18, or 78 percent, of the 23 statements on the Pain Cognitions Scale as true. Her statements suggest that her pain is all-encompassing, control-ling, and devastating in terms of its effect on her occupational, physical, psycho-logical, and social functioning. Items 1, 2, and 10 may reflect true statements about the experience of having rheumatoid arthritis. For example, given that Paulette has been refusing to take antirheumatic medications and has essentially gone untreated since her initial diagnosis, it is realistic to speculate that her increased pain is a reflection of the progressive joint degeneration that accompanies worsening RA in the absence of antirheumatic medications.

However, even if these particular cognitions do not reflect distortions, they are nonetheless low in their utility value. Moreover, Paulette has endorsed a large number of other statements that are much clearer indications of cognitive distor-tions about pain. Based on findings from this measure, the therapist determined that

TABLE 5. Paulette's responses to the pain cognitions scale at baseline. ·

The Pain Cognitions Scale	
Please answer "true" (T) or "false" (F) to the following statements	
1. My pain makes me worry that my condition is getting worse.	T
2. My pain is unpredictable.	T
3. People do not take my pain seriously.	F
4. I believe I deserve to be in pain.	F
5. When I am in pain, I think of the possibility that I might be dying.	F
6. I feel guilty because of my pain.	T
7. My doctor is not responsive to my pain.	T
8. My pain makes others feel uncomfortable around me.	T
9. My pain makes me less attractive to others.	T
10. My pain never goes away.	T
11. My pain has changed my personality.	T
12. I cannot keep my mind off my pain.	T
13. My pain will never improve.	T
14. My pain renders me useless at work.	T
15. I can no longer live with my pain.	T
16. People think my pain is "all in my head".	F
17. People think I exaggerate my pain.	F
18. I cannot control my pain.	T
19. My pain has changed who I am as a person.	T
20. I feel I have failed in life because of my pain.	T
21. I cannot do anything without feeling pain.	T
22. At times my pain makes me want to die.	T
23. I cannot cope with my pain.	T

identifying and modifying maladaptive cognitions would be a focus of Paulette's treatment. By examining Paulette's response to item 22, the therapist was alerted to the fact that Paulette might have been at risk for suicide. She endorsed the statement, "At times my pain makes me want to die."

Suicide Assessment and Prevention Plan

Based on Paulette's responses to the Pain Cognitions scale, a suicide assessment was conducted in clinical interview format. Questions were asked regarding:

- The timing and circumstances surrounding Paulette's thoughts about her own death,
- The frequency with which she has these thoughts, and
- The exact nature and description of her thoughts about death.

Paulette was also asked about plans and means for suicide, her history of any prior attempts, and whether she has ever had an intention to kill herself. Paulette consistently denied ever having any suicidal ideation outside of times when she is in so much pain that she fantasizes about her own death. She denied ever having a plan or intention to kill herself and she denied any history of self-harm or suicide attempts.

Somewhat contradictory to her responses on the pain cognitions scale, Paulette denied suicidal ideation during the initial interview. When questioned about this, Paulette explained that she only thinks about death when her pain is severe, but she never thinks about death or wanting to die when she is not in severe pain. Based on this information, the therapist proposed a suicide prevention plan. This consisted of:

- Contacting the therapist through her emergency telephone number should she ever have thoughts about harming or killing herself.
- Calling 911 directly or going directly to the local emergency room should she ever have plans or intentions to harm or kill herself.

Paulette agreed to follow this plan. She informed the therapist that, because of her two sons and the grief it would cause them, she would never attempt suicide, even if she was experiencing very severe pain.

DSM-IV Diagnostic Profile

Following completion of all of the assessments, the therapist arrived at the following diagnostic conclusions:

Axis I: Dysthymic disorder

Axis II: Personality disorder, not otherwise specified (passive-aggressive and mild borderline features)

Axis III: Rheumatoid arthritis

Axis IV (psychosocial issues): chronic pain in fingers, wrists, elbows, shoulders, back, hips, knees ankles, and feet; work performance issues; conflict with rheumatologist; couples problems; socially isolated

Axis V (global assessment of functioning): 50

Treatment Goal

Based upon the contents of her problem list, Paulette and her therapist agreed that the overarching goal of therapy would be pain reduction. The therapist then recommended corresponding objectives, or steps that Paulette would need to take to accomplish that goal. They decided to set a target date for goal attainment as the 20th session of therapy. Paulette rated her confidence level for attaining the goal by the 20th session as a "10" on a scale of 1–10 and seemed very motivated to engage in therapy. Paulette's treatment goal, corresponding objectives, and confidence rating are presented in Figure 2.

Cognitive Behavioral Case Conceptualization

By the second session, the therapist was ready to develop a cognitive behavioral case conceptualization that would guide the subsequent sessions of therapy. First, the therapist reviewed the basic aspects of the cognitive model with Paulette. This included a review of the relationships between health event triggers,

Goal Form		
Goal(s) **Target Date**	**Confidence Rating** (1-10)	**Objectives** (realistic steps I can take to achieve goal)
Goal 1: Reduce pain Target date:20th session	10	a. Identify and evaluate beliefs about pain (pain-related cognitions). b. Learn and practice specific pain management techniques (including relaxation, meditation, and distraction exercises). c. Identify and increase activities that are pleasurable and gratifying using the daily activity record. d. Decide on an appropriate course of medical treatment for RA.

FIGURE 2. Paulette's Goal Form

automatic thoughts, and emotional, behavioral, and physiological outcomes. They also reviewed the three levels of beliefs and their role in the cognitive model. Despite some mild difficulties concentrating because of her pain, Paulette was able to learn and understand the basic aspects of the cognitive model very quickly.

The case conceptualization worksheet (introduced in Chapter 4) was used to illustrate application of the cognitive model to Paulette's difficulties with her pain. Paulette understood the overarching idea of the cognitive model very quickly and her reaction to it was that she found it helpful in explaining her reactions to her pain. She stated "I never knew that beliefs were that powerful, or that they could really be changed." She felt that the diagram accurately reflected how her beliefs about her pain played a role in her emotional, behavioral, and physiological reactions to it.

Paulette's case conceptualization worksheet is presented in Figure 3. The type of core belief that was chosen as the focal point of treatment was Paulette's core belief related to her chronic condition – specifically, her core belief about pain itself. This type of core belief was chosen over other core beliefs that Paulette had about herself, others, and health-care professionals because it was the core belief around which her most problematic symptoms revolved.

As the case conceptualization illustrates, the core belief that underlies Paulette's experience of pain is that her pain is omnipotent. When Paulette experiences pain, she automatically concludes that she is no longer able to do something. Her unconditional belief is that pain always prevents her from doing things. The consequences of her beliefs are that she feels anxiety and despair, chooses not to attend work the next day, and remains at home on the couch being physically and mentally inactive.

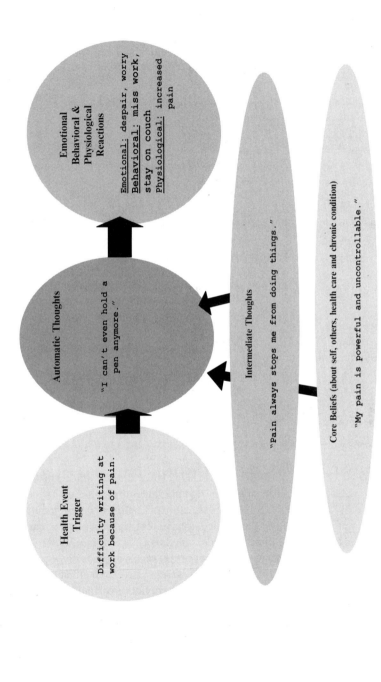

FIGURE 3. Paulette's Case Conceptualization Worksheet

Summary of the Orientation and Assessment Phase

For Paulette, six actions were of particular importance in socializing her into cognitive behavioral therapy. These included:

- Using empathic summary statements to strengthen the therapeutic relationship.
- Creating a concrete plan for Paulette to provide the therapist with both positive and negative feedback about therapy in written form.
- Recognizing that Paulette had suicidal ideation, conducting a suicide assessment, and obtaining Paulette's agreement to follow a suicide prevention plan.
- Outlining the structure, process and other essential elements of cognitive behavioral therapy.
- Defining problems, setting a goal, and setting a provisional target date for completion.
- Teaching the cognitive model as it applied to Paulette's experience of pain.

By the end of the initial assessment and orientation period, the therapist was confident that Paulette was motivated to participate in cognitive behavioral therapy and that she understood its basic structure and process.

Subsequent Sessions: Course of Treatment

Paulette received a total of 20 sessions of cognitive behavioral therapy, occurring every other week, over a one-year period. The therapy aimed to address her central goal of pain reduction. Because results of her initial assessment indicated that a significant degree of her pain experience was influenced by cognitive and emotional variables, the central emphasis of therapy was to teach Paulette to evaluate and modify her dysfunctional cognitions about pain. More information about the course of treatment is presented in the sections that follow.

Main Emphasis of the Socratic questioning

The therapist used Socratic questioning liberally throughout the course of treatment as a means of assisting Paulette in identifying and modifying her maladaptive cognitions. The main emphasis of the questioning targeted Paulette's core beliefs. Questions were designed to elicit and modify Paulette's core beliefs regarding pain (e.g., "Pain controls my life" and "Pain prevents me from doing anything"), her core beliefs related to herself (e.g., "I am worthless" and "I am unlovable"), and her core beliefs involving others (e.g., "My doctor is selfish" and "People expect reciprocity at all times"). Following sufficient practice using the response record, Paulette learned to ask herself Socratic questions when evaluating the validity and utility of her own cognitions.

In-Session Cognitive and Behavioral Activities

Using the case conceptualization worksheet (introduced in Chapter 4 and presented in Figure 3) Paulette's case conceptualization was reviewed periodically during the course of treatment. Once Paulette became knowledgeable about the nature and role of negative automatic thoughts, various thought records and worksheets that focused on identifying and modifying maladaptive cognitions (presented in Chapters 7 and 8) were introduced. These were used as the primary in-session activities during the treatment process. Because Paulette was able to recognize that many of her beliefs were maladaptive, the response record, presented in Chapter 7, was used; it will be discussed below.

Because Paulette tended not to volunteer what she was thinking and feeling during therapy until questioned, sequential questioning (presented in Chapter 7) was used frequently as a means of introducing the thought record exercises. This approach to questioning not only served to elicit Paulette's active participation but also served to elicit her negative automatic thoughts. An example of the therapist's use of sequential questioning with Paulette is presented in Table 6.

Following this exchange the therapist took out a response record form and asked Paulette to help her complete the record. The response record that was used to address the negative automatic thought that her "family [would] think she did not care" is introduced in Chapter 7 and presented in Figure 4.

In providing feedback to the therapist, Paulette reported that she found the response record exercise to be very helpful in allowing her to "distance herself from the situation" and evaluate her thinking more objectively. Given Paulette's ease in learning and her positive response to this exercise, the therapist then decided to utilize downward sequential questioning to teach Paulette how to identify her intermediate and core beliefs. An example of the therapist's application of this technique to Paulette's dilemma regarding whether to attend her niece's wedding is introduced in Chapter 7 and presented in Figure 5.

TABLE 6. Example of Paulette's responses to sequential questioning.

An Example of Paulette's Responses to Sequential Questioning

Therapist:	(noticing Paulette sitting passively and appearing unhappy) "May I ask, what are you feeling right now?"
Paulette:	"In pain... and worried."
Therapist:	"What thoughts or pictures pass through your mind as you feel this?"
Paulette:	"I am thinking that I won't be able to make my niece's wedding ... that I will be letting my family down and they will think I don't care about them. But then a part of me thinks that maybe they won't miss me that much, anyway. It might be good just to stay home and avoid it altogether."
Therapist:	"Which thought makes you feel the worst?"
Paulette:	"That my family will think I don't care about them."
Therapist:	"OK, what you have identified just now is your hot thought, or the automatic thought that makes you feel the worst. I would like to see how it would work if we used what I call a response record to look at this thought a little more closely."

Response Record

Date: Nov. 3	Health event trigger (or other triggering event): Symptom flare-up			
What am I feeling right now? (Circle all that apply.)	panicked	numb	sad	Angry
	hopeless	(worried)	Other:(pain)	

What thoughts or pictures are passing through my mind?

I won't be able to attend my niece's wedding;
I will be letting my family down;
My family will think I don't care about them;
Maybe I won't be missed, anyway.

Which of these thoughts or pictures makes me feel the worst? (Circle one above.)

What are the emotional, behavioral, and physical consequences of thinking this way?

Emotional: Feel more anxious	Behavioral: Eating too much	Physical: Increased pain, can't sleep

- What do I already know that supports this belief?
That my mother considers it rude to miss family events.
- What do I already know that does not support this belief?
My niece and brothers know me better than that and know
I would attend if I could.
- What might someone else think about this situation?
My brother knows what it is like to have to miss out on
activities because he had to miss my parents' anniversary when
he was dealing with depression.
- What advice would I give to a friend if he or she were in this situation?
Take care of yourself and explain your situation.
- What is the best possible outcome of this situation?
I could let them know how much I care by making it clear that
I really hate to miss this event.
- What is the worst possible outcome of this situation?
My mother will call me up and make me feel selfish and guilty.
- If the (worst outcome) were to happen, what could I do to minimize its impact?
I could send a message they could read or call them on a cell
phone during the event.
- Given what I know so far, how likely is [the worst outcome] to happen?
Likely, but that's ok.
- How do I benefit from keeping this belief?
I don't - I just feel guilty and sad.
- What negative consequences go along with keeping this belief?
Worry and sadness
- Is there anything else that could explain this situation?
I'm projecting my own insecurities onto the situation, but I
really doubt that knowing my mother.

FIGURE 4. Paulette's First Response Record

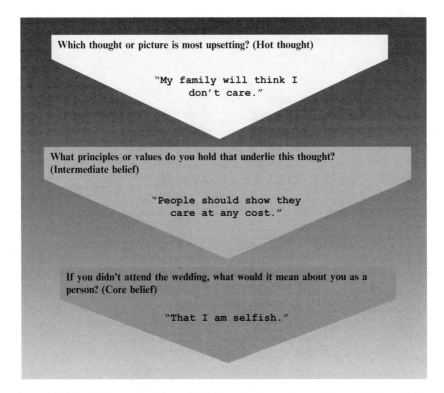

Which thought or picture is most upsetting? (Hot thought)

"My family will think I
don't care."

What principles or values do you hold that underlie this thought? (Intermediate belief)

"People should show they
care at any cost."

If you didn't attend the wedding, what would it mean about you as a person? (Core belief)

"That I am selfish."

FIGURE 5. Use of Downward Sequential Questioning to Access Intermediate and Core Beliefs

Once Paulette fully understood all three levels at which maladaptive cognitions can occur, the practicing moderation in beliefs worksheet (introduced in Chapter 7) was utilized. This offered Paulette a straightforward means of modifying all three levels of her maladaptive cognitions about a single situation using a single worksheet. Figure 6 presents an example of one of Paulette's worksheets that focuses on a statement she made in therapy that people did not want to be around her because she has RA and is no longer of much use to them.

Given that pain reduction was the central goal of therapy, education was the central strategy of therapy. Paulette was also introduced to a number of relaxation and meditation exercises. Paulette's favorites included walking meditation (presented in Chapter 8) and a diaphragmatic breathing meditation that involved body scanning and progressive muscle relaxation without muscle tensing (Taylor, Friedberg and Jason 2001). These exercises were used not only on days when Paulette's pain interfered with her concentration during therapy, but also whenever Paulette appeared to be having difficulty tolerating the more introspective demands of therapy of identifying and modifying her maladaptive cognitions.

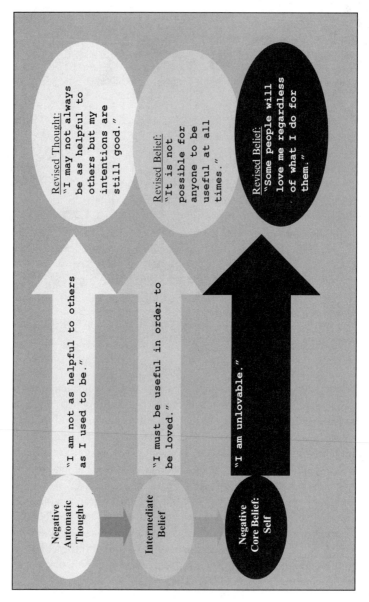

FIGURE 6. Paulette's Practicing Moderation in Beliefs Worksheet

Homework Prescribed

Paulette reacted positively to the idea of homework assignments. She completed them consistently and reported that she found them helpful in allowing her to structure her thinking and practice what she learned in therapy. In addition to the initial assessments, which Paulette completed as homework for the second session, Paulette completed the following homework assignments during the course of therapy.

- Thought records (response record and practicing moderation in beliefs worksheet)
- Daily activity record (Chapter 9)
- Self-care activities (*Woman's Comfort Book*)

When indicated, Paulette was assigned to work on thought records at home. This increased the likelihood that she would develop an increasing ability to identify and modify her maladaptive cognitions independently, without assistance from the therapist. Because Paulette was relatively inactive and had difficulty identifying activities that were important, pleasurable, and caused her to feel competent, she was also instructed to complete a daily activity record (discussed in Chapter 9) as homework. An example of a daily activity record that Paulette completed toward the end of therapy is presented in Figure 7.

Daily Activity Record			
Date: July 1	Rating 10= Best 1=Worst		
Activities Completed Today	Importance Rating	Competence Rating	Pleasure Rating
Washed and ironed clothes	10	3	3
Took son to school	10	5	5
Went to doctor	10	1	1
Watched son's soccer game	10	5	10
Read a chapter in a novel	3	5	10
Walked	10	5	8

FIGURE 7. Paulette's Daily Activity Record

The therapist also recommended that Paulette read entries from *The Woman's Comfort Book* (Louden 1992) and complete the activities that most appealed to her as homework. The activities from this book that Paulette found most useful included "creative selfishness" "comfort clothing," and "bathing pleasures." Creative selfishness is an exercise designed to facilitate assertiveness, self-care, and limit-setting. The "comfort clothing" exercise provides recommendations for evaluating the contents of one's current wardrobe and retaining only the clothing that is comfortable and/or leads to feelings of self-worth. The "bathing pleasures" exercise provides recommendations and numerous ideas for enhancing one's bathing experience.

Difficulties Encountered

The primary obstacles encountered during Paulette's therapy involved her difficulties with consistent attendance and her difficulties sustaining attention and concentration during therapy sessions. These were most pronounced in the initial stages of therapy, before Paulette began to develop and practice skills to more effectively prevent and predict pain flare-ups. In addition to these difficulties, Paulette's prior history of losses and interpersonal conflicts required that the therapist pay particular attention to issues involving the therapeutic relationship. Although she followed through with the agreement she had made with the therapist to provide written feedback to the therapist after each session, Paulette continued to have difficulty providing negative feedback to the therapist about what was not working in therapy. Instead she provided only positive feedback and selectively ignored the aspects of therapy that did not work as well. Eventually, the therapist recognized this pattern and began to help Paulette verbalize her discontent with the aspects of therapy that she selectively ignored.

Paulette's Axis I and II disorders introduced additional complexities. Paulette's negative emotions and difficulties regulating her emotional reactions to therapy were often accompanied by an increase in her physical pain during and following therapy. Initially, Paulette had difficulties tolerating exercises that involved introspection, such as thought records and worksheets that encouraged her to identify and evaluate her cognitions. She reported that she often felt tremendous sadness, guilt, and shame each time she realized that her beliefs were dysfunctional or unrealistic. She reported that she would often dwell on these feelings for days following therapy and that her pain would be very severe during those times.

In addition, Paulette occasionally made demonstrative comments alluding to the fact that she could no longer live with her pain, or that she wished that she would die rather than suffer through the pain. This led to interruptions of the therapy process, in which the therapist made periodic suicide assessments to ensure that Paulette was not at any risk for suicide. Although Paulette acknowledged feeling depressed and accepted the idea that her pain did increase when her depressive symptoms worsened, it was clear to the therapist that Paulette's central motivation in therapy was pain reduction.

In addition, on a number of occasions Paulette appeared concerned about the therapist's opinion about her. Paulette was fearful that the therapist would judge her for having beliefs that she knew were irrational. In addition, she continued to avoid providing the therapist with negative feedback out of fear that the therapist would abandon her emotionally. It was clear to the therapist at the outset of therapy that the ongoing use of empathically based summary statements would be required to facilitate trust and open communication in therapy. This liberal use of empathy allowed Paulette to eventually recognize that her concerns about her therapist's opinion of her paralleled her concerns about other people's opinions of her, including those of her husband and family members. Eventually she was able to evaluate her concerns about others' opinions of her as they related to her underlying fears of abandonment and to one of her core beliefs that she was unlovable.

Use of Related Knowledge as a Supplemental Approach

As mentioned earlier, the therapist drew heavily upon related knowledge of empathy and self psychology throughout Paulette's therapy. For example, Chapter 11 presents a dialogue between Paulette and her therapist that illustrates the use of empathy with Paulette in discussing her concerns about her husband. Because of Paulette's difficulties with consistent attendance and her reluctance to provide the therapist with any negative feedback following each therapy session, the therapist had occasional concerns about whether the therapy was truly reaching Paulette. These concerns were heightened by the unpredictable nature of Paulette's approach to the therapeutic relationship. Paulette tended to alternate between two emotional styles during therapy. One style was characterized by emotional intensity and positive affect and the other was characterized by emotional disengagement and passivity. When Paulette became emotionally disengaged during therapy, her concentration difficulties became worse. This made it more difficult for the therapist to involve her in a collaborative relationship.

The therapist's knowledge of self psychology (introduced in Chapter 11) allowed her to manage these reactions toward Paulette outside of the therapeutic relationship so that she could develop an effective cognitive behavioral strategy for managing Paulette's style and behaviors within the therapeutic relationship. The therapist worked hard to understand Paulette's emotional behavior and reluctance to relate to the therapist in an honest and trusting way from a more developmental, object-relations perspective. For example, the therapist understood that Paulette's early relationships with her biological mother and with her adoptive mother involved an actual experience of abandonment from her biological mother and the threat of abandonment from her adoptive mother. Moreover, Paulette's relationship with her adoptive mother was characterized by what she described as a "hot and cold" relationship that involved repeated experiences of a developmentally inappropriate level of idealization followed by rejection. The next significant relationship in Paulette's life was her relationship with her ex-husband.

This relationship was also characterized by instability, rejection, and physical and emotional abuse. Based on Paulette's description of the significant relationships in her life, the therapist came to understand Paulette's emotional style in therapy and her concerns about being judged, rejected, and abandoned. This allowed the therapist to form a complex understanding of Paulette's psychological development from an empathic perspective.

Through the use of empathically based summary statements, the therapist conveyed this more complex level of understanding of Paulette's history to Paulette. The therapist described the more difficult interpersonal aspects of her history in terms of injuries to her core sense of self. This provided a rationale for their work together on Paulette's maladaptive core beliefs. The development of understanding of Paulette's core beliefs in relation to her past significant relationships reduced Paulette's sense of shame about having maladaptive core beliefs. In addition, when it became clear that Paulette was having difficulty tolerating too much emphasis on the examination of her own cognitions, the therapist varied her emphasis and introduced relaxation exercises into the therapy sessions and provided Paulette with other educational information about self-care.

Over time, Paulette eventually began to trust the therapist enough to work on her maladaptive core beliefs. The "Core Beliefs Time line," presented in Figure 8 and originally introduced in Chapter 7, was used as a means of allowing Paulette to revisit key events within her life that led to the development of the negative core belief that she was unlovable. In addition, the time line allowed her to work toward countering those beliefs with alternative examples of events that disconfirmed the evidence for her unlovability. Without the use of these strategies, it is

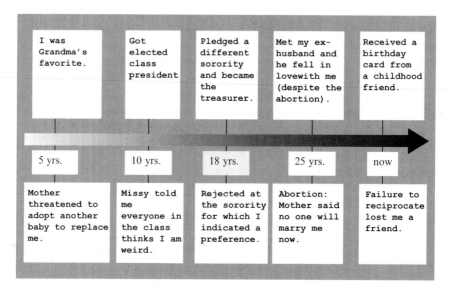

FIGURE 8. Paulette's Core Beliefs Timeline

very likely that Paulette would not have developed as complex an understanding of the cognitive model as it related to her pain experiences.

Treatment Outcome: Termination and Relapse Prevention

By the 20th session, Paulette reported that she felt she had made substantial progress toward her goal of learning how to manage and reduce her pain. She reported that her work on modifying her beliefs about her pain and about herself were the most helpful aspects of therapy. By the end of therapy, Paulette had joined a therapeutic health club that was affiliated with her local hospital. She began to participate in classes and activities offered for individuals with chronic illnesses at the club, including water therapy classes. Through participation in these therapeutic exercise classes, Paulette met a few individuals with shared interests and concerns and began to socialize with them on a periodic basis. In addition, she completed a behavioral experiment, which allowed her to begin to take the prescribed antirheumatic medications. She also began to take an antidepressant medication, which she found helpful in managing her mood and her pain. It also helped with her occasional sleep difficulties.

Because she was not always sure whether Paulette's feedback adequately reflected her experience with therapy, the therapist decided to have Paulette complete two outcomes assessments – the short form of the McGill Pain Questionnaire (Melzack 1987) and the Pain Cognitions Scale. Paulette's final scores on the pain questionnaire are included in Table 7 and her responses on the pain cognitions scale are shown on Table 8. Both tables compare her final scores with those she assigned in her initial assessment. Together they indicate that her experiences of pain and pain-related cognitions have improved.

Learning from Paulette: Unique Features of Individuals with Pain

Like many individuals with chronic conditions involving chronic pain of moderate to severe intensity, Paulette named relief from pain as her first priority. With

TABLE 7. Paulette's final and initial scores on the McGill pain questionnaire – short form.

		Final Score	Initial Score
Part I (items 1–11)	Sensory Pain Rating Index	5/33 = 15%	12/33 = 36%
Part I (items 12–15)	Affective Pain Rating Index	2/12 = 17%	11/12 = 92%
Part I (items 1–15)	Total Pain Rating Index	7/45 = 16%	23/45 = 51%
Part II	Overall Pain Rating – Visual Analog Scale	5/10 = 50%	8/10 = 80%
Part III	Evaluative Rating of Present Pain Intensity from 0–5	2/5 = Discomforting = 40%	2/5 = Horrible = 80%

TABLE 8. Paulette's current and past responses on the pain cognitions scale.

The pain cognitions scale		
Please answer "true" (T) or "false" (F) to the following statements.		
	Current	Initial
My pain makes me worry that my condition is getting worse.	T	T
My pain is unpredictable.	T	T
People do not take my pain seriously.	F	F
I believe I deserve to be in pain.	F	F
When I am in pain, I think of the possibility that I might be dying.	F	F
I feel guilty because of my pain.	T	T
My doctor is not responsive to my pain.	F	T
My pain makes others feel uncomfortable around me.	F	T
My pain makes me less attractive to others.	F	T
My pain never goes away.	F	T
My pain has changed my personality.	F	T
I cannot keep my mind off my pain.	F	T
My pain will never improve.	F	T
My pain renders me useless at work.	F	T
I can no longer live with my pain.	F	T
People think my pain is "all in my head".	F	F
People think I exaggerate my pain.	F	F
I cannot control my pain.	F	T
My pain has changed who I am as a person.	F	T
I feel I have failed in life because of my pain.	F	T
I cannot do anything without feeling pain.	F	T
At times my pain makes me want to die.	F	T
I cannot cope with my pain.	F	T

the exception of periodic corticosteroid injections and the use of NSAIDs, Paulette had left the underlying cause of her pain, RA, untreated for several years. This resulted in a more pronounced level of impairment and more severe pain. During times when her pain was severe (particularly in the initial stages of therapy), Paulette was distracted by it and frequently had difficulty maintaining concentration. Alternatively, she took heavier dosages of prescribed painkillers and failed to attend therapy because she had to remain at home. This influenced the consistency and pacing of the therapy process. However, as Paulette gained more of an ability to prevent or at least predict flare-ups, she was more able to attend therapy consistently.

Another issue that Paulette faced that is common among individuals with chronic pain is conflict with her health-care provider regarding the appropriate course of treatment for her pain. In addition to these issues, Paulette was unsure how to communicate her needs for self-care to others in a way that would be effective and assertive. She vacillated between trying to maintain a façade of health, not asking for any help, and feeling powerless and overly dependent on others.

In summary, there are six unique considerations to bear in mind when conducting cognitive behavioral therapy with individuals with chronic pain:

- If an individual is facing moderate or severe chronic pain, finding relief from the pain is usually the first priority for therapy.
- Individuals with chronic pain often feel misunderstood by health-care providers or may be in conflict with their care providers about the appropriate course of treatment for their pain.
- Pain and pain medications can interfere with cognition and limit an individual's ability to participate in therapy consistently. This can slow the therapy process.
- If left untreated, chronic pain typically worsens with time and affects all aspects of life and functioning, including activities of daily living, intimate relationships, social interactions, work performance, role performance, and sleep.
- Individuals with pain may have difficulty communicating their needs to others because of pain-related cognitions that involve shame, guilt, or embarrassment about the pain.
- Interactions with family, friends, coworkers, and health care providers may involve others minimizing a client's pain, accusing the individual of dwelling or exaggerating, abandoning the individual emotionally and/or physically, or otherwise blaming the individual for "having done too much," for "not exercising enough," or for some other lifestyle error. Sometimes a less direct insinuation of blame by a friend or family member can be equally painful. In many cases, a client's perceptions of these kinds of interactions as negative and hurtful may be grounded in genuine experience. Typically, clients with chronic pain do not view this kind of feedback or advice from others as helpful. In many cases, it only serves to perpetuate feelings of stigma, low self-worth, and isolation. When this dynamic appears to be occurring in a client's relationships, therapists can coach clients in terms of how to respond to others in assertive or otherwise self-protective ways. Occasionally, therapists may find it beneficial to invite family, partners, or friends to join a therapy session so that they can learn how to respond to the client's pain complaints or behaviors in ways that are less blaming, less stigmatizing, and ultimately more effective.

Appendix

Published pain Assessments covered in chapter 17.

Title	Description	Reference	How to obtain
Short-Form McGill Pain Questionnaire	A three-part self-report measure of the perception of the nature and intensity of pain. Part I requires the client evaluate pain according to 15 adjectives. Part II requests an overall rating of average pain intensity on a visual-analogue scale. Part III requests a rating of present pain intensity according to a 0-5 scale.	Melzack, R. (1987). The short-form of the McGill Pain Questionnaire. *Pain, 30*, 191–197.	The questionnaire is printed in the referenced article. Permission for use may be obtained without charge by writing to the author.

Pain assessment developed by the author.

The pain cognitions scale

Please answer "true" (T) or "false" (F) to the following statements.
1. My pain makes me worry that my condition is getting worse.
2. My pain is unpredictable.
3. People do not take my pain seriously.
4. I believe I deserve to be in pain.
5. When I am in pain, I think of the possibility that I might be dying.
6. I feel guilty because of my pain.
7. My doctor is not responsive to my pain.
8. My pain makes others feel uncomfortable around me.
9. My pain makes me less attractive to others.
10. My pain never goes away.
11. My pain has changed my personality.
12. I cannot keep my mind off my pain.
13. My pain will never improve.
14. My pain renders me useless at work.
15. I can no longer live with my pain.
16. People think my pain is "all in my head".
17. People think I exaggerate my pain.
18. I cannot control my pain.
19. My pain has changed who I am as a person.
20. I feel I have failed in life because of my pain.
21. I cannot do anything without feeling pain.
22. At times my pain makes me want to die.
23. I cannot cope with my pain.

18

Sleep Dysfunction: Diagnostic Categories, Prevalence, and Associated Conditions

Sleep dysfunction is associated with a wide range of chronic conditions. Insomnia, the most prevalent of all reported sleep problems, is estimated to occur in between 20 percent and 40 percent of adults within the general population and is even more prevalent among individuals with chronic illness and impairments (Morin 1993). Excessive daytime sleepiness, which involves daytime sleep episodes at inappropriate and unexpected times, is estimated to occur in 12 percent of the general population and to result in significant cognitive, emotional, and accident-risk consequences (Happe 2003). Excessive daytime sleepiness may accompany a wide range of sleep disorders, including narcolepsy and various forms of insomnia. One study found that over half of individuals with severe insomnia reported two or more heath problems during a past 12-month period (Mellinger, Balter, and Uhlenhuth 1985). A second longitudinal study reported a strong association between poor health status among aging subjects and severe sleep dysfunction (Rodin, McAvay, and Timko 1988).

Some suggest that the physical symptoms reported by individuals with chronic sleep dysfunction tend to be nonspecific and indicative of underlying stress, depression, or anxiety. For example, one study found that individuals with sleep dysfunction tend to report gastrointestinal problems, generalized aches and pains, tension headaches, and allergies (Kales et al., 1984). Other studies have found that individuals with sleep dysfunction tend to be more preoccupied with their health (Ford and Kamerow 1989; Kales et al., 1984; Morgan et al., 1988). One study found that sleep problems were twice as prevalent in men that regularly sought medical care as compared with those that did not regularly seek care (Gislason and Almqvist 1987).

There are a number of potential explanations for these observed linkages between sleep dysfunction, help-seeking behavior, and an increased number of health complaints. These include the possibility of a physiological basis for sleep dysfunction, the possibility of a psychological basis for sleep dysfunction, and the possibility of a combined physiological and psychological basis for sleep dysfunction. The extent to which physiological versus psychological variables contribute to a given sleep problem likely varies depending on the nature of the role of sleep in the specific condition under consideration.

This chapter provides an overview of basic sleep facts and a general description of the most prevalent types of sleep dysfunction and disorder. The chapter also describes role of sleep in the chronic conditions that most commonly involve disordered sleep. This chapter is not intended to provide an exhaustive, systematic, or detailed review of the epidemiology and characteristics of sleep for each condition covered. Basic information about a number of conditions that involve sleep dysfunction is offered to provide therapists with general guidelines and information about the role of sleep in some of the more common chronic illnesses. When working with clients with a chronic illness for which sleep dysfunction is a primary symptom, therapists will inevitably need to seek out additional information about the role of sleep in that specific condition from collaborating physicians and research-related resources.

Basic Information about Sleep

Before initiating any cognitive behavioral intervention targeted toward improving sleep, therapists must first be familiar with some basic information about the nature of normal sleep, the factors that determine and regulate the sleep/wake cycle, and the consequences of sleep disruption. Basic information about sleep can be shared with clients for educational purposes and can aid in assessment and collaborative treatment planning. Clients with chronic conditions that also experience sleep dysfunction will generally have a number of questions about sleep and its potential role in their condition and its symptoms. Thus it is important for therapists to be educated about these issues.

What Characterizes a Healthy Sleep Cycle?

Sleep can be classified into two major categories: non-rapid-eye-movement sleep (NREM) and rapid-eye-movement sleep (REM) (Morin 1993). During normal sleep, these two types of sleep comprise a highly organized and structured cycle. This is often referred to as sleep architecture. In a healthy young adult, sleep begins with an initial stage of drowsiness followed by four stages of NREM sleep that reflect different brain wave patterns:

- Stage 1 NREM sleep typically lasts approximately five minutes and represents a transitional phase between being awake and more definite sleep. It is the lightest form of sleep, when individuals are most vulnerable to arousal.
- Stage 2 NREM sleep lasts between 10 and 15 minutes and represents definitive physiological sleep.
- Stages 3 and 4 of NREM sleep (slow wave or delta sleep) are the deepest stages of sleep, when individuals are not as vulnerable to arousal. Together, these stages last between 20 to 40 minutes in the first cycle.

Taken together, all stages of NREM sleep are characterized by a slowing down of most physiological functions and a minimal level of cognitive activity. At the same time, periodic body movements typically accompany shifts from one sleep stage to another in NREM sleep. Once stage 4 NREM sleep is reached, the individual cycles backward through stages 3 and 2 sleep and ultimately experiences the first cycle of REM sleep. This lasts approximately 5 to 15 minutes (Morin and Espie 2003). REM sleep reveals a paradoxical brain wave pattern that is similar to NREM stage 1 sleep and reflects activation. During REM sleep, rapid eye movements occur under the eyelids, vivid hallucinatory dreams occur, and the body is essentially paralyzed (Morin 1993). In healthy young adults, the entire duration of a single NREM to REM sleep cycle may last between 70 to 120 minutes. Sleep dysfunction is characterized by alternations in the amount and proportion of time spent in each stage of sleep, which occur independently of advancing age.

Classifying and Describing Sleep Dysfunction

According to the DSM-IV, (American Psychiatric Association, 1994) there are two broad types of sleep dysfunction: dyssomnias and parasomnias. Dyssomnias are characterized by abnormalities in the quality, amount, or timing of sleep. Parasomnias are characterized by abnormal behavioral or physiological events that occur during sleep or in conjunction with specific sleep stages or sleep-wake transitions. Insomnia, the most common dyssomnia, is defined as a subjective complaint of difficulties initiating sleep, maintaining sleep, and/or experiencing sleep as refreshing and restorative. This complaint must persist for at least one month and the symptoms must cause marked distress or impairment in occupational, social, and other areas of functioning. In the case of primary insomnia, the insomnia must not occur exclusively as an aspect of a diagnosed sleep disorder or as a symptom of a psychiatric disorder. In addition, it must not result from the direct physiological effect of substance use or a chronic illness. By contrast, secondary insomnias are those that are caused by a specific underlying condition, such as a chronic illness, a psychiatric disorder, substance abuse, or a sleep disorder other than primary insomnia.

Primary Insomnias

According to the International Classification of Sleep Disorders, there are three subtypes of primary insomnia:

- Psychophysiological insomnia
- Sleep-state misperception
- Idiopathic (childhood onset) insomnia

Psychophysiological insomnia

Psychophysiological insomnia is the equivalent of DSM-IV defined primary insomnia. It involves two central components: learned sleep-preventing habits and somatized tension. Learned sleep-preventing habits are established by pairing sleeplessness with location (bed/bedroom), time (expected bedtime), and behavioral stimuli (e.g., bedtime rituals) that are normally associated with sleep. As a result, a conditioned response develops as a result of pairing wakefulness with typical sleep triggers.

Somatized tension is thought to involve internalization or suppression of daily stress, anxiety, and psychological conflicts that are not directly acknowledged by the individual but at the same time are incompatible with sleep. Thus, there is a fair degree of variability in terms of the extent of insomnia from night to night.

Sleep-state misperception

Sleep-state misperception is defined as an individual's perception of poor sleep that is not corroborated by abnormal polysomnographic findings nor is a reflection of psychopathology or malingering.

Idiopathic insomnia

Idiopathic insomnia is of unknown origin and usually has its onset in childhood and persists throughout adulthood. This form of insomnia is associated with objective measures of sleep disturbance and daytime consequences, including difficulties with memory, concentration, and motivation that are significant enough to interfere with occupational and social functioning. It is one of the most difficult forms of insomnia to treat. Unlike the other primary insomnias, it is not characterized by temporal variability and is not associated with observations of somatization, or with significant amounts of emotional distress. It occurs in the absence of psychological trauma during childhood and it is not associated with a specific medical disorder. Some have speculated that this type of insomnia may be associated with an underlying neurological abnormality that affects sleep/wake mechanisms, since this condition has been observed in individuals with diagnoses of learning disabilities, attention-deficit hyperactivity disorder, and similar conditions that have a neurological basis.

Secondary Insomnias

Secondary insomnias are defined as insomnias that arise as a result of a condition other than primary insomnia. These can involve sleep disorders other than primary insomnia as well as psychiatric disorders, substance abuse, and chronic illnesses. The sleep disorders that involve secondary insomnias include:

- Circadian rhythm disorders
- Narcolepsy
- Sleep apnea
- Periodic limb movements
- Restless leg syndrome
- Parasomnias

Circadian rhythm disorders

Circadian rhythms are the biological and behavioral functions of the body that occur in a distinctive pattern within an approximate time frame of 24 hours. These biological and behavioral rhythms are reflected in daily variations in sleep, waking, body temperature, and the secretion and regulation of hormones that are critical to sleep, such as cortisol, melatonin, and growth hormone. An individual's ability to sleep, as well as the quality and efficiency of his or her sleep, are intimately linked to these biological and behavioral rhythms. Circadian rhythms are regulated by the hypothalamus, which aids in the secretion and regulation of sleep hormones and responds to environmental cues that predispose an individual toward sleep (Morin and Espie 2003). One of the strongest of these cues is the light-dark cycle. Daily visual exposure to direct sunlight reminds the brain to be wakeful during daytime hours, whereas darkness signals the brain to sleep (Hickie and Davenport 1999). Other environmental cues include physical activity levels, social interactions, and work schedules. These should peak during midday hours and decline into the evening to allow for a drop in body temperature (a prerequisite for sleep). The relationship between meal times and sleep is an additional environmental cue that is incorporated into the sleep-wake cycle.

Other variables that serve to disrupt or maintain regular homeostasis within the body can also contribute to the onset and maintenance of sleep. As just mentioned, body temperature varies according to a circadian rhythm and is closely linked to the sleep-wake cycle (Hickie and Davenport 1999). Body temperature begins to rise in the early morning (e.g., between 3:00 and 5:00 am). It typically peaks during the midday, drops slightly in late afternoon, and peaks again during the early evening hours (Hickie and Davenport 1999). Peaks in body temperature generally correspond to the time of maximal cognitive alertness (Monk et al. 1983). As mentioned, a drop in body temperature during the evening hours is a prerequisite for sleepiness and sleep. It is important to keep in mind that body temperature is closely linked to physical activity levels. As physical activity increases, so does body temperature. Once elevated, it can take time for body temperature to drop. This is why it is typically recommended that clients with sleep onset difficulties engage in maximal activity levels or exercise during midday hours rather than during evening hours.

In addition to body temperature, the amount of sleep experienced during an individual's most recent sleep cycle can affect sleep onset and maintenance within the current sleep cycle (Morin 1993). Individuals that have slept for a longer-than-usual period of time the previous night will have greater difficulty falling asleep at the usual time the following evening. Individuals that have been deprived of sleep will demonstrate an increasingly strong drive to sleep as deprivation continues. Once they initiate sleep, these individuals experience a rebound effect characterized by a shorter time required to fall asleep, an increase in total sleep time, and a greater degree of time spent in stages 3 and 4 of NREM sleep (Morin and Espie 2001). Disruption in circadian rhythms can explain a large proportion of sleep dysfunction that occurs within the general population. When circadian rhythms are violated, the total length and continuity of the sleep episode are affected (Morin 1993). Both the speed of sleep onset and the likelihood of entering or remaining in certain sleep stages are affected (Morin 1993).

Circadian rhythm disorders are biobehavioral disorders characterized by a mismatch between an individual's sleep-wake schedule and the typical schedule that is considered normative within society (Morin 1993). One of the central features of these disorders is that the individual desires to engage in sleep or remain awake during the times consistent with a normal schedule, but he or she simply cannot do so. There is a sense of lack of control over the sleep-wake schedule (Morin 1993). Once an individual reaches sleep, he or she typically does not have a problem maintaining sleep. Circadian rhythm disorders may be caused by night-shift work, changing time zones, or an intrinsic chronobiological process (e.g., phase-delay syndrome or phase-advance syndrome). Phase-delay syndrome is defined as an inability to fall asleep until late night or early morning hours (e.g., 3:00 am). Phase-advance syndrome is defined as an inability to stay awake during earlier evening hours (e.g., 8:00 or 9:00 pm) coupled with early-morning awakening. Circadian rhythm disorders can be differentiated from psychophysiological insomnia in that they do not involve a learned component and there is typically no evidence of accompanying somaticized tension (Morin 1993). Circadian rhythm disorders are typically treated by making adjustments to an individual's peak times of maximal physical, occupational, and social activity and adjusting the amount of exposure to direct sunlight (e.g., light therapy).

Narcolepsy

Narcolepsy is a disabling sleep disorder characterized by excessive daytime sleepiness (100 percent of individuals), fragmented nighttime sleep (90 percent of individuals), cataplexy (80 percent of individuals), hypnagogic hallucinations (70 percent of individuals), sleep paralysis (60 percent of individuals), and automatic behaviors (50 percent of individuals) (Feldman 2003). Excessive daytime sleepiness is defined as daytime sleep episodes that occur at inappropriate and unexpected times. Fragmented nighttime sleep is characterized by disruption in healthy sleep architecture and frequent awakenings. Cataplexy involves a sudden loss of muscle tone that may be reflected in a sagging jaw, inclined head, slurred speech, buckling of the knees, or even collapse. Hypnagogic hallucinations are bizarre or frightening visual experiences, which sometimes have auditory and sensory components. Sleep paralysis is characterized by an inability to move for seconds or minutes during sleep onset or when transitioning to wakefulness. Automatic behaviors occur when sleep has partially overtaken the brain, but the body continues to perform familiar tasks. It is accompanied by reterograde amnesia and manifests itself in terms of brief lapses during conversation or during routenized activities, like walking or driving. Narcolepsy is estimated to occur in approximately one in every 2,000 individuals residing within the United States (Feldman 2003). It is thought to be associated with a deficiency of the neurotransmitter hypocretin.

Sleep apnea

Sleep apnea both exists as a primary sleep disorder and is comorbid with a number of chronic illnesses. It is a condition characterized by impaired breathing during sleep. Individuals with sleep apnea experience snoring, abrupt and temporary cessation of breathing during sleep, frequent awakenings during sleep, and excessive daytime sleepiness (Morin 1993). There are three main types sleep apnea, which are classified according to causal factors:

- Central
- Obstructive
- Mixed

Central sleep apnea is caused by a disruption in the regulation of airflow and a ceasing of respiratory movements that is linked to neurological dysfunction. Obstructive sleep apnea does not involve a cessation of respiratory activity but instead involves obstruction of effective airflow. Mixed sleep apnea involves both central (cessation of respiration) and obstructive (blockage of adequate airflow) processes. Generally, the cycle begins with a brief cessation of breathing that lasts at least 10 seconds. This is followed by arousal (a state of near-wakefulness), a period of breathing that involves snoring and gasping, and a return to sleep (Morin 1993). Sleep apnea is diagnosed by polysomnography according to criteria that involve the frequency and duration of the episodes of apnea. The presence of complications arising from the apnea, such as the lack of adequate oxygen in red blood cells, cardiac arrythmias, and memory and concentration difficulties, is also considered. Sleep apnea is estimated to occur in between 4 percent and 9 percent of women and between 9 percent and 24 percent of men (Friedman et al., 2001; Kutty 2004). Rates are higher in individuals with chronic illnesses.

Periodic limb movements

Periodic limb movements are defined as repetitive and stereotypic movements of the legs and arms lasting up to 5 seconds and occurring repeatedly every 20–40 seconds (Morin 1993; Montplaisir and Godbout 1989). Periodic limb movements are associated with sleep onset difficulty, arousals with fragmentation of the sleep profile, nocturnal awakenings, associated daytime sleepiness, and leg cramps (Happe 2003). They typically occur during stages 1 and 2 of NREM sleep and may be associated with arousal or awakening (Comella 2002). Periodic limb movements are common in individuals with chronic illnesses that involve lower extremity pain, renal disease, and other conditions characterized by poor circulation, such as diabetes (Morin 1993). Periodic limb movements are experienced only during sleep and most individuals with this condition are unaware that they have it unless notified by a bed partner.

Restless leg syndrome

Restless leg syndrome is experienced when an individual is awake during the day and, in particular, just prior to sleep. It is characterized by pain and aching in the calves and a compelling desire to move one's legs. This pain and urge to move may also occur in the feet, knees, thighs, and arms (Morin 1993). Walking or stretching usually reduces the pain, at least on a temporary basis. Approximately 94 percent of individuals with restless leg syndrome report symptoms of sleep-onset insomnia, prolonged sleep latency, reduced total sleep time, frequent night-time awakenings, and excessive daytime sleepiness (Comella 2002; Happe 2003). Objective findings typically reveal decreased slow wave sleep and decreased overall sleep efficiency. Restless leg syndrome is frequently associated with periodic limb movements in sleep (Comella 2002).

Parasomnias

Parasomnias reflect excessive or abnormal central nervous system activation and typically involve changes in autonomic or skeletal muscle activity. They include nightmares, sleep terrors, sleepwalking, and other abnormal behaviors during sleep, such as rhythmic movement disorders (e.g., head banging or rocking). Depending upon when they occur during the sleep cycle, parasomnias may involve excessive states of arousal, difficulties with sleep-wake transition, or dysfunctions of REM sleep. Parasomnias are more common in childhood than in adulthood.

Chronic Illnesses Involving Secondary Insomnia

In addition to the specific sleep disorders reviewed in the previous section, secondary insomnia is a key symptom of a wide range of other chronic illnesses. In individuals with chronic illness, sleep dysfunction is associated with a number of variables, including:

- Features of the illness itself,
- Secondary symptoms or conditions associated with the illness,
- Side effects of treatments and medications, and
- Psychological, behavioral, and lifestyle variables that occur in tandem with the chronic illness (Morin 1993).

This section will provide a general overview of the prevalence and nature of sleep dysfunction in some of the more common chronic illnesses. The conditions that will be covered in this review were selected because they are among the more prevalent conditions that involve sleep dysfunction as a primary symptom. They include:

- Asthma and other pulmonary diseases
- Arthritis
- Cancer
- Chronic Fatigue Syndrome
- Epilepsy
- Fibromyalgia
- Gastroesophageal reflux disease (GERD, acid reflux)

- Head injury
- Heart and cardiovascular diseases
- HIV/AIDS
- Myasthenia gravis
- Parkinson's disease
- Renal (kidney) disease
- Sjogren's syndrome
- Thyroid disease

Asthma and Other Pulmonary Diseases

Asthma and other pulmonary diseases, described in Chapter 14, are almost invariably associated with sleep dysfunction (Morin 1993; Williams 1988; Wooten 1989). Approximately 74 percent of individuals with asthma wake up during the night at least once a week because of asthma and roughly 64 percent wake up at least three times per week (Lewis 2001). Individuals with asthma are twice as likely to report difficulties initiating sleep, early morning awakenings, and excessive daytime sleepiness than those without asthma (Lewis 2001). The sleep difficulties observed in people with asthma have been linked to an increased tendency to have asthma symptoms (e.g., cough, wheezing, chest tightness) and a decline in lung function at nighttime, with the worst symptoms occurring in the early morning hours (Lewis 2001). These changes in airway resistance at nighttime may be associated with circadian rhythm changes (Lewis 2001).

Similar to findings in studies of asthma, studies of stable outpatients with chronic obstructive pulmonary disease (COPD) demonstrate a high prevalence of reported sleep dysfunction. More than 40 percent of individuals with COPD report difficulty sleeping always or almost always (Lewis 2001). Difficulty initiating or maintaining sleep, and nonrestorative sleep in COPD has been attributed to disordered sleep architecture, hypoventilation, disturbed gas exchange, and medication-related sleep deprivation (Kutty 2004). In addition to pulmonary symptoms, common treatments for pulmonary conditions, many of which contain steroids, also cause insomnia, nonrestorative sleep, and excessive daytime sleepiness. The link between bronchodilators and insomnia is discussed in more detail later.

Arthritis

Information on osteoarthritis and rheumatoid arthritis is provided in Chapters 14 and 16. Any disorder involving chronic musculoskeletal pain, including all forms of arthritis, is likely to be associated with sleep dysfunction (Follick, Smith, and Ahern 1985; Morin 1993). Up to two-thirds of individuals with rheumatoid arthritis report chronic sleep difficulties (Nicassio and Wallston 1992; Taibi, Bourguignon, and Taylor 2004). Approximately 57 percent report that their sleep is restless most of the time, 60 percent report that arthritis interferes with their sleep on a mild-to-moderate level, and 14 percent report that arthritis interferes with their sleep on a severe or very severe level (Nicassio and Wallston 1992).

Awakening during the night is often accompanied by getting out of bed to stretch and move around in order to relieve the joint stiffness and pain that has occurred sleep (Nicassio and Wallston 1992). Research indicates that individuals with rheumatoid arthritis are more likely to have difficulties maintaining sleep than initiating sleep (Nicassio and Wallston 1992). Various aspects of arthritis can contribute to sleep dysfunction, including chronic pain that interferes with the ability to sleep, disruption of normal circadian rhythms, increased likelihood of having a primary sleep disorder, and disrupted immune function (i.e., excessive production of proinflammatory cytokines) (Taibi, Bourguigon, and Taylor 2004).

Cancer

A brief description of cancer is presented in Chapter 14. Irrespective of the stage, type, or means by which cancer is being treated, sleep dysfunction is frequently and consistently experienced by individuals with cancer. One study of veterans with cancer found that 45 percent reported symptoms of sleep-onset insomnia (Chang et al. 2000). Of the 45 percent that reported insomnia, 13 percent rated this symptom as moderate, 18 percent rated it as severe, and 20 percent described severe distress resulting from insomnia. In another study, between 30 percent and 50 percent of individuals newly diagnosed with cancer or recently treated for cancer reported insomnia (Savard and Morin 2001). High rates of insomnia persisted in 23 percent to 44 percent of the sample two-to-five years following treatment (Savard and Morin 2001). These findings suggest that insomnia assumes a chronic course in many individuals with cancer (Savard and Morin 2001).

Chronic Fatigue Syndrome

Chronic fatigue syndrome is described in Chapter 14. Primary sleep disorders that are not being effectively treated, such as narcolepsy or sleep apnea, can exclude an individual from receiving a diagnosis of chronic fatigue syndrome (Fukuda et al., 1994). However, nonspecific symptoms of sleep dysfunction are common among individuals with this syndrome and do not prevent an individual from receiving a CDC-defined diagnosis of chronic fatigue syndrome (Fukuda et al., 1994).

Nonrestorative sleep is one of the key diagnostic symptoms of the condition (Fukuda et al., 1994). In addition to nonrestorative sleep, roughly 53 percent of individuals with chronic fatigue syndrome report sleep-onset insomnia, and 19 percent report early morning awakenings (Komaroff et al., 1996). The causes and functional implications of sleep-related symptoms in chronic fatigue syndrome are currently unknown.

Epilepsy

Virtually any disorder affecting the central nervous system, including epilepsy, will involve sleep dysfunction (Morin 1993). Epilepsy describes a range of neurological disorders characterized by recurrent seizures that are caused by abnormal electrical activity in the brain. Seizures may arise for a variety of reasons, including damage to the brain caused by infection, injury, birth trauma, tumor, stroke, drug use, and chemical imbalance. In epilepsy, sleep is most commonly disrupted by seizures and/or symptoms of sleep apnea (Bazil 2000). One study found that approximately 54 percent of individuals with epilepsy also have a diagnosis of sleep apnea (Bazil 2000).

Fibromyalgia

A brief description of fibromyalgia is presented in Chapter 14. Perhaps because its etiology remains unknown, the role of sleep as a potential etiological variable in fibromyalgia has been studied extensively. Sleep dysfunction and primary sleep disorders are highly prevalent among individuals with fibromyalgia. Unrefreshing sleep has been described as an important component of fibromyalgia (Moldofsky 2002). In addition to unrefreshing sleep, between 29 percent and 33 percent of individuals with fibromyalgia have a primary sleep disorder (Manu et al. 1994; Moldofsky, 2002). The most prevalent disorders observed include sleep apnea, periodic limb movements, restless leg syndrome, and narcolepsy (Manu et al. 1994; Moldofsky, 2002).

Some argue that primary sleep disorders (e.g., restless leg syndrome, periodic limb movements, sleep apnea) serve as the underlying cause of fibromyalgia (Harvey, Cadena, and Dunlap 1993). However, this hypothesis is not well established nor is it uniformly accepted within the research community. The precise explanation for the sleep difficulties observed in fibromyalgia is currently unknown. However, research on human growth hormone suggests that some individuals with fibromyalgia have a clinically significant deficiency in growth hormone (Moldofsky 2002). Other research suggests that immunological variables may serve as the primary contributors (Moldofsky 1993).

Other disorders that involve chronic pain of unknown origin are also strongly associated with sleep dysfunction. One study of 170 individuals with chronic pain found that 75 percent reported that a disruption in their sleep had occurred within the past one to two weeks and 59 percent reported that they felt direct negative consequences of their sleep disturbance on their health and well-being the following day (Iverson and McCracken 1997).

Gastroesophageal Reflux Disease (GERD, Acid Reflux)

Gastroesophageal reflux disease, commonly referred to as "acid reflux" or "GERD," is described in Chapter 20. Research indicates that GERD causes sleep onset insomnia, frequent nighttime awakenings, and excessive daytime sleepiness. GERD during sleep, which often involves waking up with acid or vomit in the mouth, can be exacerbated when individuals drink milk or eat a meal close to bedtime. Approximately 75 percent of individuals with acid reflux report that their symptoms interfere with their sleep (Shaker et al. 2003).

Head injury

Though various forms of head injury exist, all head injuries directly involve injury to the brain. Sleep dysfunction is the most common symptom of minor head injury and often persists for up to one month following the injury (Haboubi et al., 2001). In addition, excessive daytime sleepiness occurs in approximately one-third of individuals with head injury and sleep apnea is diagnosed in approximately 12 percent. Sleep disturbance in individuals with head injury is centrally mediated. Chronic headache and pain also contribute to sleep difficulties in individuals with head injury.

Heart and Cardiovascular Diseases

Information on heart and cardiovascular diseases is provided in Chapter 14. Among individuals with congestive heart failure, approximately 11 percent have a diagnosis of obstructive sleep apnea and 40 percent have a diagnosis of central sleep apnea (Javaheri et al. 1998). Similarly, approximately 50 percent of individuals with coronary heart disease show evidence of clinically significant obstructive sleep apnea (Parish and Sommers 2004). Among individuals with heart and cardiovascular diseases, the development of obstructive sleep apnea is attributable to hypertension and its effects on left ventricular function (Sin et al., 1999).

Sleep dysfunction is also prevalent among individuals that have experienced a stroke. Individuals that have experienced a hemispheric stroke are significantly more likely to have sleep dysfunction than individuals of similar age that have not experienced a stroke (Parish and Somers 2004). Approximately 80 percent of individuals that have had a stroke develop obstructive sleep apnea (Parish and Somers 2004). In addition to the diseases themselves, antihypertensive medications used to treat heart and blood pressure problems also contribute to higher rates of sleep dysfunction.

HIV/AIDS

HIV/AIDS is described in Chapter 14. Individuals with HIV/AIDS experience a wide range of sleep difficulties and disorders. Approximately 73 percent of individuals with HIV have at least one symptom of sleep dysfunction (Rubinstein and Selwyn 1998). Immunological variables and opportunistic infections that affect the central nervous system are hypothesized to be responsible for a significant proportion of sleep dysfunction among individuals with HIV/AIDS (Rubinstein and Selwyn 1998).

Myasthenia Gravis

Myasthenia Gravis is described in Chapter 14. Sleep dysfunction is highly prevalent among individuals with this condition. It is characterized by frequent arousals, awakenings, and symptoms of excessive daytime sleepiness. Sleep apnea is responsible for a significant degree of sleep dysfunction in individuals with myasthenia gravis, occurring in up to 75 percent of individuals with this condition. In this condition, sleep apnea is thought to be of central type and to occur almost exclusively during REM sleep (Happe 2003).

Parkinson's Disease

Parkinson's disease is a neurodegenerative disorder that affects movement. Primary motor symptoms include bradykinesia/akinesia (slow or absent movement), rigidity (stiffness of the limbs and joints), tremor (involuntary rhythmic shaking of a limb, the head, mouth or tongue; or the entire body), and postural instability (impaired balance and coordination). Parkinson's disease is caused by a degeneration of dopaminergic cells in the substantia nigra, which leads to loss and deficit of dopamine. Individuals with Parkinson's disease are seven times more likely to experience unexpected sleep attacks as compared with healthy controls (Happe 2003). Other sleep symptoms include other symptoms of narcolepsy, sleep apnea, and REM sleep behavior disorder (Happe 2003). Because this disease is centrally mediated, the neurodegenerative process itself affects elements of the reticular activating system (Happe 2003). In addition to disease progression, mood disorders and higher dosages of medications that affect dopamine levels also contribute to sleep dysfunction in Parkinson's disease.

Renal (Kidney) Disease

General information about renal diseases was provided in Chapter 16. Approximately 65 percent of individuals with end-stage renal disease report at least one problem with sleep (Mucsi et al. 2004). Restless sleep is reported by approximately 56 percent of individuals with renal disease, restless leg syndrome is reported by approximately 15 percent, and periodic limb movements are reported by approximately 30 percent (McCann and Boore 2000; Mucsi et al., 2004). These symptoms and disorders are linked to the circulatory problems and pain characteristic of renal disease.

Sjogren's Syndrome

Sjogren's syndrome is described in Chapter 14. Sleep disturbance in Sjogren's syndrome primarily involves difficulties initiating and maintaining sleep due to symptoms of muscular tension and restless leg syndrome (Gudbjornsson et al. 1993).

Thyroid Disease

General information about thyroid disease is provided in Chapter 14. Insomnia is one of the primary symptoms of primary hyperthyroidism, or overactive thyroid. Hyperthyroidism can be secondary to other thyroid diseases in that it can arise from irregularities or changes in the dosages of medications used to treat hypothyroidism.

Other Variables Affecting Healthy Sleep Architecture

In addition to chronic illness, there are a number of other variables that can interfere with or alter the sleep architecture ideal described above. These include:

- Aging
- Lifestyle and habit patterns
- Environmental contributors
- Psychiatric disorders and stress
- Prescribed medications, other drugs, and alcohol

Aging

As individuals age, their sleep patterns change gradually but dramatically (Morin 1993). Newborns require approximately 16 to 18 hours of sleep per day (Hauri 1982). As an individual progresses through childhood and into adolescence, he or she requires approximately 9.5 hours of sleep (Morin and Espie 2001). In early adulthood, sleep time decreases to between 7 and 8.5 hours per night (Morin and Espie 2001). As an individual ages, REM sleep time decreases from 50 percent in newborns to 25 percent in young adults (Hauri 1982). In addition, time spent in stages 3 and 4 of NREM sleep decreases and the number of awakenings during sleep increases. After the age of 40, the total amount of nocturnal sleep continues to be reduced to approximately 7 hours per night, the number of nocturnal awakenings increase, there is greater reduction of time spent in stages 3 and 4 of NREM sleep, and more time spent in stages 1 and 2 of NREM sleep (Morin and Espie 2001). To compensate for this disruption, older adults may nap during the day or spend more time in bed awake. This can lead to decreased sleep efficiency and a greater likelihood of overall sleep dysfunction (Morin and Espie 2001).

Habit Patterns

A number of habit patterns can have significant sleep-related consequences, in part because of their effects on normal circadian rhythms. These include: napping during the day, exercising too close to bedtime (e.g., later than early evening hours), use of caffeine, nicotine, and alcohol late in the evening, and eating a heavy meal late in the evening.

Environmental Contributors

There are myriad features within an individual's physical environment that can contribute to sleep difficulties, including room temperature, light, sound or noise, an uncomfortable mattress, or a bed partner that moves or snores. Individuals differ widely in the extent to which their sleep is affected by environmental contributors such as these.

Psychiatric Disorders and Stress

There is a well-supported association between psychiatric disorders and sleep dysfunction (Morin and Espie 2004). Despite this linkage, the distinction between psychiatric disorders and sleep dysfunction is not always clear and the causal relationship between psychiatric symptoms and sleep dysfunction is not yet known. Research indicates that more than three-quarters of individuals with currently active psychiatric disorders also have sleep dysfunction (Sweetwood et al. 1980). Likewise, studies of individuals with insomnia have found that approximately 30 percent to 40 percent also have at least one psychiatric disorder (Coleman et al., 1982; Ford and Kamerow 1989; Jacobs et al., 1988; Kales, et al., 1983; Mellinger et al., 1985; Morin 1993; Tan et al., 1984).

Various forms of sleep dysfunction, including sleep-onset insomnia, sleep-maintenance insomnia, hypersomnia, nightmares, night terrors, nocturnal panic attacks, and early-morning awakenings, all represent symptoms of a wide range of psychiatric disorders. Mood disorders (e.g., major depressive disorders, bipolar disorders) anxiety disorders (e.g., generalized anxiety disorder, post-traumatic stress disorder, panic disorder) and substance abuse are the three psychiatric disorders most likely to involve sleep dysfunction.

Psychotic disorders and dementia also involve sleep dysfunction that is characterized by a reversal of the sleep-wake cycle, frequently awakenings during nighttime sleep, and frequent intrusive sleep episodes during the day. The "sundowner's syndrome," characterized by nighttime wanderings and confusion, is experienced by approximately 45 percent of individuals with Alzheimer's disease (Happe 2003). It is one example of a reversal in the sleep-wake cycle that may relate to a centrally mediated circadian rhythm disturbance (Volicer et al., 2001).

In addition to psychiatric disorders, sleep is highly sensitive to stressful life events and to acute states of emotional distress. Morin, Rodrigue and Ivers (2003) found that both major life events (e.g., death of a loved one, divorce) and minor daily stressors (e.g., pressure at work, interpersonal conflict) were linked to a higher state of arousal prior to sleep onset and during nighttime awakenings. Dysfunctional cognitions about sleep, such as undue anxiety about the consequences of not getting enough sleep, can exacerbate existing sleep dysfunction.

Prescribed Medications, Other Drugs, and Alcohol

A wide range of prescribed medications, other drugs, and alcohol can affect the sleep cycle. One study found that side effects of medications were responsible for 68 percent of complaints of insomnia in an inpatient sample (Berlin et al., 1984). Some medications and drugs cause insomnia (difficulties getting to sleep and/or sleeping too little). Others can induce sleep, help maintain sleep, or cause daytime drowsiness. Others exert effects on certain stages of sleep by either suppressing them or shortening them (Morin 1993). Some of these effects are temporary and only accompany short-term administration of the medications. When some of these medications or drugs are used on a long-term basis, their effects on sleep may be attenuated or they may disappear altogether as the body adapts to them over time. For example, long-term use of hypnotic drugs for the treatment of insomnia ultimately produces tolerance and a decrease in overall effectiveness in initiating and maintaining sleep. This can lead individuals to increase their intake of hypnotics, but this eventually results in secondary symptoms of daytime drowsiness and sedation. Withdrawal from hypnotics can lead to an increase in the severity of insomnia that far exceeds that experienced before the client began taking the hypnotics. This cycle is commonly referred to as "drug-dependent insomnia" (Morin 1993).

When working with and educating individuals with sleep dysfunction related to medication usage, knowledge of which drugs are most likely to have acute side effects on sleep that gradually disappear with time, versus drugs that are likely to have a continued impact on sleep, is important. In addition, the time of day during which certain medications and drugs are taken can affect the degree to which a particular substance will influence sleep. Medications, drugs, and alcohol that are taken closer to bedtime will have the greatest effect on sleep. If a client has difficulty with sleep onset or maintenance, medications that are likely to induce or sustain sleep are most appropriately administered close to bedtime. Accordingly, medications that are likely to produce insomnia as a side effect or are likely to interfere with the overall quality or maintenance of sleep should not be taken close to bedtime.

Many psychotropic medications used to treat mood disorders, anxiety disorders, and psychotic disorders also have effects on sleep. Because of this feature, some benzodiazepines, other drugs with antianxiety properties, and some antidepressants are prescribed in the absence of a primary psychiatric disorder and for the sole purpose of treating a sleep disorder. However, these medications invariably affect healthy sleep architecture. As such, they should not be regarded as a substitute for healthy sleep. In some cases, they can become addictive, cause daytime drowsiness, be associated with rebound effects or paradoxical effects (e.g., insomnia upon withdrawal), and/or lose their effectiveness over time (Gillin, Spinweber, and Johnson 1989; Kales and Kales 1984; Morin 1993). For example, benzodiazepines, which are commonly prescribed to promote sleep continuity, generally serve to decrease the amount of time spent in deep (stage 3 and 4) sleep and increase the amount of time spent in lighter (stage 1 and 2) sleep (Morin and Espie 2001). Some antidepressant medications (particularly those that are used to treat symptoms of anxiety or mixed anxiety-depressive disorders) have sedating features and are commonly prescribed for insomnia. Certain mood stabilizers commonly used to treat bipolar disorders can also serve to induce and maintain sleep. Other antidepressants that are used to treat more vegetative sub-types of depression are designed to stimulate energy and can cause insomnia.

A number of other medications used to treat chronic illnesses have sleep-related side effects. For example, bronchodilators and steroids prescribed for the treatment of pulmonary conditions (e.g., asthma) are known to cause insomnia, particularly when administered close to bedtime. One study found that individuals with chronic pulmonary disease that were treated with bronchodilators reported twice as many sleep disturbances than those who were not treated with bronchodilators (Gislason and Almqvist 1987). Other steroids and medications containing steroids used to treat a wide range of conditions that involve inflammatory processes (e.g., Crohn's disease, multiple sclerosis) can serve as stimulants and can cause insomnia. Certain medications used to treat high blood pressure (i.e., antihypertensives), particularly certain beta blockers, may produce feelings of sedation during the day and yet may also produce difficulties with sleep onset and maintenance at night (Betts and Alford 1983; Morin 1993; Rosen and Kostis 1985). Diuretics and certain thyroid medications have also been linked to insomnia (Morin 1993).

Alcohol, which serves as a depressant to the central nervous system, can lead to an initial period of sedation and deeper sleep earlier in the night, followed by an increased number of awakenings throughout the night, REM rebound effects, and early-morning awakening (Morin 1993). Many individuals use alcohol as a sleep aid, restricting their use to the period just before sleeping for the specific purpose of promoting sleepiness and sedation prior to bedtime. Ultimately, this leads to disruption in the continuity of the sleep cycle. If used daily to promote sleep for three weeks or longer, a condition known as "alcohol-dependent insomnia" may be diagnosed. Many individuals are not aware that they have this condition at first because of the initial, sedating effects of the alcohol in the earlier phases of sleep. In addition to alcohol use, stimulants that affect the central nervous system (e.g., caffeine, cocaine, amphetamines, appetite suppressants, and nicotine) can interfere with sleep onset and/or maintenance and can suppress REM sleep.

This section provided only general guidelines for thinking about the potential effects of certain prescribed medications, other drugs, and alcohol on sleep. Before cognitive behavioral treatment of sleep dysfunction begins, it is essential for the therapist to gather the client's medical records, obtain a history of current and past medication, other drug, and alcohol usage, and consult actively with all prescribing physicians from whom the client is currently receiving care. Active communication with the client about his or her perception of drug side effects, in addition to ongoing collaboration with physicians that are knowledgeable about the pharmacological properties of medications and their side effects, are important adjunctive elements of cognitive behavioral treatment for sleep dysfunction.

Consequences of Sleep Dysfunction: Implications for Cognitive Behavioral Therapy

The consequences of sleep dysfunction depend on the extent of sleep deprivation and its duration. They can be physiological (changes in key hormone levels), physical (impairment in motor skills), cognitive (impairment in attention, judgment, creativity, short-term memory, and concentration), and emotional (mood swings, depression, and anxiety). Acute sleep deprivation is short-term in nature (e.g., one night) and may be caused by a voluntary need to continue working to complete a task or by insomnia related to a stressful life event, illness, or injury. Total acute sleep deprivation has been found to result in an increased drive to sleep and day-time drowsiness. In addition, as the time period of total sleep deprivation increases beyond one night, individuals experience daytime micro-episodes of sleep, difficulties sustaining attention and concentration, slowed reaction times, decreased judgment, creativity, and mental flexibility, and an increased risk for major accidents (Dinges 1995; Happe 2003; Morin and Espie 2003). Individuals may also become more irritable and demonstrate decreased motivation. When it occurs on a regular basis, partial sleep deprivation, or sleeping fewer hours than necessary, is associated with similar outcomes.

The consequences of insomnia are distinct from the consequences of total and partial sleep deprivation. In most cases of chronic insomnia, subjective reports of sleep loss are not typically correlated with objective evidence of excessive day-time sleepiness, such as daytime micro-episodes of sleep at unexpected or inappropriate times (Morin and Espie 2003). Although insomnia is associated with symptoms of severe daytime fatigue, people with insomnia, most typically, are unable to sleep or nap during the daytime. Instead, insomnia is thought to be characterized as a chronic state of arousal or hypervigilance (Morin and Espie 2003). In addition, the subjective reports of severe and significant difficulties with attention, short-term memory, and concentration are not always corroborated by objective evidence of these types of cognitive impairment (Vignola et al., 2000). Although chronic forms of insomnia may have limited or minimal effects on cognitive functioning, individuals with insomnia do experience significant limitations to overall quality of life. These limitations stem from the fatigue, mood disturbances, and impaired occupational and social functioning that are often associated with insomnia.

In terms of physical health, insomnia appears to have no significant effects on health and mortality. Though it has been suggested that individuals with unusually short (i.e., four hours or less) or unusually long (i.e., 10 hours or more) sleep duration have higher rates of mortality, insomnia itself is not associated with increased mortality (Morin and Espie 2003). Moreover, the nonspecific physical and cognitive symptoms commonly reported by individuals with insomnia have not been linked to the development of any specific diseases or chronic illnesses. Some research has found that chronic sleep deprivation is associated with changes in endocrine (e.g., growth hormone, cortisol, and melatonin levels) and immune (e.g., immune suppression) function (Savard et al., 2003). However, the long-term effects and clinical implications of these consequences are not known.

Conveying to clients that the physical health consequences of insomnia are not significant is a key educational piece of the cognitive behavioral therapy process. Some individuals with insomnia tend to report fears that their sleep difficulties will have profound consequences for their physical health. Some may interpret the nonspecific physical symptoms that often accompany their insomnia as indicators that the insomnia is exerting long-lasting and damaging effects on the body. This may lead to an increase in dysfunctional cognitions about sleep and sleep-related anxiety. Accordingly, it is important that therapists be knowledgeable about the distinctions between the consequences of insomnia (e.g., fatigue, mood changes, and decreased quality of life) and the consequences of total and partial sleep deprivation (e.g., objectively measurable signs of excessive daytime sleepiness, cognitive and motor dysfunction) is critical when designing cognitive behavioral therapy interventions for sleep dysfunction (Morin and Espie 2003).

Conclusion

This chapter provided an overview of the prevalence of sleep dysfunction and sleep disorders within the general population and among individuals with various chronic illnesses. It described common ways in which sleep dysfunction is sub classified and experienced. In addition, basic information about a number of conditions for which sleep dysfunction is a primary symptom was provided, and the role of sleep in each condition was described. The next chapter provides a case study of Curtis, who has difficulties with insomnia secondary to his cancer and depression. It will also highlight some assessment and intervention considerations for the person with insomnia.

19

Cognitive Behavioral Assessment and Treatment Outcomes for Sleep Dysfunction: The Case of Curtis

Chapter 18 described normal sleep and presented sleep disorder as a major symptom category. It discussed the prevalence of sleep disorders, and some of their causes. It also overviewed common chronic conditions associated with sleep dysfunction. This chapter will illustrate the application of cognitive behavioral therapy to Curtis, who was introduced in Chapter 1 and periodically discussed throughout the text.

The aim of this case presentation is twofold. First, it will synthesize the earlier examples of Curtis, discussing the case as a whole and illustrating outcomes. Second, this chapter will illustrate unique assessment and intervention approaches that can be incorporated into cognitive behavioral therapy with the person who has a sleep disorder. In this regard, the chapter will illustrate assessments that in the author's experience are useful for the client with a sleep disorder. Copies of the assessments developed by the author for use with persons who have sleep disorders are reproduced in the Appendix of this chapter. It should also be noted that this chapter will illustrate cognitive behavioral strategies that are specific to the treatment of the person with a sleep disorder. The chapter will close with an overview of the unique considerations in treating individuals with sleep disorders.

As noted in Chapter 1, Curtis is a 60-year-old man with advanced prostate cancer (Stage T3, Gleason Score = 8) and secondary insomnia. Curtis was referred for cognitive behavioral therapy by his urologist to address his sleep difficulties. Curtis initially felt he did not need therapy. However, after he discovered that his cancer was inoperable, he accepted the referral with a hope that he would learn how to manage his difficulties with sleeping. Detailed information about Curtis' background and health history was presented in Chapter 1.

Initial Orientation, Approach to Assessment and Assessment Findings

Curtis completed the initial orientation and assessment within two sessions. Medical records and verbal information from Curtis' urologist, oncologist, and sleep specialist were collected. In addition, the following assessments were completed:

- Semistructured clinical interview
- Problem list
- Sleep rating form
- Sleep behavior and cognitions scale
- Occupational self assessment

These assessments were administered in the order listed. The semistructured interview and problem list were administered during the first session. Following instructions from the therapist, the sleep rating form, sleep behavior and cognitions scale, and occupational self assessment were administered as homework due the second session. Curtis completed all of the initial assessments without any difficulties. Findings from these assessments are presented in the sections that follow.

Orientation and Rapport-Building

At the beginning of therapy, Curtis appeared pleasant, relaxed, task-focused, and business-like. He occasionally made jokes with the therapist that reflected a degree of cynicism and dark humor about his health. He listened carefully to the therapist's introduction to the structure, process, and expectations of cognitive behavioral therapy. Although he was relatively quiet and did not ask many questions, he responded to the therapist's questions readily and appeared motivated to participate in a collaborative relationship.

Semistructured Clinical Interview

Because Curtis appeared comfortable and ready to begin the formal tasks of therapy, the therapist conducted the semistructured clinical interview during the first session. Interview questions were used to elicit information about the client's physical health history, present symptoms, level of impairment, adjustment to cancer, psychosocial history, and family background (reviewed in Chapter 1). Because the referral information suggested that Curtis had been experiencing depression, the therapist asked Curtis more detailed questions about his depressive symptoms. Curtis was not at risk for suicide. His depression appeared to be in partial remission at the time of the interview. Curtis reported that he found the new antidepressant medication that he was taking helpful in reducing his anxiety and improving his mood.

A semistructured interview format was selected so that the therapist could obtain additional information about Curtis' psychological and social functioning and his adjustment to having cancer. The therapist's rationale for dedicating an entire session to the interview was that this interview would allow Curtis to discuss other aspects of his life and concerns he might be having apart from his sleep difficulties. A goal of this initial interview was to allow him to feel more comfortable with self-disclosure so that he would be more likely to report any negative automatic thoughts and emotions during the course of therapy. It also served to set a precedent for a collaborative relationship. During this interview, the therapist made a point to actively understand and empathize with Curtis's sleep difficulties, ask basic psychiatric interview questions, validate his current emotional experience, and normalize his reactions to having cancer.

Problem List

During the initial clinical interview, Curtis completed a problem list. His highest priority problems were as follows:

- Difficulties sleeping
- Concerns about death and dying
- Economic problems
- Feeling a sense of distance from his wife and daughter
- Falling behind on household upkeep and chores

The therapist's selection of subsequent assessments was based on this problem list.

Sleep Rating Form

Curtis' top priority for therapy was to improve his sleep. Curtis had already completed a sleep study and the sleep specialist concluded that the exact cause of his secondary insomnia was unknown. Because the therapist had insufficient information about Curtis' daily sleep patterns, she requested that he complete a sleep rating form. This form was designed by the author to gather basic information about a client's daily sleep-wake cycle and sleep-related behaviors over a seven-day period. In the first column, the client writes the date or day of the week. The second column elicits a client's daily waking time. In the third column, the client documents the time at which he or she first got into bed and attempted to go to sleep. The fourth column requires the client to estimate the number of times he or she recalled waking from sleep that night. For the fifth column, the client is asked to estimate the total amount of time he or she spent sleeping that night. In the sixth column, the client documents any behaviors he or she engaged in when he or she could not sleep. The final column requires the client to document the number of naps taken during the day and to estimate the total amount of time spent in daytime sleep. Curtis' baseline responses are shown in Figure 1.

Curtis confirmed that the form was an accurate reflection of his daily sleep patterns. Results of this assessment indicated that, before therapy officially began, Curtis had an irregular sleep-wake cycle. For example, he was not waking up at the same time each day and he was spending more time in bed on weekends in an attempt to compensate for lost and disrupted sleep during the week. Similarly, Curtis was not going to bed at a consistent time each night. Though he was typically spending 8–11 hours in bed each night, his sleep efficiency was very poor and he was only sleeping an average of four to five hours per night.

Sleep Rating Form

Day	Wake-up Time	Time of first attempt to sleep	# times awoke from sleep	Total estimated hours of night sleep	What did I do if I could not sleep?	Number of naps & total day sleep
Mon.	6:00 am	11:00 pm	1	2	Went to living room to watch TV	1 (3 hrs.)
Tues.	7:30 am	9:00 pm	3	4	Lay in bed trying to sleep	2 (2 hr.)
Wed.	7:00 am	10:00 pm	2	3	Went to living room to watch TV	2 (4 hr.)
Thurs.	6:00 am	9:00 pm	3	3	Lay in bed trying to sleep	1 (30 min.)
Fri.	7:30 am	11:30 pm	1	5	Lay in bed trying to sleep	1 (15 min.)
Sat.	10:00am	11:30 pm	4	7	Lay in bed trying to sleep	0
Sun.	9:30 am	10:00 pm	1	9	Lay in bed trying to sleep	0

Consistent bed time?   ___ yes   X **no**   **Consistent waking time?**   ___ yes   X **no**

Average hours of sleep per night = 5 hours   **Average hours of nap time** = 1 ½ hours

FIGURE 1. Curtis' Sleep Rating Form at Baseline

When Curtis could not sleep, many times he would lie in bed feeling anxious and wondering when he would fall asleep. He reported that his wife did not like it when he left the bed at night because she often worried about him. In part, he remained in bed in order to ensure that his wife would not worry about him and also to lead her to believe that he was sleeping. Additionally, Curtis was sleeping quite a bit during his daytime work hours at the furniture store. He reported that he would often "steal time" on a bed in the lower level when no customers were around. When he would hear the door chime signal that a customer had entered, it would typically wake him up and give him time to get to the upper level. When he began therapy, Curtis did not realize that all of these behaviors only exacerbated his insomnia.

Sleep Behavior and Cognitions Scale

The therapist chose to administer the sleep behavior and cognitions scale in order to obtain more information about the nature and extent of Curtis' negative sleep cognitions and behaviors. The scale is a 23-item clinical measure developed by the author for use in practice. It contains 10 items that measure negative or dysfunctional attitudes, beliefs, and attributions about sleep (items 1, 2, 3, 6, 16, 17, 18, 19, 20, 23), eight items that measure dysfunctional behaviors related to sleep (items 4, 5, 7, 8, 9, 10, 11, 21) and five miscellaneous items that measure sleep-related anxiety and functional consequences of lost sleep (12, 13, 14, 15, 22). Because it is brief and offers an easy "true" or "false" response format, it can be administered rapidly during a session or assigned for homework. Generally, the number and nature of statements that a client endorses as "true" reflect the degree to which a given client's cognitions about sleep and behavioral responses to insomnia are dysfunctional.

A second strength of this scale is that it allows therapists and their clients (when appropriate) to use clinical judgment and contextual information about the client's illness to determine whether and how to address a potentially dysfunctional sleep behavior. For example, in some cases it may be appropriate for a client to take medications that serve to initiate and/or sustain sleep. Similarly, in certain circumstances it may be appropriate for some clients to nap during the day. Curtis' responses to this scale are presented in Figure 2.

Occupational Self Assessment

Given that Curtis had concerns about the effects of his sleep dysfunction on various aspects of his everyday social and occupational functioning, the therapist decided to administer the occupational self assessment (introduced in Chapter 13). This was followed by open-ended interview questions about his volition, since Curtis had described a number of recent situations that suggested he had lost the motivation to function in many areas of his life. Findings from this part of the assessment (See Figure 3) indicated that Curtis was having difficulty completing some very basic activities of daily living. These findings were con-

Sleep Behavior and Cognitions Scale	
Please answer "true"= T or "false"= F to the following statements`.	
1. If I miss sleep at night, I try to sleep in the next morning if I can	T
2. Even if I cannot sleep, the more time I spend resting in bed, the better	T
3. Napping during the day is a good way to make up for lost sleep	T
4. If I don't get enough sleep, my health will only get worse	T
5. I can never sleep at night	F
6. When I cannot sleep, I look at the clock frequently during the night	T
7. I feel like my sleep problems will never improve	T
8. When I can't sleep at night, I can't keep my mind off not being able to sleep	T
9. Other kinds of worries keep me awake at night	T
10. When I miss sleep, I wonder how I will get through the next day	T
11. When I miss some sleep at night, I tend to think that I haven't slept at all	F
12. I cannot sleep at night because thoughts race through my head	F
13. I cannot sleep at night because I feel keyed up or on edge	T
14. When I cannot sleep, I often ask myself why I have not been able to fall asleep yet	T
15. I cannot sleep at night because I feel nervous	T
16. Eating or drinking something just before bed helps me get to sleep	F
17. Eating or drinking something in the middle of the night helps me get to sleep	F
18. I watch television in bed when I cannot sleep at night	F
19. I try to catch up on lost sleep by sleeping longer on weekends	T
20. I take sleeping pills or other medicines or drugs to get to sleep at night	T
21. I worry that lack of sleep will shorten my life span	T
22. My difficulties getting to sleep or staying asleep interfere with my ability to function at home, at work, or socially	T
23. When I have difficulties sleeping, I decrease my level of physical activity the following day	F

FIGURE 2. Curtis' Baseline Responses to the Sleep Behavior and Cognitions Scale

sistent with the problem areas Curtis identified on his problem list. They included difficulties taking care of himself, difficulty ensuring that his wife and daughter would be economically stable if he should die, difficulty managing his current day-to-day responsibilities, and difficulty being involved in his work and family activities. These findings enabled him to identify four secondary goals for therapy, which are presented in the section of this chapter entitled "Treatment Goals." More information about the findings from Curtis's occupational self assessment is presented in Chapter 13.

DSM-IV Diagnostic Profile

Following the assessment process the therapist arrived at the following DSM-IV diagnoses.

Axis I: Dyssomnia, not otherwise specified; current major depressive disorder, single episode, moderate, in partial remission

Axis II: No diagnosis

Axis III: Prostate cancer

Myself	Priority	Competence				Values		
		Lot of problems	Some difficulty	Well	Extremely well	Not so important	Important	Extremely important
Concentrating on my tasks.			X					X
Physically doing what I need to do.		X					X	
Taking care of the place where I live.		X					X	
Taking care of myself.	1	X						X
Taking care of others for whom I am responsible.		NOT APPLICABLE						
Getting where I need to go.				X			X	
Managing my finances.	3	X						X
Managing my basic needs (food, medicine).				X				X
Expressing myself to others.				X			X	
Getting along with others.				X			X	
Identifying and solving problems.					X		X	
Relaxing and enjoying myself.		X				X		
Getting done what I need to do.			X					X
Having a satisfying routine.		X				X		
Handling my responsibilities.	2	X						X
Being involved as a student, worker, volunteer, and/or family member.	4	X						X
Doing activities I like.		X				X		
Working towards my goals.		X					X	
Making decisions based on what I think is important.				X				X
Accomplishing what I set out to do.				X				X
Effectively using my abilities.			X					X

FIGURE 3. Curtis's Occupational Self Assessment

Axis IV: Psychosocial issues: economic problems
Axis V: Global assessment of functioning = 65

Treatment Goals

Curtis' first goal for therapy, which was to improve his sleep, was established at the end of the first session. The 15th session was set as the target date for attaining this goal, and Curtis' initial confidence rating was a "5" on a scale of 1 to 10. The client's confidence rating was low in the initial phase of therapy because of the strength of his conviction that, irrespective of what he did or tried, he would not be able to control his ability to sleep. Figure 4 shows this goal and the steps that Curtis agreed to take to accomplish that goal.

Findings from the occupational self assessment also enabled Curtis to identify the following secondary goals. These secondary goals were established without a specific target date and with the understanding that they would not be a focus of treatment until sufficient progress was made on Curtis' initial goal to improve his sleep.

- To assume more autonomy in taking his medication, scheduling physician appointments and managing other aspects of his health care that he had defaulted to his wife.
- To focus on getting his finances in order, so that his wife and daughter would be taken care of.
- To do some of the chores around the house and yard that he had not attended to.
- To become reinvolved in his old roles, particularly being a more involved father and husband.

Once these goals were established, the final step of orientation involved establishing a cognitive behavioral case conceptualization.

Goal Form		
Goal(s) **Target Date**	**Confidence Rating** **(1–10)**	**Objectives** (realistic steps I can take to achieve goal)
Goal 1: Improve Sleep 15th session (on 9/6/03)	5	a) Learn and practice sleep hygiene techniques b) Identify and modify negative sleep cognitions using sleep reversal record c) Identify and modify negative sleep behaviors using sleep reversal record

FIGURE 4. Curtis's Goal Form

Cognitive Behavioral Case Conceptualization

During the second session, Curtis was introduced to the cognitive model. The therapist explained the relationships between health event triggers, automatic thoughts, and emotional, behavioral, and physiological outcomes. She also explained the three levels of beliefs and their role in the cognitive model. Curtis accepted and understood the cognitive model relatively quickly. By the end of the second session he was ready to work with the therapist to try to understand his sleep dysfunction according to the cognitive model. Because Curtis's expectations of therapy were that it would be brief and informative, the therapist accommodated his style by briefly educating him about the role of negative sleep cognitions and negative sleep behaviors in preventing sleep. Together, they completed the "case conceptualization worksheet" to develop a case conceptualization that explained the cognitive, behavioral, and emotional aspects of Curtis' insomnia. Curtis was satisfied with this conceptualization, which is presented in Figure 5.

As illustrated in Figure 5, the core belief that underlies Curtis' sleep difficulties is that he is unable to control his ability to sleep. When the client is reminded of his cancer sometime during the day, thoughts of cancer typically come to mind as he is trying to sleep. This triggers an automatic thought that relates to sleep, such as, "If I keep thinking about this, I will never be able to sleep." This results in an up-regulation of Curtis' nervous system that includes feeling terrified, not being able to sleep, and experiencing a rapid heartbeat. The intermediate belief underlying Curtis' automatic thoughts about sleep is that sleep is required in order to keep his body strong. Because his core belief is that he is not able to control his ability to sleep, this sparks a vicious cycle of sleep-related anxiety, negative sleep cognitions and behaviors, and resulting insomnia.

Summary of the Orientation and Assessment Phase

In summary, the following five steps were important in socializing Curtis into cognitive behavioral therapy. They included:

- Establishing an empathic understanding of his sleep-related difficulties and overall experience with cancer.
- Outlining the structure, process and other essential elements of cognitive behavioral therapy.
- Defining problems, establishing goals, and setting a provisional target date for completion of his primary goal.
- Teaching the cognitive model.
- Examining the relationship between Curtis' sleep dysfunction, his volition, and his everyday functioning.

By the end of the initial assessment and orientation period, it appeared as though Curtis understood the basic structure and process of cognitive behavioral therapy and was motivated to work toward his primary goal of improving his sleep.

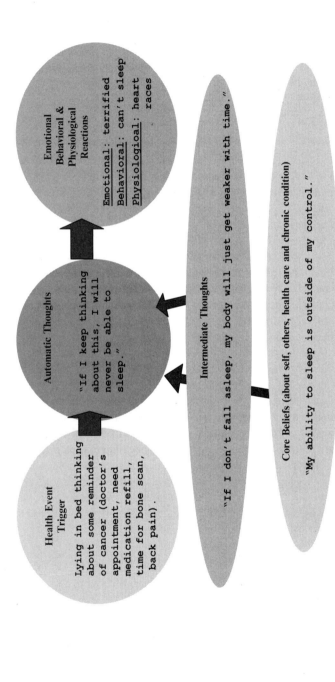

FIGURE 5. Curtis' Case Conceptualization

Subsequent Sessions: Course of Treatment

Curtis received a total of 53 sessions of cognitive behavioral therapy over a
1½ year period. The first 15 sessions focused specifically on reducing his insomnia and improving his overall sleep hygiene. Subsequent sessions addressed his
secondary goals of assuming more independence in his own health care, making
appropriate financial arrangements for his wife and daughter, completing household upkeep responsibilities and chores, and reestablishing open communication
and more of an emotional connection with his wife and daughter.

Main Emphasis of the Socratic Questioning

During the first 15 sessions of therapy, Socratic questioning focused on questions
that probed evidence for and against the client's core belief that his insomnia
was uncontrollable. As therapy progressed, a wider range of Socratic questions
were introduced to address cognitions about cancer and feelings of anticipatory
anxiety about his death. Increasingly, Curtis' cognitions reflected concerns about
role changes and about abandoning his wife and daughter. For example, as Curtis'
cancer progressed, he was no longer able to join his daughter in physical activities. Socratic questioning allowed him to consider alternative ways he had served
as a parent to his daughter and to modify cognitions that led him to believe he was
no longer useful as a father.

Curtis' concerns about role changes and about the possibility of dying were
accompanied by feelings of tremendous guilt and shame. Curtis was worried that
he would never live to see his daughter get married or to see his grandchildren
being born. He was concerned that he did not have enough money in his savings
account to cover the rising costs of inflation and anticipated financial needs
that his wife and daughter might have in the future. Rather than merely empathizing with Curtis or making reassuring comments, the therapist decided to use
Socratic questions that prompted Curtis to consider alternative perspectives on
these issues. This approach facilitated Curtis' reliance on his own strengths
(which included strong religious beliefs) to resolve some of his concerns about
dying and gave him the opportunity to consider alternative perspectives in the
presence of the therapist, who served as an objective, silent, and nonjudgmental
observer on these occasions.

In-Session Cognitive and Behavioral Activities

The first 15 sessions of therapy focused on teaching Curtis to identify, evaluate,
and correct the negative sleep cognitions and behaviors that he had been engaging in on a daily basis. The case conceptualization worksheet (See Figure 5) was
reviewed periodically to reinforce Curtis's awareness of the relationship between
his thoughts, feelings, and behavioral reactions to insomnia. The reversal record
was utilized to teach Curtis to identify, evaluate, and respond to realistic but

negative automatic thoughts. Curtis learned to engage in activities that would distract him from dwelling on his cancer or on his sleep difficulties. An example of one of Curtis's reversal records is presented in Figure 6. Curtis agreed to use the reversal record to help him control his anxiety and fear around dying and focus on living in the here and now. He completed the reversal record shown in Figure 6 in response to a frequent trigger (i.e., receiving a bill from the hospital, or notice form his insurance company or his doctor). As the reversal record shows, Curtis's reversal activity was to go out and spend some time in the garden, which he subsequently found to be both anxiety reducing and enjoyable. Curtis's use of this reversal record is discussed in more detail in Chapter 8.

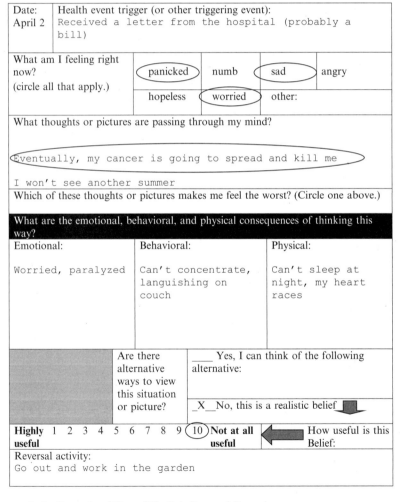

FIGURE 6. An Example of One of Curtis's Reversal Records

In addition to learning to identify negative sleep cognitions and behaviors, Curtis received basic sleep hygiene training. During a single session, background information about circadian rhythms and a rationale for sleep hygiene was provided. Curtis was coached and quizzed until it was clear he had memorized the following main points about sleep hygiene:

- Regardless of whether you are able to sleep or not, total time spent in bed should be gradually restricted to no more than 8 hours per 24-hour period.
- Gradually, daytime naps should be reduced to 20 minutes at a time. Ideally, daytime naps should be eliminated entirely.
- Engage in physical activity each day during midday or early evening hours (no later than 7 p.m.). When possible, outdoor activities, such as walking in a grassy area or gardening, are recommended to ensure adequate exposure to daylight.
- Daily exposure of the eyes to natural daylight and daily exposure of the body to natural sunlight are recommended whenever possible.
- Reduce stress, particularly before bedtime.
- Limit eating after 7 p.m.
- Limit caffeine intake. No caffeine after 2 p.m.
- Limit alcohol intake. No alcohol after 7 p.m.
- Your bedroom environment should be appropriate for sleep [e.g., absent of bothersome sounds or noise; appropriate room temperature (e.g., 65–70 degrees Fahrenheit); dark; comfortable mattress, pillow, sheets, and clothing].

Curtis was reminded that he should practice these guidelines daily unless health-related considerations presented an exception (e.g., he was forced to remain in bed or to sleep during the day following an acute illness-related episode or medical procedure). With daily practice of these techniques and modification of his negative sleep cognitions, Curtis's sleep efficiency had increased significantly by the 15th session.

The remaining sessions of therapy focused on maintaining Curtis's sleep-related achievements and working toward his secondary goals. For example, Curtis reported that he began experiencing spontaneous episodes of anxiety that did not appear to be linked to a specific negative health event trigger or to any identifiable thought. Curtis was coached to observe the time of day when these episodes were at their worst and to observe where he was and what he was doing. He was able to identify that he felt most anxious in the mornings, and was able to modify his activities to help him cope with his morning anxiety. The details of this procedure as it applied to Curtis are presented in Chapter 8.

During the course of therapy, Curtis began chemotherapy. Shortly after beginning chemotherapy, Curtis reported that riding in a car following chemotherapy exacerbated his nausea and made him vomit. As a result, he developed a specific aversion to riding in a car, and at one point during the course of his therapy, began to experience nausea even before setting foot in a car, regardless of where he was going or what he was doing. Systematic desensitization, reviewed in more detail in Chapter 9, was used effectively to address Curtis's aversion.

In addition to periodic episodes of anxiety, Curtis reported a significant amount of guilt and shame about the possibility that he would die and leave his wife and daughter with limited financial resources. The responsibility jigsaw, presented in Figure 7, was utilized as a means of encouraging Curtis to view the family's financial situation from a broader perspective (i.e., recognizing the multiple factors contributed to their financial situation). Details about the use and outcomes of this technique are provided in Chapter 8.

Homework Prescribed

In addition to the assessments that Curtis initially completed as homework following the first session, the following homework assignments were recommended:

- Sleep rating form
- Reversal record
- Sleep reversal record
- Problem-solving worksheet

The sleep rating form was assigned as homework to expose disruptions in Curtis's sleep-wake cycle and to allow him to observe the effects of his dysfunctional sleep behaviors on his insomnia. Examples of Curtis's initial and final responses on this form are presented in Figures 1 and 8. As will be discussed later and illustrated by comparing the two forms, Curtis was able to achieve significant improvement in his sleeping.

Curtis was also instructed to continue completing reversal records as weekly homework. He was informed that this record could be completed at any time of the day or night whenever he felt overwhelmed by negative thoughts. This included nighttime, which he identified as the time he was most likely to think about his cancer or worry about his family.

After Curtis had memorized the cognitive model of insomnia, had learned how to complete a reversal record and to identify negative sleep cognitions and behaviors, a sleep reversal record was assigned as weekly homework. The "sleep reversal record," which is a form that was developed by the author to address sleep dysfunction, should be distinguished from the "reversal record," which is a form that was developed to address realistic negative cognitions.

The sleep reversal record not only allowed Curtis to document his sleep-related cognitions and behaviors, but also enabled him to apply the basic sleep hygiene techniques that he learned in therapy in his efforts to modify his sleep-wake cycle. An example of one of Curtis's sleep reversal records is presented in Figure 9. As illustrated in the figure, Curtis had already begun reducing the time he was spending in bed awake. Leaving the bedroom when he was unable to sleep and using only the bedroom for sleep, increased the likelihood that being in the bedroom would trigger a conditioned sleep response.

In addition, the form indicates that Curtis was slowly reducing the number of naps taken per day and was responding more adaptively to worries about his

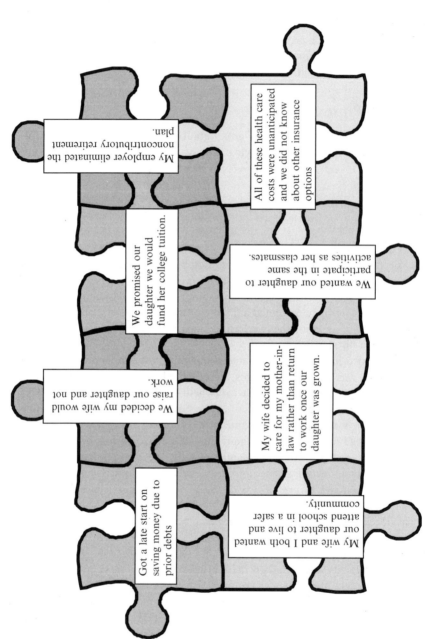

FIGURE 7. Curtis's Responsibility Jigsaw–Situation: Financial Crisis

Sleep Rating Form

Day	Wake-up time	Time of first attempt to sleep	# times awoke from sleep	Total estimated hours of night sleep	What did I do if I could not sleep?	Number of naps & total day sleep
Mon.	6:00 am	11:00 pm	4	5	Went to living room to watch TV	1 (20 min.)
Tues.	7:30 am	9:00 pm	1	8	Lay in bed trying to sleep	0
Wed.	7:00 am	10:00 pm	3	6	Went to living room to watch TV	1 (20 min.)
Thurs.	6:00 am	9:00 pm	2	7	Lay in bed trying to sleep	0
Fri.	7:30 am	11:30 pm	0	8	Lay in bed trying to sleep	0
Sat.	10:00am	11:30 pm	3	5	Lay in bed trying to sleep	1 (20 min.)
Sun.	9:30 am	10:00 pm	1	9	Lay in bed trying to sleep	0

Consistent bed time?   X yes   ___ no

Consistent waking time?   X yes   ___ no

Average hours of sleep per night = 7 hours

Average hours of nap time = less than 1 hour

FIGURE 8. Curtis' Final Responses to the Sleep Rating Form

Sleep Reversal Record

Date Day	Wake-up time	Time of first attempt to sleep	# times awake from sleep	Total estimated hours of sleep	Sleep thoughts (positive and negative)	Reversal activities (What did I do when I could not sleep?)
Mon.	7:00 am	11:00 pm	4	4 (night) 1 (nap)	Positive: "Get up and do something if you can." Negative: "Tomorrow will be a very long day." "I hope I'll sleep sometime soon."	Went to the living room to watch television.
Tues.	7:00 am	9:00 pm	5	3 (night) 2 (nap)	Positive: "I will sleep when I need to." Negative: "I have my bonescan tomorrow." "When will my cancer spread? " "How bad will the pain be?" "I can't let my family know."	Completed a thought reversal record to deal with negative thoughts about my cancer. Tried to read some magazines. Did an online search about painkillers. Started a long letter to my wife. Bought my wife and daughter gifts online.
Wed.	6:00 am	10:00 pm	2	7 (night) 0 (nap)	Positive: "I did not nap today; it should be easier tonight". "Try to calm down." Negative: "I wonder if I will be able to sleep."	Took deep breaths. Meditation and relaxation.

FIGURE 9. One of Curtis's Sleep Reversal Records

health and concerns about his insomnia, which often kept him awake at night. He wrote down a number of positive self-statements and coaching statements on the record. Moreover, when he could not sleep he engaged in a "sleep reversal activity" that distracted him from dwelling on negative cognitions and took him out of the bedroom environment. Examples of sleep reversal activities that can be provided to clients as suggestions for things to do when they are unable to sleep are presented in the Appendix to this chapter.

Once Curtis obtained his goal of reducing his insomnia, the therapist continued to recommend that he complete reversal records for the remaining sessions that he participated formally in cognitive behavioral therapy. The focus of these records was to address his secondary goals for therapy. In addition, one supplemental homework assignment included completing a problem-solving worksheet (originally introduced in Chapter 8). Curtis completed this worksheet (presented in Figure 10) early in therapy, when he was contemplating changing urologists. More information about Curtis' use of this worksheet is provided in Chapter 8. Once Curtis decided to continue treatment under the care of his original urologist, he was assigned to take the "weighing medical treatment options" worksheet to his urologist and to his other doctors in order to gather information about the best course of treatment given his stage of cancer. This worksheet is found in Chapter 8.

Difficulties Encountered

There were few difficulties encountered during the course of therapy. Curtis naturally preferred the highly structured nature of cognitive behavioral therapy, provided honest feedback when appropriate, and reported that he found therapy very helpful in improving his sleep and helping him manage his experience with cancer. Until his disease progressed, he enjoyed participating fully in therapeutic activities and homework assignments.

The only difficulties encountered were those that arose in relation to his cancer, and these occurred during the final stages of therapy. As the cancer progressed, it spread to his kidneys, bones, bladder, and brain. Eventually, his pain and cognitive impairment became so severe that therapy had to be discontinued. Curtis was placed on increasingly higher dosages of pain medication. Possibly in conjunction with the brain metastasis, these medications caused him to experience confusion, delusions, and hallucinations. He was hospitalized and died within approximately one month of his final therapy session.

Use of Related Knowledge as a Supplemental Approach

At different time points throughout the course of Curtis' therapy, the therapist drew upon knowledge of empathy, volition, and hope. Although the therapist sought to achieve an empathic understanding of Curtis' difficulties throughout the

Problem-Solving Worksheet					
Problem: Difficulty finding a competent urologist				Date: 5/6/02	
Goal: Find a competent urologist					
Steps I can take?	List what is important to me in a doctor.	Internet search of top urologists in my state	Check whether the doctor accepts my insurance.	Call hospitals or offices and ask nurses to provide their opinions about nominated physicians.	
Potential consequences of these steps?	Time and energy to find a good doctor, but I might find a good doctor.				
What will I do?	Follow all the steps in sequence.				
Alternate action if it does not work	Use the same process to develop a new list of doctors. Consider traveling to see a urologist and expanding the search to other states or regions of the country.				
What did I do? Followed all the steps.			Was it effective?	X Yes __No	
What happened? I identified three potential doctors and I made an appointment with the one that was closest to my home.					

FIGURE 10. Curtis's Problem-Solving Worksheet

course of therapy, the use of empathy became particularly important to Curtis toward the end of his life. Although Curtis appeared comfortable participating in the therapeutic relationship, he was not as comfortable interacting with other health-care providers, including the urologist that originally diagnosed him. In part, his discomfort stemmed from feeling misunderstood by his providers. In addition, he reported that he found many of his medical examinations and treatments to be not only painful but also dehumanizing.

Once Curtis began to consider the possibility that he would not survive his cancer, he began to see many of the therapeutic activities, and particularly the homework assignments, as relatively futile (with a few exceptions). He requested that the therapist serve as a witness to his pain and experience, and he asked her to just listen while he reflected upon his life, mourned his own death, read journal entries and letters he had written to family and friends, and described the plans he made for the care of his wife and daughter.

In addition to empathy, volitional issues were an ongoing consideration throughout the course of therapy with Curtis. These issues became particularly important as Curtis' cancer progressed and he continued to lose the ability to participate in many of the activities that had once been important to him. Using the occupational self assessment, the therapist worked with Curtis to develop short-term goals that were possible for him to accomplish during his illness. Focusing on self-care and on providing for the needs of others, such as his wife and daughter, enabled him to sustain hope and find value and meaning in present-time activities.

In addition to volitional work, the use of hope theory was fundamental to the therapy process. Toward the end of his life, Curtis was having difficulties achieving satisfaction with some parts of his past. His main regret was that he did not have enough time to contribute to others in his life, and to humanity in general, in what he considered to be a significant way. The therapist was highly vigilant about introducing elements of hope and optimism into as many aspects of the therapy process as possible. The excerpt from Curtis' therapy session, presented in Chapter 12, illustrates how the therapist relied upon hope theory to structure her questioning and to ultimately allow Curtis to see his contributions to others on a broad public level.

Treatment Outcome: Termination and Relapse Prevention

Because the therapist was aware of Curtis' stage of cancer and prognosis from the beginning of therapy, therapy was time-structured but not time-limited. In addition, the therapist used related knowledge more liberally toward the end of treatment because Curtis was facing issues that are unique to the process of death and dying. Curtis continued in therapy for 53 sessions until he became so impaired that he was no longer able to participate in therapy.

At the 15th session, Curtis completed the sleep rating form and the sleep behavior and cognitions scale as measures of his attainment of Goal 1. As evident from the sleep rating form (presented in Figure 8), Curtis's sleep efficiency increased significantly as a result of his efforts to learn and practice basic sleep hygiene techniques. He learned the value of restricting the amount of time he spent in bed to eight hours per night, and was successful in limiting his nap time to a maximum of 20 minutes per day.

In addition, Curtis learned the importance of maintaining consistency in his sleep and wake times and not allowing himself to sleep in on weekends for longer than one hour after his usual wake time. His progress in this area is also evident from his responses to the sleep behavior and cognitions scale (presented in Table 1). His responses demonstrate that he no longer endorsed dysfunctional sleep cognitions and no longer engaged in many behaviors that only serve to exacerbate insomnia.

In addition to his progress on his primary goal, Curtis made significant progress on his secondary goals. He became more independent in self-care activities, such as taking his medication on schedule and scheduling and attending medical appointments on time. He also made as many provisions for the financial well-being of his family as possible. He remortgaged his home, updated his will, and met with an accountant to complete as much of the anticipated tax-related tasks that would involve the transfer of his estate as he could prior to his death.

He made detailed specifications and preparations for his wife and daughter to donate his personal property or sell it at a garage sale. He completed as many of the household upkeep tasks and chores as he could, and hired a handyman to complete the remaining tasks. In addition, to assure his wife and daughter that he loved them, he wrote each of them an extensive letter and prepared a scrapbook that contained memories, pictures, advice, and other loving statements.

TABLE 1. Curtis' final and initial responses to the sleep behavior and cognitions scale.

Sleep Behavior and Cognitions Scale T= true F=false	Initial	Final
1. If I miss sleep at night, I try to sleep in the next morning if I can.	T	F
2. Even if I cannot sleep, the more time I spend resting in bed, the better.	T	F
3. Napping during the day is a good way to make up for lost sleep.	T	T
4. If I don't get enough sleep, my health will only get worse.	T	F
5. I can never sleep at night.	F	F
6. When I cannot sleep, I look at the clock frequently during the night.	T	F
7. I feel like my sleep problems will never improve.	T	F
8. When I can't sleep at night, I can't keep my mind off of not being able to sleep.	T	F
9. Other kinds of worries keep me awake at night.	T	F
10. When I miss sleep, I wonder how I will get through the next day.	T	F
11. When I miss some sleep at night, I tend to think that I haven't slept at all.	F	F
12. I cannot sleep at night because thoughts race through my head.	F	F
13. I cannot sleep at night because I feel keyed up or on edge.	T	F
14. When I cannot sleep, I often ask myself why I have not been able to fall asleep yet.	T	F
15. I cannot sleep at night because I feel nervous.	T	F
16. Eating or drinking something just before bed helps me get to sleep.	F	F
17. Eating or drinking something in the middle of the night helps me get to sleep.	F	F
18. I watch television in bed when I cannot sleep at night.	F	F
19. I try to catch up on lost sleep by sleeping longer on weekends.	T	F
20. I take sleeping pills or other medicines or drugs to get to sleep at night.	T	T
21. I worry that lack of sleep will shorten my life span.	T	F
22. My difficulties getting to sleep or staying asleep interfere with my ability to function at home, at work, or socially.	T	F
23. When I have difficulties sleeping, I decrease my level of physical activity the following day.	F	F

Learning from Curtis: Unique Features of Individuals with Insomnia

Like many individuals with insomnia, Curtis held an underlying core belief that he had no control over his ability to sleep at night. As is common among individuals with insomnia that is secondary to both a chronic illness and a comorbid psychiatric disorder, the exact cause of Curtis' sleep symptoms was not clear. Knowing this, the therapist had less ability to predict up front the extent to which modifying negative sleep cognitions and behaviors and teaching sleep hygiene techniques would be effective in resolving the sleep difficulties. However, by the 15th session it became clear that the cognitive behavioral approaches were effective in reducing Curtis's insomnia.

In addition to the direct work on Curtis's sleep-related behaviors and cognition, it is possible that his additional work on his secondary goals may have contributed to the improvements in his sleep indirectly. For example, Curtis worked to assume more autonomy in managing his medical care, to make plans to improve the family's financial situation, to become more involved in household chores and upkeep, and to participate more actively in his relationships with his wife and daughter. Work toward these secondary goals may have led to increased physical activity, feelings of mastery, and increased social support. In conjunction with his antidepressant medication, work toward these secondary goals may have led to decreased feelings of anxiety and depression, which, in turn, served to improve sleep. In summary, the following are unique considerations to bear in mind when conducting cognitive behavioral therapy with individuals with insomnia:

- Individuals with insomnia often hold underlying core beliefs that they cannot control their ability to sleep.
- If the role of physiological variables in the sleep disorder is unknown, it can be more difficult to predict the extent to which cognitive behavioral interventions will be effective in resolving the sleep difficulties. However, clinicians can be confident that these interventions will, in many cases, help to improve sleep on some level.
- A client's work toward secondary goals that aim to decrease symptoms of anxiety and depression may have indirect effects on sleep.

In addition to these unique issues involving sleep, this case also highlighted the importance of adjusting the goals and techniques of therapy to a client's needs and illness stage. In the later stages of the therapy process, Curtis was facing severe pain and cognitive difficulties. It became evident immediately that he was no longer interested in following along with the traditional structure and activities of cognitive behavioral therapy. At that point, Curtis wanted only support and empathy from the therapist as he prepared for the process of dying. Exercising judicial flexibility in circumstances where individuals are facing a terminal illness is an important consideration to keep in mind regardless of the therapeutic orientation being applied.

Appendix

Sleep Rating Form

Day	Wake-up time	Time of first attempt to sleep	# times awoke from sleep	Total estimated hours of night sleep	What did I do if I could not sleep?	Number of naps and total day sleep

Consistent bed time?   ___yes   ___no   Consistent waking time?   ___yes   ___no

Average hours of sleep per night = ___   Average hours of nap time = ___

Sleep Behavior and Cognitions Scale

Please answer "true"= T or "false"= F to the following questions.

1. If I miss sleep at night, I try to sleep in the next morning if I can.
2. Even if I cannot sleep, the more time I spend resting in bed, the better.
3. Napping during the day is a good way to make up for lost sleep.
4. If I don't get enough sleep, my health will only get worse.
5. I can never sleep at night.
6. When I cannot sleep, I look at the clock frequently during the night.
7. I feel like my sleep problems will never improve.
8. When I can't sleep at night I can't keep my mind off of not being able to sleep.
9. Other kinds of worries keep me awake at night.
10. When I miss sleep, I wonder how I will get through the next day.
11. When I miss some sleep at night, I tend to think that I haven't slept at all.
12. I cannot sleep at night because thoughts race through my head.
13. I cannot sleep at night because I feel keyed up or on edge.
14. When I cannot sleep, I often ask myself why I have not been able to fall asleep yet.
15. I cannot sleep at night because I feel nervous.
16. Eating or drinking something just before bed helps me get to sleep.
17. Eating or drinking something in the middle of the night helps me get to sleep.
18. I watch television in bed when I cannot sleep at night.
19. I try to catch up on lost sleep by sleeping longer on weekends.
20. I take sleeping pills or other medicines or drugs to get to sleep at night.
21. I worry that lack of sleep will shorten my life span.
22. My difficulties getting to sleep or staying asleep interfere with my ability to function at home, at work, or socially.
23. When I have difficulties sleeping, I decrease my level of physical activity the following day.

Examples of Positive Sleep Reversal Activities (what to do when you cannot sleep).

1) Leave the bedroom area
2) Distract yourself by nonstimulating mental or physical activities. These may include:
    a. Reading a book or magazine that does not contain upsetting content
    b. Watching a television show or movie that does not contain upsetting content
    c. Doing a relatively sedentary chore, such as sorting laundry or cleaning out a drawer
    d. Writing a letter to a friend
    e. Writing in a diary
    f. Practicing relaxation or meditation exercises
    g. Playing a card game or a computer game
    h. Doing a hobby or an arts and crafts activity
    i. Surfing the Internet or browsing stores on the Internet

Sleep Reversal Record

Date Day	Wake-up time	Time of first attempt to sleep	# times awoke from sleep	Total estimated hours of sleep	Sleep thoughts (positive and negative)	Reversal activities (What did I do when I could not sleep?)

20

Gastrointestinal Dysfunction: Diagnostic Categories, Prevalence, and Associated Conditions

Gastrointestinal dysfunction includes a wide range of symptoms, syndromes, and disorders of the gastrointestinal (GI) tract. Non-food-borne gastroenteritis, the most prevalent of all GI disorders, is estimated to occur at a rate of 135 million cases per year. Food-borne GI illnesses are estimated at 76 million cases per year. In terms of chronic conditions, gastroesophageal reflux disease (acid reflux) is estimated to occur at a rate of 19 million new cases per year. Irritable bowel syndrome (IBS) is close behind at a rate of 15 million per year. In addition, GI dysfunction is a symptom and/or consequence of a number of prevalent chronic illnesses.

This chapter provides an overview of basic facts about the gastrointestinal (GI) tract and about normal and abnormal GI function. In addition, a general description of the most prevalent types of GI disorders is provided. The chapter also describes the role of GI dysfunction in other chronic conditions that are not considered to be primary diseases of the GI tract. This chapter is not intended to provide an exhaustive review of the epidemiology and characteristics of GI dysfunction for each condition covered. However, basic information about a number of conditions that involve GI dysfunction is offered to provide therapists with general guidelines and information about the role of the GI tract in some of the more common chronic illnesses. When working with clients with a chronic illness for which GI dysfunction is a primary symptom, therapists will inevitably need to seek out additional information about the role of the GI tract in that specific condition from collaborating physicians and research-related resources.

Basic Information about the GI Tract

Because GI dysfunction is so prevalent within the general population and even more likely to accompany the experience of chronic illness for many individuals, it is important for therapists to have a basic working knowledge of the components and functions of the GI tract. When appropriate, basic information about the GI tract and about normal and abnormal GI function can be shared with clients for educational purposes. In addition, it can aid in assessment and collaborative treatment planning. Clients with chronic conditions that involve GI dysfunction, and particularly those that tend to focus on somatic symptoms, will generally have a number of questions about the GI tract and its potential role in their conditions. Thus it is important for therapists to be educated about these issues.

There are two components of the GI tract that form a continuous tube:

- The upper GI tract
- The lower GI tract

The upper GI tract begins with the mouth, which is connected to the esophagus and extends down into the stomach, into the duodenum (which connects the stomach to the small intestine), and eventually into the small intestine. The lower GI tract begins with the small intestine, which is approximately 20 feet long and ends with the ileum. The ileum connects the small intestine to the cecum, which is the dilated pouch that forms the first part of the large intestine, or colon. The colon is the part of the large intestine from the cecum to the rectum. The rectum is the last four-to-five inches of the digestive tract, ending with the anal canal or opening. The organs within the GI tract allow digestion to occur.

The liver, gallbladder, and pancreas are three other organs that are associated with the GI tract and are key to healthy GI function. The liver is a large gland located in the upper part of the abdomen that serves many vital functions within the body, one of which is to produce bile for digestion. The liver also stores and filters blood, excretes bilirubin and other substances formed in the body, and serves numerous metabolic functions. The gallbladder is a sac located under the liver. The gallbladder stores approximately one-half pint of bile, which is released through the bile ducts into the duodenum. Bile is a complex digestive fluid that functions to digest fats and is used to process other nonsoluble wastes. The pancreas is a two-part (endocrine and exocrine) gland. The exocrine part of the pancreas secretes juices that are fundamental to the digestion of protein. The pancreas is situated next to the duodenum and behind the stomach.

What Characterizes Healthy GI Function?

In healthy GI function, the organs within the upper and lower GI tracts work together, along with the liver, gallbladder and pancreas, to allow digestion to occur. Digestion refers to the process of breaking food down into more basic chemical components for eventual release into the bloodstream. Following the initial digestive processes that occur with chewing and the secretion of saliva in the mouth, food travels down the esophagus and enters the stomach. Once in the stomach, food mixes with digestive juices and is passed into the small intestine in small amounts as it is processed. While it travels through the small intestine, energy-producing nutrients and other by-products that are essential to healthy bodily functioning are absorbed by the wall of the small intestine and released into the bloodstream.

Once the food reaches the large intestine, extraction of the nutrients has taken place and only wastes are left behind. Through a series of involuntary muscle contractions called peristalsis, the waste material passes through the colon and water is absorbed from the waste material by the large intestine. Once the waste reaches the end of the colon it is passed out of the body down the rectum and out the anal cavity.

A certain level of gas production is a normal and necessary aspect of digestion. Normal bowel function is defined broadly as bowel movements that occur at a frequency that ranges from three times per day to three times per week. There is also a wide range in the interpretation of what is considered a normal consistency and color of stool. Because bowel habits vary considerably between individuals and are highly sensitive to subtle changes in diet, exercise, lifestyle and stress, normal bowel function is a relative concept that should be interpreted in light of an individual's lifelong bowel habits and daily routines.

Gastrointestinal Dysfunction

In this chapter, GI dysfunction will be described according to four categories:

- Nonspecific GI symptoms
- Chronic GI disorders
- Functional GI disorders (chronic GI disorders of unknown cause)
- Other chronic illnesses and treatments involving GI dysfunction

Acute gastrointestinal disorders, such as acute bacterial, viral, or parasitic gastroenteritis, food-borne GI illnesses, and acute pancreatitis, will not be emphasized in this chapter since the focus of this book is on chronic conditions.

Nonspecific GI Symptoms

From time to time and depending on the symptom, everyone is likely to experience nonspecific GI symptoms. Nonspecific GI symptoms may occur independently of any known pathological process, chronic condition, medication, or treatment, or they may occur as a part of a chronic GI condition or other chronic illness. The most common categories of nonspecific GI symptoms include:

- Bloating
- Constipation
- Diarrhea
- Gas
- Nausea and vomiting
- Abdominal pain

Bloating

Bloating is defined as a feeling of fullness and/or distention of the abdomen. Bloating often increases throughout the day and is most prominent following mealtime in the evening. Abdominal bloating may be accompanied by gas pains, gas sounds, belching, and the passage of gas through the rectum. As such, bloating and distention can be caused by an excess of intestinal gas that has not been expelled. However, abdominal bloating and distention can also occur in the absence of excessive gas. In this circumstance, bloating is most commonly caused by a loss of abdominal muscle tone.

Constipation

Constipation is defined as infrequent bowel movements (e.g., fewer than three per week) and stool that is frequently dry and hard. Dry and hard stool results from the excess absorption of water by the large intestine due to the prolonged time period in which the waste remains in the colon. Individuals with constipation often report feeling bloated or full in their abdominal region. Other symptoms may involve excessive gas, abdominal distention, and the feeling that the bowels have not been completely emptied following a bowel movement. Some of the most common causes of constipation include GI disorders and other chronic illnesses, a diet low in fiber, lack of exercise, and stress. The likelihood of constipation also increases with age. Other causes include, but are not limited to, side effects of certain antidepressant medications, narcotic analgesics, antihypertensive medications, and iron supplements.

Diarrhea

Diarrhea refers to the abnormal frequency and urgency of the passage of loose or watery stool. Because there is wide variation between individuals in terms of their tolerance for changes in the frequency and consistency of their bowel movements, the definition of diarrhea is, in large part, subjective and depends on the individual's definition of what he or she considers to be abnormal. Common causes of diarrhea include gastroenteritis due to viral or food-borne pathogens, chronic GI disorders and other chronic illnesses, side effects of various treatments and medications, intolerance to specific contents within certain foods, caffeine, artificial sweeteners, a diet low in fiber, lack of exercise, and stress.

Gas

Gas collects in the stomach and intestinal tract and is expelled by the body through burping or flatus. Gas that results in belching is generated from swallowed air, which mixes with stomach content and is returned in belching. Individuals are more likely to swallow air if they chew gum, smoke, suck on hard candy, have ill-fitting dentures, or have nasal allergies or an upper respiratory infection. Drinking carbonated beverages and eating too quickly are also likely to produce stomach gas.

Swallowed air that is not returned in belching enters the small intestine, where it is either absorbed or enters into the large intestine to be passed rectally as flatus. In addition to nitrogen found in the air that is swallowed, the other sources of flatus include difficult-to-digest foods and poorly absorbed carbohydrates. Though most food by-products are absorbed by the small intestine, high-fiber foods such as broccoli, cabbage, beans, cauliflower, bran, and foods high in sugar and carbohydrates are not well absorbed by the small intestine and must be further processed by bacteria within the large intestine. Flatus is the result of gases that are produced by the interaction between bacteria and foods within the large intestine.

Having a certain amount of gas in the GI tract that needs to be expelled is a normal part of digestion. However, certain individuals develop excessive amounts of gas and/or are particularly sensitive to the accumulation of gas in the stomach and intestinal tract.

Nausea and vomiting

Nausea refers to an unpleasant sensation in the upper abdomen and/or esophagus region that often culminates in vomiting. Vomiting refers to the expulsion of contents of the stomach through the mouth. In less common circumstances of bowel obstruction, appendicitis, or when bacterial overgrowth has occurred in the upper intestine, fecal matter may also be vomited. Similar to diarrhea, nausea and vomiting may be chronic or acute. Nausea and vomiting may be caused by a wide range of acute and chronic conditions involving the GI tract and surrounding organs, other chronic illnesses, intoxication with alcohol or street drugs, and side effects of various treatments and medications.

Abdominal pain

Broadly, abdominal pain refers to any type of pain or discomfort experienced in any location within the lower and/or upper abdominal regions. Most individuals experience brief episodes of abdominal pain that are not associated with a specific cause and are not of serious concern. However, when pain persists for hours or days, a physician should always be consulted. The two most prominent types of abdominal pain are abdominal cramping and constant abdominal pain. Abdominal cramping is sometimes referred to as colic. It occurs in a cyclical or wave-like pattern characterized by an increase in intensity followed by a gradual decrease in intensity.

Generally, any stretching, pressure, or squeezing within the intestines can cause cramping pain, since this type of pain reflects an abnormal increase in intestinal muscle contractions (peristalsis). Causes can include, but are not limited to, excessive gas collection in pockets of the intestine, and irritation of the intestines from infection, inflammation, blockage or obstruction, or stress.

Constant abdominal pain is characterized by a less fluctuating pain that can be described as sharp, gnawing, burning, aching, or hunger pain. This type of pain most commonly reflects a deeper inflammatory process within the abdominal cavity or in any of the organs that comprise the GI tract. Constant abdominal pain may be located anywhere in the abdomen and is caused by a wide range of variables. These include, but are not limited to, gallstones, ulcers, local infections or abscesses, irritation of the inner lining of the esophagus, and irritation of the outer lining of the intestines from the leakage of blood, wastes, and bile.

Chronic GI Disorders

The following section describes the symptoms, complications, and causes of six of the most prevalent chronic GI disorders within the U.S. population. These include:

- Food intolerance
- Gallstones
- Gastroesophageal reflux disease
- Gastrointestinal cancers
- Inflammatory bowel disease
- Peptic ulcer disease

Food intolerance

Food intolerance is diagnosed when it is clear that consumption of a certain food or food by-product leads to GI dysfunction. The most common symptoms of food intolerance include abdominal pain, gas, bloating, nausea, and diarrhea. Less frequent symptoms include shock, welts, rash, difficulty breathing, inflammation of the sinuses and eyes, vocal cord swelling, and headache. The food by-products that are most frequently associated with food intolerance include certain sugars (lactose, fructose, and sorbitol) and gluten (the protein of wheat and other grains). Monosodium glutamate, sulfites, and histamines are also known to cause symptoms in a smaller number of people. The two most widely recognized forms of food intolerance include lactose intolerance and celiac disease.

Lactose is the primary sugar in milk. Lactose intolerance is a chronic condition characterized by the inability to digest lactose. Unlike other food by-products that are absorbed through the walls of the small intestine and passed into the bloodstream, lactose is not digested within the small intestine. As a result, it is passed into the large intestine, where it interacts with bacteria and produces symptoms of bloating, gas, diarrhea, cramping pain, and nausea. Lactose intolerance is caused by an absence or shortage of lactase, an enzyme produced by cells within the small intestine that breaks down lactose into smaller by-products to be absorbed into the bloodstream.

Celiac disease is a chronic condition that involves the inability to digest gluten. Gluten describes a group of proteins found in all forms of wheat and related grains, rye, barley, and tritcale. Gluten is present in a number of foods, including wheat breads and other baked goods, cereals, and pasta? It is also present in numerous processed foods and medications. Symptoms of celiac disease include abdominal pain, gas, bloating, chronic diarrhea, constipation, oily stools, and an increased appetite that is associated with a change in weight (either weight loss or weight gain) (Collin et al., 2002; Dahl 2000). Other symptoms may include fatigue, weakness, bone and joint pain, dental enamel defects, infertility, and depression. When individuals with celiac disease consume gluten, damage to the lining of the small intestine occurs, causing the body to have difficulty absorbing key nutrients, such as proteins, carbohydrates, vitamins, minerals, water, and bile salts. If left untreated, celiac disease can result in long-term complications, such as anemia, osteopenia or osteoporosis, vitamin deficiencies, central and peripheral nervous system disorders, cancers of the GI tract, and other food intolerances.

The cause of celiac disease is currently unknown. Research suggests that it may involve an autoimmune process that involves genes that are involved in the regulation of the body's immune response to gluten proteins. Celiac disease may occur in conjunction with other autoimmune diseases, such as diabetes, thyroid disease, and lupus.

Gallstones

Gallstones are hardened masses of cholesterol crystals or bile salts (bilirubin) that form within the gallbladder. Gallstones comprised of cholesterol crystals are the most common form of gallstones, representing 90 percent of gallstone formation. These form when there is an excess of cholesterol that is not dissolved in the bile. Approximately 80 percent of individuals with gallstones do not experience symptoms. Symptoms occur when the stones block one or more of the biliary ducts. They include abdominal pain, jaundice, gas, and inflammation of the gallbladder, bile ducts, liver, and/or pancreas. Within the U.S. gallstones are highly prevalent. Up to 20 percent of women and 10 percent of men will develop gallstones before the age of 60. Gallstones are three times more common in women than in men. Risk factors include multiple pregnancies, age, and obesity.

Gastroesophageal reflux disease (GERD, acid reflux)

Gastroesophageal reflux disease, commonly referred to as "acid reflux" or "GERD," can include symptoms of acid reflux with or without symptoms of esophagitis. Acid reflux involves the leakage of stomach acid upward into the esophagus. Esophagitis is defined as an inflammation of the lining of the esophagus. The symptoms of GERD include heartburn, nausea, an acid taste in the mouth, bloating, belching, abdominal pain, chest pain, and a burning pain when swallowing hot drinks. These symptoms may wax and wane and tend to worsen after eating.

Gastrointestinal cancers

There are five common types of gastrointestinal cancers: colorectal, esophageal, gastric, liver, and pancreatic. Among these, colorectal cancer, or "colon cancer," is the most prevalent. Colorectal cancer is defined as cancer of the two major organs within the large intestine, the colon and the rectum. More than 138,000 new cases are diagnosed within the U.S. each year. Colorectal cancer is responsible for an estimated 55,000 deaths each year and has the second highest mortality rate among all forms of cancer. Colorectal cancer begins with polyps, which are abnormal growths on the intestinal wall. If they are not removed, these polyps may become cancerous over time. Symptoms of colorectal cancer include frequent gas pains, blood in or on the stool, diarrhea or constipation, and a feeling that the bowel has not been emptied after a bowel movement. Colorectal cancer is equally prevalent among women and men and is most common after the age of 50. Individuals with nonfunctional chronic digestive diseases or those with close relatives that have had colorectal cancer are at an increased risk for developing this disease.

There are two main types of esophageal cancer, or cancer of the esophagus: squamous cell carcinoma and adenocarcinoma. Squamous cell carcinoma usually develops in the upper or middle part of the esophagus and adenocarcinoma usually develops in the lower region. In its initial stages, esophageal cancer is usually asymptomatic. It begins with very small tumors. As the tumors grow, individuals develop difficulty swallowing solid foods such as meats, breads, or raw vegetables. With continued tumor growth and narrowing of the esophagus, individuals also develop difficulty swallowing liquids. Other symptoms include indigestion, heartburn, vomiting, weight loss, choking, coughing, and hoarseness of the voice. Esophageal cancer typically develops after the age of 55 and is twice as common in men as in women. Though the cause is unknown, risk factors include smoking, obesity, and alcohol use. Esophageal cancer has also been linked to Barrett's esophagus, a condition resulting from severe cases of gastroesophageal reflux disease (GERD). In Barrett's esophagus, irritation of the lining of the esophagus by stomach acids can cause changes in esophageal cells, and these cells may become cancerous over time.

Gastric cancer, commonly referred to as stomach cancer, is cancer that develops in any part of the stomach. This cancer can spread throughout the stomach into the small intestine, colon, lymph nodes, liver, and pancreas. In its early stages, the disease may be asymptomatic. Symptoms of advanced disease include abdominal pain, feeling full after eating relatively small amounts of food, fatigue and weakness, nausea and vomiting, vomiting blood or passing blood in stool, loss of appetite, and weight loss. Gastric cancer is twice as common in men as in women and it tends to occur after the age of 55. The causes of gastric cancer are unknown. Risk factors include a past history of stomach surgery, pernicious anemia, and gastric atrophy.

Liver cancer (hepatocellular carcinoma) is cancer that forms in the liver. It is the fifth most prevalent form of cancer in the world, and it is becoming more prevalent within the U.S. There are no symptoms of early disease. Symptoms of advanced disease include abdominal pain from tumor growth, weight loss, fever, sudden appearance of abdominal swelling, jaundice, and muscle wasting. The most frequently cited cause of liver cancer is chronic infection with the hepatitis B or hepatitis C viruses. Other diseases that lead to an increased risk for liver cancer include cirrhosis of the liver from alcoholism, hemochromatosis (a condition associated with abnormal iron metabolism), and alpha-1-antitrypsin deficiency (deficiency of a plasma protein produced in the liver that is associated with emphysema).

Pancreatic cancer is cancer that forms in the pancreas. There are no symptoms of early disease. Symptoms of advanced disease include jaundice, abdominal pain, nausea, loss of appetite, and weight loss. Cancer of the pancreas is curable only if it is detected in its early stages. The causes of pancreatic cancer are unknown. Risk factors include smoking, alcohol consumption, chronic pancreatitis, a diet rich in animal fat, and genetic vulnerability.

Inflammatory bowel disease

There are two main categories of inflammatory bowel disease: ulcerative colitis and Crohn's disease. Ulcerative colitis is defined as chronic, recurrent inflammation and ulceration of the inner lining of the large intestine, or colon. Symptoms include cramping, abdominal pain, weight loss and anorexia, rectal bleeding, and loose discharges of blood, pus, and mucus among few stools or stool particles. Complications can include hemorrhoids (i.e., swollen or stretched veins in the anal canal), abscesses (localized pockets of pus), anal fistulas (i.e., abnormal connections or tunnels near the anus that do not communicate with the rectum), perforation of the colon (i.e., abnormal hole in the colon wall), polyp-like growths of mucus membrane (caused by ulceration), and cancer.

Crohn's disease has both similarities to and differences from ulcerative colitis. Similarities include already-described common symptoms and complications resulting from the inflammatory process. One key difference is that the inflammatory process in Crohn's disease involves a deeper level penetration of the intestinal lining (i.e., deeper into the lining of the intestinal wall). A second difference is that Crohn's disease primarily affects the small intestine, while ulcerative colitis primarily affects the large intestine. Crohn's disease can also affect any other part of the GI tract spanning from the mouth to the anus. Typically, Crohn's disease affects the terminal ileum (i.e., lowest part or end of the small intestine) and involves scarring and thickening of the bowel wall. This results in a progressive narrowing of the small intestine and increased pain in the lower right quadrant near the belt line. Crohn's disease frequently leads to bowel obstruction, and this tends to reoccur after surgery or other treatment. It may also involve chronic fever, elevated white blood cell count, persistent diarrhea, and bleeding.

The definitive cause of inflammatory bowel disease is currently unknown. However, some findings suggest that an infectious or allergic process may lead to a chronic inflammation of the small or large intestine. Genetic variables may increase an individual's vulnerability or predisposition to develop antibodies that chronically attack the organs within the GI tract, leading to an ongoing cycle of inflammation. There is little evidence to suggest that stress plays a role in the development or perpetuation of these conditions.

Inflammatory bowel disease differs from irritable bowel syndrome (IBS) in that inflammatory bowel disease involves a detectable inflammation of the GI tract with other structural abnormalities that can be observed through barium X ray or colonoscopy. Moreover, IBS does not typically involve fever, internal bleeding, or an elevated white blood cell count.

Peptic ulcer disease

Peptic ulcer disease is characterized by an ulcer or ulcers within the esophagus, stomach, or duodenum (i.e., beginning of the small intestine). An ulcer is a localized area of the mucus membrane that has been destroyed by stomach acid and digestive juices. It is typically no larger than the size of a pencil eraser. Ulcers are common within the U.S. population. Approximately 20 million individuals in the U.S. will experience an ulcer at some point during their lives. The primary symptom of an ulcer is a burning or gnawing pain in the upper abdominal region that lasts for minutes or hours. This pain typically worsens between meals and during sleep. It may be relieved with eating or by taking antacids. Other less common symptoms and complications may include loss of appetite and weight, nausea, vomiting, bleeding, perforation (a hole in the intestinal lining), and obstruction (caused by scarring close to the outlet of the stomach that prevents food from passing into the small intestine).

Although it was initially thought that stress contributed to the development of ulcers, this hypothesis is no longer valid. There are two main causes of ulcers. One is infection with the bacteria, Helicobacter pylori (H. pylori) in a genetically vulnerable individual. The other involves regular use of the nonsteroidal class of antiinflammatory pain medications (NSAIDs), including aspirin and ibuprofen.

Functional GI Disorders (GI Disorders of Unknown Cause)

By definition, functional GI disorders are those of unknown etiology. They do not involve anatomical or structural defects, the presence of pathogenic agents, or any other signs of disease that can be seen or measured. However, it is clear that in these disorders, different organs within the GI tract are not functioning normally. It has already been established that attributing these disorders solely to stress and psychological variables is neither useful nor completely accurate (Toner et al., 2000). However, a certain level of evidence suggests that these disorders are stress-sensitive (Toner et al., 2000). Given this information, the task of the therapist is to work with the patient and his or her physician to determine the *extent* to which stress and other psychological variables play a role in symptoms. The five disorders that will be covered in this section include:

- Functional constipation
- Functional diarrhea
- Functional abdominal bloating
- Functional abdominal pain syndrome
- Irritable bowel syndrome

Functional constipation

Functional constipation is a chronic condition characterized by the persistence of difficult and infrequent bowel movements. After all other potential explanations for constipation are excluded, functional constipation is diagnosed when an individual reports two or more of the following six symptoms for a period of three months or longer.

- Straining with bowel movements a minimum of 25 percent of the time
- Hard or lumpy stools a minimum of 25 percent of the time
- Fewer than three bowel movements per week
- A feeling that the bowel has not been emptied completely a minimum of 25 percent of the time
- A sensation that the bowel is blocked or obstructed a minimum of 25 percent of the time
- Using a hand or finger to help pass stool a minimum of 25 percent of the time

Functional constipation can be distinguished from irritable bowel syndrome (IBS) in that, unlike IBS, it is typically characterized by an absence of abdominal pain. The causes of functional constipation are not known. However, poor bowel habits, lack of exercise, and a lack of dietary fiber may contribute.

Functional diarrhea

Functional diarrhea is characterized by chronic diarrhea, or the frequent and urgent passage of loose and watery stool. It generally occurs on a fairly regular basis over a period of months or years. Though many GI disorders, chronic illnesses, treatments, and medications can cause diarrhea, there are no known causes or contributors to functional diarrhea. After ruling out all other possible explanations, functional diarrhea is diagnosed according to the following three criteria set forth by the American College of Gastroenterology:

- Presence of unformed bowel movements
- Diarrhea must be present more than 75 percent of the time
- Absence of abdominal pain

Functional abdominal bloating

Functional abdominal bloating involves an increase in bloating and abdominal distention throughout the day that is often at its worst following the evening meal. It is typically relieved by lying down or by sleeping. The causes of this syndrome are unknown, but may involve a combination of excessive gas and weakness or thinning of the abdominal muscles.

Functional abdominal pain syndrome

In functional abdominal pain syndrome, individuals experience unexplained pain and discomfort anywhere within the abdominal region. The pain may be cyclical or constant, and it may not always be triggered by eating or by having a bowel movement. In this way, it can be distinguished from the pain that is characteristic of irritable bowel syndrome, which is usually related to diarrhea, constipation, and/or bloating. Though the exact etiology of this syndrome is not known, in some cases pain appears following a series of painful abdominal conditions, surgeries, or after a distressing life event. Repeated injury or inflammation can cause abdominal nerves to become hypersensitive. This pain can be exacerbated by stress or by past negative experiences involving pain.

Irritable bowel syndrome

As presented in Chapter 14, irritable bowel syndrome (IBS) is the most widely known and prevalent of the functional bowel disorders, occurring in up to one in every five individuals residing in the U.S. (Drossman et al., 1982; Drossman et al., 1993; Sandler 1990). IBS is a cluster of symptoms that persists for three or more months and includes abdominal pain, bloating, diarrhea, and constipation. There is inconsistency in terms of the frequency of defecation, changes in stool consistency, and changes in the way that the stool is passed (Drossman et al., 1994). Many individuals report alternating episodes of constipation and diarrhea. IBS may also involve the passage of mucus within and around the stool (Drossman et al., 1994).

IBS is two-to-five times more prevalent in women than in men (Toner et al., 2000). It is a stress-sensitive condition that is often comorbid with other disorders of unknown etiology, such as chronic fatigue syndrome and fibromyalgia (Taylor, Friedberg, and Jason 2001). Typically, it begins in late adolescence or early adulthood. First onset of IBS symptoms after the age of 50 is rare. Though it is chronic and can cause significant impairment, IBS is not fatal and does not lead to other serious diseases or conditions.

Other Chronic Illnesses and Treatments Involving GI Dysfunction

In addition to the specific GI disorders reviewed in the previous section, GI symptoms accompany a number of other chronic illnesses and/or treatments for these conditions. In individuals with non-GI chronic illnesses, GI dysfunction is most commonly linked to side effects of treatments and medications. This section will provide a general overview of the nature and causes of GI dysfunction that accompany some of the more common chronic illnesses and their treatments. It should be noted that this review is unsystematic. As a result, it excludes many other chronic illnesses, medications, and treatments that involve or result in GI dysfunction. The limited number of conditions that will be covered in this review were selected because they are among the more prevalent conditions that involve GI dysfunction as a primary symptom. They include:

- Addison's disease
- Asthma and other pulmonary diseases
- Cancer (non-GI cancers)
- Diabetes
- Heart and cardiovascular diseases
- HIV/AIDS and other infectious diseases

In addition to these chronic illnesses, nonsteroidal antiinflammatory drugs (NSAIDs) that are often used to treat diseases and disorders that involve chronic pain and inflammation are known to irritate the stomach by weakening the ability of the lining to resist stomach acids. In some cases, this irritation may lead to inflammation of the stomach lining (gastritis), to ulcers, bleeding, or perforation of the stomach lining. Use of NSAIDs, including aspirin and ibuprofen, can produce severe stomach cramps and pain or burning in the stomach or back. In addition, use of NSAIDs may result in black, tarry, or bloody stools; diarrhea; bloody vomit; severe heartburn; and indigestion.

Addison's disease

Addison's disease is a chronic illness characterized by abnormally low blood pressure, weight loss, anorexia, weakness, and a bronze-like pigmentation of the skin. These symptoms reflect a chronic deficiency in the hormones secreted by the adrenal glands, aldosterone and cortisol. In the absence of medications designed to replace these deficiencies, the condition can be fatal. There are two widely recognized causes of Addison's disease. The first is an autoimmune-induced destruction of the adrenal cortex (outer layer of the adrenal glands). The second is a tuberculosis-induced destruction of the adrenal cortex. Abdominal pain, nausea, vomiting, and diarrhea are present in approximately 50 percent of cases of Addison's disease (McConnell 2002; National Institute of Diabetes and Digestive and Kidney Diseases 2000).

Asthma and other pulmonary diseases

Asthma and other pulmonary diseases are described in Chapter 18. A number of medications used to treat asthma and other pulmonary diseases are known to produce gastrointestinal side effects. For example, common side effects of systemic corticosteroids, bronchodilators, and leukotriene receptor antagonists include nausea and/or vomiting, diarrhea, and abdominal pain (Kemp 1999).

Cancer (non-GI forms)

A brief description of the general characteristics of cancer is presented in Chapter 14. GI dysfunction in other forms of cancer typically arises as a side effect of medications or certain cancer treatments. For example, nausea, vomiting, constipation, and diarrhea are common side effects of chemotherapy medications. Up to 80 percent of individuals treated with chemotherapy experience nausea and 40 percent have at least one episode of vomiting (Matteson et al., 2002). These medications tend to irritate the lining of the stomach and esophagus. Diarrhea, constipation, and abdominal pain can also occur as common side effects of radiation to the stomach or other parts of the abdominal region (American Cancer Society 2004). Certain hormone therapies, including those used to treat breast cancer, are also associated with nausea and vomiting. However, some women develop a tolerance to the hormone therapies over time and symptoms can disappear within a few weeks.

Diabetes

Diabetes is described in Chapter 14. A wide range of medications used to treat Type II diabetes, including biguanides (e.g., Metformin), sulfonylureas, alpha-glycosidase inhibitors, and meglitinides, can cause GI dysfunction. For example, up to 30 percent of individuals taking Metformin report experiencing nausea, diarrhea, gas, and abdominal cramping (DeFronzo 1999).

Heart and cardiovascular diseases

Information on heart and cardiovascular diseases is provided in Chapter 14. GI dysfunction that is associated with heart and cardiovascular diseases is most commonly the result of side effects from the medications used to treat these conditions. For example, common side effects of digitalis (a medication frequently used to treat congestive heart failure, most supraventricular tachy-cardias, cardiogenic shock, and other heart conditions) include diarrhea, loss of appetite, lower abdominal pain, nausea, and vomiting (U.S. National Library of Medicine, National Institutes of Health 1999). The side effects of angiotensin converting enzyme (ACE) inhibitor (a medication used to treat cardiovascular diseases) may include abdominal pain, abdominal distention, nausea, vomiting, and diarrhea. The side effects of beta blockers (frequently used to treat high blood pressure) include nausea or vomiting, constipation, and diarrhea. Nitrates, which are used to treat chest pain, may also produce nausea and vomiting as side effects. Similarly, thrombolytic agents (medica-tions that dissolve clots in the arteries) can produce nausea, vomiting, and abdominal pain.

HIV/AIDS and other infectious diseases

HIV/AIDS is described in Chapter 14. In addition to GI dysfunction that can occur in conjunction with opportunistic infections and other immune-related abnormalities, certain medications used in the treatment of HIV/AIDS are also known to produce GI symptoms. Four classes of medications used in the treat-ment of HIV/AIDS can cause gastrointestinal side effects. These include:

• Nonnucleoside reverse transcriptase inhibitors
• Nucleoside reverse transcriptase inhibitors
• Protease inhibitors
• Fusion inhibitors

To varying degrees, all of these drugs and their combinations may produce nau-sea, vomiting, diarrhea, abdominal pain, and/or abdominal pain to varying degrees in up to 27 percent of individuals (Friedland et al., 1999; Fung and Guo 2004; Nadler 2003; Pollard et al., 1998).

   In addition to the side effects produced by anti-HIV/AIDS medications, vari-ous antibiotics used to treat common infections and other infectious diseases may produce diarrhea and abdominal cramping.

Conclusion

This chapter provided an overview of the prevalence of GI dysfunction within the general population and among individuals with various chronic illnesses. It described common ways in which GI dysfunction is subclassified and experienced. In addition, basic information about a number of conditions for which GI dysfunction is a primary symptom was provided. The next chapter will present case study of Alex, who has Crohn's disease. This chapter will also illustrate some special considerations of assessment and intervention with persons who have gastrointestinal dysfunction.

21

Cognitive Behavioral Assessment and Treatment Outcomes for Gastrointestinal Dysfunction: The Case of Alex

Chapter 20 covered gastrointestinal problems as a major symptom category. It provided an overview of common chronic conditions that involve gastrointestinal symptoms and reviewed issues related to the etiology and prevalence of common gastrointestinal disorders. This chapter will illustrate the application of cognitive behavioral therapy to Alex, who was introduced in Chapter 1 and periodically discussed throughout the text.

The first objective of this case example is to synthesize the earlier examples that focused on Alex, discussing the case as a whole and summarizing therapy outcomes. The second objective of this chapter is to illustrate unique intervention approaches that can be incorporated into cognitive behavioral therapy with clients that have gastrointestinal symptoms or disorders. The chapter will close with an overview of the unique considerations in treating individuals with gastrointestinal symptoms and disorders.

As described in Chapter 1, Alex is a 23-year-old graduate student with Crohn's Disease. He was referred for cognitive behavioral therapy by his school advisor because he was having difficulty adjusting to a recent progression of his Crohn's disease and appeared unusually concerned about his academic performance.

Initial Orientation, Approach to Assessment and Assessment Findings

Alex completed the initial orientation and assessment within a single session. Medical records and verbal information from Alex's colorectal surgeon and school advisor were collected. In addition, the following assessments were completed during the first session:

- Semistructured clinical interview
- Problem list

Findings from these assessments are presented in the sections that follow.

Orientation and Rapport-Building

Alex approached therapy seriously and listened actively to the therapist's introduction to the structure, process, and expectations of cognitive behavioral
therapy. Although he appeared anxious, it was clear that he was social, open, and
comfortable with self-disclosure. Alex responded well to the therapist's efforts to
establish rapport and create a collaborative working relationship.

Semistructured Clinical Interview

The therapist conducted the semistructured clinical interview to elicit information
about Alex's physical health history, present GI symptoms, level of impairment,
psychosocial history, family background, current psychiatric symptoms, and recent
difficulties adjusting to the progression of Crohn's disease (reviewed in Chapter 1).

The therapist included questions that were specific to Alex's GI problems to
obtain more information about Alex's reactions to the recent change in his health
status. These questions and Alex's responses are presented in Table 1.

From this exchange the therapist was able to establish that Alex was generally
compliant in taking prescribed medications but he was not as committed to
managing his illness through exercise. The therapist was also able to obtain more
background information about the origin of Alex's current health, academic, and
social (dating) concerns.

Problem List

During the initial clinical interview, Alex completed a problem list. This list consisted of two problems:

- Worries about the effects of his recent health problems (e.g., severe diarrhea,
  abdominal pain, occasional mild fevers, and fatigue) on his academic performance.
- Concerns about the implications recent progression of his Crohn's disease in
  terms of his future plans for career and family.

Because Alex requested to complete his therapy within five sessions, the therapist did not administer any additional assessments. Based on findings from the
semistructured clinical interview and problem list, the therapist felt comfortable
making the following diagnostic conclusions.

DSM-IV Diagnostic Profile

Axis I: Adjustment disorder with anxiety
Axis II: No diagnosis
Axis III: Crohn's disease
Axis IV: Psychosocial issues: educational problems
Axis V: Global assessment of functioning = 75

TABLE 1. Alex's responses to supplemental clinical interview questions for clients with GI difficulties.

Therapist:	"Right now, what are your main concerns about Crohn's?"
Alex:	"That it will interfere with my ability to attend class, study, and keep up my social life. I'm also worried about my future. If this disease continues to progress, I may lose my colon and have to wear a colostomy bag. I just can't fathom that right now."
Therapist:	"Have you asked your doctor how likely it would be that you would lose your colon?"
Alex:	"Well he said that they only remove it after all other attempts have been made to reduce the number of obstructions and complications with medications, diet, and exercise."
Therapist:	"How many of these options have you tried?"
Alex:	"Well, not all the options, but I do watch my diet and take any medications that the doctor prescribes pretty regularly – some of them cause my face to swell up and stuff but I take them anyway. That's why I'm worried about what's going on with this right now. It doesn't make sense that it's happening again."
Therapist:	"Have you noticed that making changes to your diet and activity levels have been helpful in the past?"
Alex:	"Yes and no. I've never been a big exerciser. Grad school has made it more difficult for me to be active. Plus, it's more stressful now. I suppose there are some things I could do to improve my overall health. Maybe exercise would help."
Therapist:	"Tell me more about your academic concerns. When your Crohn's was severe in the past were you not able to attend class and study?"
Alex:	"Yes. The first time it happened, it interrupted everything. I had to go have surgery and take incompletes in all my classes. This girl I was dating stopped dating me at that time. I didn't think about it much then because she wasn't that great, but looking back on it now, it was a very dark time."
Therapist:	"What do you anticipate is your situation right now—with your classes?"
Alex:	"I did poorly on a midterm in one class and so I have to get an A on the final. Otherwise, I'm doing OK in all the other classes, but if I fail the finals, my grade point average could really plummet."
Therapist:	"Are you dating anyone right now?"
Alex:	"Not seriously, but I am interested in this one girl, Judy."
Therapist:	"Any concerns about Judy?"
Alex:	"Well, she doesn't really know I have Crohn's and it might scare her away."

Treatment Goals

Alex's main goal for therapy was to reduce his feelings of anticipatory anxiety. Alex was worried about his performance on upcoming final exams at school and concerned about the recent progression of his Crohn's disease. His goal was established at the end of the first session, and the 5th session was set as the target date for attaining this goal. Alex's confidence rating that he would be able to reduce his anxiety was an "8" on a scale of 1 to 10. Figure 1 shows this goal and the steps that Alex agreed to take to accomplish that goal.

Once these goals were established, the final step of orientation involved establishing a cognitive behavioral case conceptualization.

Goal Form		
Goal(s) **Target date**	**Confidence rating** (1–10)	**Objectives** (realistic steps I can take to achieve goal)
Goal 1: Reduce anxiety about academic performance and recent disease progression 5th session on 11/22/03	8	a) Identify and dispute pessimistic beliefs using ABCDE method. b) Increase physical activity before and after surgery as a means of managing stress and building endurance.

FIGURE 1. Alex's Goal Form

Cognitive Behavioral Case Conceptualization

During the first session, a very basic overview of the cognitive model was provided. The therapist explained the relationships between health event triggers, automatic thoughts, and emotional, behavioral, and physiological outcomes. The therapist did not include information about the three levels of belief because she knew that Alex would not be spending enough time in therapy to begin work on his intermediate and core beliefs. Alex accepted and understood the basic aspects of the cognitive model relatively quickly and was ready to work with the therapist to try to understand his anxiety according to the cognitive model. Together, they completed the "case conceptualization worksheet" to develop a case conceptualization that explained the cognitive, behavioral, and emotional aspects of his anticipatory anxiety. Alex was satisfied with this conceptualization, which is presented in Figure 2.

Alex identified his health-event trigger as one of any number of GI symptoms. In this case, he chose to identify diarrhea as the triggering event. When Alex has an episode of diarrhea, he automatically wonders about its potential impact on some aspect of his academic performance. In this example he is concerned that his diarrhea at school might interfere with his ability to remain present during his next class. This thought is accompanied by worry, inactivity, eating the wrong foods, and worsening GI symptoms.

Summary of the Orientation and Assessment Phase

In summary, Alex's socialization into cognitive behavioral therapy was brief and straightforward. The following four steps were covered:

- Rapport-building and the establishment of a collaborative empirical relationship.
- Outlining the structure, process and other essential elements of cognitive behavioral therapy.

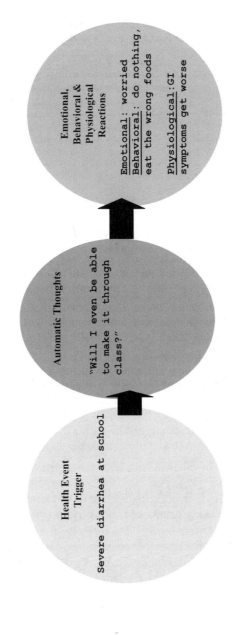

FIGURE 2. Alex's Case Conceptualization.

- Defining problems, establishing goals, and setting a provisional target date for completion of his primary goal.
- Teaching the cognitive model.

By the end of the first session, Alex understood the basic structure and process of cognitive behavioral therapy and was motivated to work toward his primary goal of anxiety reduction. He asked the therapist to recommend a self-help book that he might read between sessions. In choosing a recommended book, the therapist considered the fact that many of Alex's worries stemmed from a loss of optimism about his future. The therapist postulated that increasing Alex's sense of optimism would allow him to build upon his existing psychological strengths and coping skills following therapy. Therefore she recommended Seligman's (2002) book, *Authentic Happiness*. Alex purchased the book and had nearly completed it by the second session.

Subsequent Sessions: Course of Treatment

Alex received a total of 5 sessions of cognitive behavioral therapy over a 3-month period. The sessions focused specifically on reducing his anticipatory anxiety related to his academic performance and to the recent progression of Crohn's disease.

Main Emphasis of the Socratic Questioning

For Alex, Socratic questioning focused on probing evidence for and against the following dysfunctional cognitions:

- His fear that he might lose bowel control during classes, exams, or social outings (dates)
- His belief that he was not intelligent enough to continue graduate school
- His feelings of shame and self-disgust about his illness
- His belief that Judy would leave him if she knew about his illness

In-Session Cognitive and Behavioral Activities

In an effort to improve Alex's sense of control over his overall health, physical activity was recommended as one of the objectives for anxiety reduction. The therapist's rationale was that this recommendation would be important in terms of enhancing Alex's mood and body image, particularly following surgery. In this vein, Alex learned to complete a daily activity schedule. An example of the recommended daily activity schedule that Alex and the therapist developed together one week following surgery was originally presented in Chapter 9. For convenience, it is presented again in Figure 3.

Using this schedule, Alex was coached to list all activities planned during a single 24-hour period. He was then instructed to allocate a certain number of

Week 1: April 15th – April 21st				
Activities scheduled	**Minutes/day**	**Importance**	**Competence**	**Pleasure**
Walking meditation	10 min 3x/day	10	5	5
Watching movies	4 hours	3	3	10
Reading	2 hours	10	10	10
Contact with friends	1 hour	10	5	8
Eating	2.5hours	10	1	3
Hygiene and wound Care	1 hour	10	10	1
Rest/sleep	13 hours/day	10	1	10

FIGURE 3. Alex's Daily Activity Schedule One Week Following Surgery

minutes to each activity per day. It was recommended that the number of minutes allocated to each activity correspond to the extent to which each activity was important to Alex, pleasurable, and engendered feelings of competence. It was recommended that Alex include at least one physical activity in this schedule per week. For the first week following surgery, the therapist recommended the "walking meditation" activity (Kabat-Zin 1990), originally presented in Chapter 8.

Although initially Alex's schedule indicated that he was engaging in an appropriate level of physical activity, it was not pleasurable for him. Once his postoperative pain had subsided, Alex found a way to make physical activity more pleasurable by socializing during a vigorous walk. He increased his activity progressively following surgery and eventually saw that there were health-related and mood-related benefits to exercising. A more detailed description of how this process evolved is provided in Chapter 9.

The second recommended objective for anxiety reduction involved teaching Alex to use Seligman's (2002) ABCDE model as a means of identifying and disputing his pessimistic beliefs and worries about the future implications of Crohn's disease on his life and functioning. More information about Alex's use of this model is provided in the section of this chapter entitled "Use of Related Knowledge as a Supplemental Approach."

Homework Prescribed

Three homework assignments were recommended during the course of therapy.

- Reading Seligman's (2002) book, *Authentic Happiness*
- Completing the daily activity schedule
- Practicing Seligman's (2002) ABCDE model

Alex completed all homework assignments successfully and on time. He reported that he found them to be helpful in reducing anxiety, improving self-confidence, and allowing him to reprioritize his activities.

Difficulties Encountered

There were no significant difficulties encountered during the course of therapy. To maintain consistency in contact, one session was conducted in Alex's hospital room when he was recovering from surgery.

Use of Related Knowledge as a Supplemental Approach

From the initial interview, it was clear to the therapist that Alex possessed a number of existing psychological resources and coping mechanisms. His recent, unanticipated health crisis prompted him to experience concerns about his future. These concerns appeared to stem from a fundamental lack of optimism. The therapist relied on hope theory and other elements of positive psychology to augment Alex's existing psychological resources and to facilitate his adjustment to his recent health crisis. Specifically, Alex practiced and memorized the ABCDE model so that he could use this model to identify and dispute dysfunctional and pessimistic beliefs. One example of how he used the ABCDE model to dispute a belief related to self-disgust about his illness was originally presented in Chapter 12. For convenience, it is presented again in Table 2.

Treatment Outcome: Termination and Relapse Prevention

By the fifth session, Alex reported that, although his concerns about his future had not dissipated entirely, he felt less anxious and more equipped to manage his illness. He managed to complete all of his scheduled final exams before his surgery and reported that he received three Bs and one C in his classes. Although he was not satisfied with his grades, he was able to view his performance as situational and specific to his recent health problems. In addition, he used the ABCDE

TABLE 2. Alex's sse of Seligman's (2002) ABCDE model.

Adversity:	Had to stop at the gas station to use the toilet on a first date.
Belief:	I am disgusting.
Consequence:	I'm feeling ugly and inferior and making the situation even worse. I'm feeling depressed and can't have a good time.
Disputation:	It's embarrassing to have to run to a toilet every time I eat, but it does not mean I am disgusting. If Judy doesn't accept my disease, I'll find someone else who does.
Energization:	I'm feeling more empowered and in control with respect to my relationship with Judy. I feel good that I can advocate for myself instead of allowing fears of what others might think to make me feel uncomfortable.

model to dispute his fundamental beliefs that he was not smart enough to continue graduate school. By the end of therapy, he increased his physical activity significantly and was continuing his dating relationship with Judy. Plans for relapse prevention included:

- Reviewing what he had learned from Seligman's (2002) book whenever necessary
- Utilizing the daily activity record whenever he felt the need to prioritize his activities and maintain consistency in physical activity
- Practicing the ABCDE model to dispute pessimistic beliefs

Alex reported that he felt confident that he could rely upon any of these strategies if his anxiety became overwhelming.

Learning from Alex: Unique Features of Individuals with Gastrointestinal Difficulties

Like many individuals with gastrointestinal difficulties, Alex was concerned about the unanticipated of loss of bowel control in public and in social and occupational situations. He also worried about the effects of his lack of bowel control on the perceptions of others. In addition, he experienced significant feelings of shame and self-disgust related to his own bodily functions. These considerations are important to keep in mind when working in therapy with any individual with gastrointestinal problems.

References

Ader, R. (2003) Conditioned immunomodulation: Research needs and directions. *Brain Behavior and Immunity, 17,* S51–S57.

Ader, R. (1980). Psychosomatic and psychoimmunologic research. *Psychosomatic Medicine, 42,* 307–321.

Affleck, G., and Tennen, H. (1996). Construing benefits from adversity: Adaptational significance and dispositional underpinnings. *Journal of Personality, 64,* 899–922.

Affleck, G., Tennen, H., Croog, S., and Levine, S. (1987). Causal attribution, perceived benefits, and morbidity following a heart attack: An 8-year study. *Journal of Consulting and Clinical Psychology, 55,* 29–35.

Ajzen, I., and Fishbein, M. (1977). Attitude-behavior relations: A theoretical analysis and review of empirical research. *Psychological Bulletin,84,* 888–918.

Alan, R. (2004). Burlington, MA (August, 2004); *Symptoms of epilepsy.* Retrieved September 29, 2004, from *http://healthinfo.healthgate.com/GetContent.aspx?token= b6097602-42e3-44e8-89c8-c88ab799256b&chunkiid=19407*

American Academy of Family Physicians. (2000). Leawood, KS (November, 2001); *Familydoctor.org: Angina and heart disease.* Retrieved September 30, 2004, from *http://familydoctor.org/x1606.xml*

American Academy of Orthopaedic Surgeons (AAOS). (2000). *Low back pain.* Retrieved July 27, 2004, from *http://orthoinfo.aaos.org/brochure/thr_report.cfm?Thread_ID= 10&topcategory=Spine*

American Cancer Society, Inc. (2004). Atlanta, GA (2004); Retrieved October 18, 2004, from *http://www.cancer.org/docroot/home/index.asp?level=0*

American College of Rheumatology. (2003). Atlanta, GA (October, 2003); *American College of Rheumatology facts sheets: Fibromyalgia.* Retrieved September 29, 2004, from *http://www.rheumatology.org/public/factsheets/fibromya.asp*

American Heart Association. (1984). *Heart facts, 1984.* Dallas, TX: American Heart Association.

American Heart Association. (1988). *1989 heart facts.* Dallas, TX: American Heart Association.

American Heart Association. (2004). Dallas, TX (2004); *Heart attack and angina statistics.* Retrieved September 30, 2004, from *http://www.americanheart.org/presenter. jhtml?identifier=4591*

American Heart Association. (2004). (March 19, 2004); *Heart Disease and Stroke Statistics: 2004 Update.* Retrieved July 16, 2004 from *http://www.americanheart.org/ downloadable/heart/1079736729696HDSStats2004UpdateREV3-19-04.pdf*

American Psychiatric Association. (1994). *Diagnostic and Statistical Manual of Mental Disorders* (4ᵗʰ ed.). Washington, D.C: American Psychiatric Association.

Anemia Lifeline. (2002). *Anemia Lifeline: Understanding anemia.* Retrieved September 20, 2004, from *http://www.anemia.com*

Antoni, M.H., Lehman, J.M., Kilbourn, K.M., Boyers, A.E., Culver, J.L., Alferi, S.M., et al. (2001). Cognitive-behavioral stress management intervention decreases the prevalence of depression and enhances benefit finding among women under treatment for early-stage breast cancer. *Health Psychology, 20*(1), 20–32.

Aras, M.D., Gokkaya, N.K., Comert, D., Kaya, A., and Cakci, A. (2004). Shoulder pain in hemiplegia: Results from a national rehabilitation hospital in Turkey. *American Journal of Physical Medicine and Rehabilitation, 83*(9), 713–719.

Arnkoff, D.B. (1983). Common and specific factors in cognitive therapy. In M.J. Lambert (Ed.), *Psychotherapy and patient relationships* (pp. 85–125). Homewood, IL: Dorsey Press.

Arthritis Foundation. (2004). *Rheumatoid Arthritis.* Retrieved July 27, 2004, from *http://www.arthritis.org/conditions/DiseaseCenter/ra.asp*

Ashley, F.W., Jr, and Kannel, W.B. (1974). Relation of weight change to changes in atherogenic traits: The Framingham Study. *Journal of Chronic Diseases, 27*(3), 103–114.

Asmundson, G.J.G. and Wright, K.D. (2004) Biopsychosocial Approaches to Pain. In T. Hadjistavropoulos and K.D.Craig, (Eds.) *Pain: Psychological Perspectives.* Mahwah, New Jersey: Lawrence Erlbaum Associates (p. 35–58)

Asmundson, G.J.G., Norton, P.J., and Norton, G.R. (1999) Beyond pain: The role of fear and avoidance in chronicity. *Clinical Psychology Review, 19,* 97–119.

Aspinwall, L.G., and Staudinger, U.M. (Eds.). (2003). *A psychology of human strengths: Fundamental questions and future directions for a positive psychology.* Washington, DC: APA Books.

Atkinson, J.H., Slater, M.A., Patterson, T.L., Grant, I., and Garfin, S.R. (1991). Prevalence, onset, and risk of psychiatric disorders in men with chronic low back pain: A controlled study. *Pain, 45*(2), 111–121.

Badani, K.K., Hemal, A.K., and Menon, M. (2004). Autosomal dominant polycystic kidney disease and pain—A review of the disease from aetiology, evaluation, past surgical treatment options to current practice. *Journal of Postgraduate Medicine, 50,* 222–226.

Bajwa, Z.H., Gupta, S., Warfield, C.A., and Steinman, T.I. (2001). Pain management in polycystic kidney disease. *Kidney International, 60*(5), 1631–1644.

Bandura, A. (1986). *Social foundations of thought and action: A social cognitive theory.* Englewood Cliffs, NJ: Prentice-Hall.

Bandura, A. (2001). Social cognitive theory: An agentive perspective. *Annual Review of Psychology, 52,* 1–26.

Banks, S., and Kerns, R. (1996). Explaining high rates of depression in chronic pain: A diathesis-stress framework. *Psychological Bulletin, 119,* 95–110

Baron, K., Kielhofner, G., Iyenger, A., Goldhammer, V., and Wolenski, J. (2002). *Occupational Self Assessment (OSA)* (Version 2.1). Chicago, IL: Model of Human Occupation Clearinghouse, Department of Occupational Therapy, College of Applied Health Sciences, University of Illinois at Chicago.

Barrowclough, C., Haddock, G., Tarrier, N., Lewis, S.W., Moring, J., O'Brien, R., et al. (2001). Randomized controlled trial of motivational interviewing, cognitive behavior therapy, and family intervention for patients with comorbid schizophrenia and substance use disorders. *American Journal of Psychiatry, 158*(10), 1706–1713.

Bazil, C.W. (2000). Sleep and epilepsy. *Current opinion in neurology, 13,* 171–175.

Beck, A.T. (1964). Thinking and depression: II. Theory and therapy. *Archives of General Psychiatry, 10*, 561–571.

Beck, A.T. (1991). Cognitive therapy as the integrative therapy. *Journal of Psychotherapy Integration, 1*(3), 191–198.

Beck, A.T. (1996). Beyond belief: A theory of modes, personality, and psychopathology. In P. Salkovskis (Ed.), *Frontiers of Cognitive Therapy* (pp. 1–25). New York: Guilford Press.

Beck, A.T. (1999). *Prisoners of hate: The cognitive basis of anger, hostility, and violence.* New York: Harper Collins Publishers.

Beck, A.T., Beck, R., and Kovacs, M. (1975). Classification of suicidal behaviors: I. Quantifying intent and medical lethality. *American Journal of Psychiatry, 132*(3), 285–287.

Beck, A.T., and Emery, G. (with Greenberg, R.L.). (1985). *Anxiety disorders and phobias: A cognitive perspective.* New York: Basic Books.

Beck, A.T., Freeman, A., et al. (1990). *Cognitive therapy of personality disorders.* New York: Guilford Press.

Beck, A.T., Kovacs, M., and Weissman, A. (1979). Assessment of suicidal intention: The Scale for Suicide Ideation. *Journal of Consulting & Clinical Psychology, 47*(2), 343–352.

Beck, A.T., Rush, A.J., Shaw, B.F., and Emery, G. (1979). *Cognitive therapy of depression.* New York: Guilford Press.

Beck, A.T., Steer, R.A., and Brown, G.K. (1996). *Manual for Beck Depression Inventory— II.* San Antonio, TX: Psychological Corporation.

Beck, A.T., Weissman, A., Lester, D., and Trexler, L. (1974). The measurement of pessimism: The Hopelessness Scale. *Journal of Consulting and Clinical Psychology, 42*, 861–865.

Beck, J. (1995). *Cognitive therapy: Basics and beyond.* New York: Guilford Press.

Beck, S.L., and Falkson, G. (2001). Prevalence and management of cancer pain in South Africa. *Pain, 94*, 75–84.

Beck, A.T., Guth, D., Steer, R.A., and Ball, R. (1997). Screening for major depression disorders in medical inpatients with the Beck Depression Inventory for primary care. *Behavior Research and Therapy, 35,* 785–791.

Beisecker, A., Cook, M.R., Ashworth, J., Hayes, J., Brecheisen, M., Helmig, L., et al. (1997). Side effects of adjuvant chemotherapy: Perceptions of node-negative breast cancer patients. *Psycho-Oncology, 6*(2), 85–93.

Bekkelund, S.I., and Salvesen, R. (2002). Prevalence of head trauma in patients with difficult headache: The North Norway Headache Study. *Headache, 43*, 59–62.

Belmont, H.M. (1998). New York (1998); *Lupus clinical overview.* Retrieved December 6, 2004, from *http://cerebel.com/lupus/overview.htm*

Bergin, A.E. and Garfield, S.L. (1994). *Handbook of Psychotherapy and Behavior Change* (4th ed.). Oxford: John Wiley and Sons.

Berlin, R.M., Livovitz, G.L., Diaz, M.A., and Ahmed, S.W. (1984) Sleep disorders on a psychiatric consultation service. *American Journal of Psychiatry, 141*, 582–584.

Bets, T.A., and Alford, C. (1983) Beta-blocking drugs and sleep. *Drugs, 25,* 268–272.

Beutler, L.E., Harwood, T.M., and Caldwell, R. (2001). Cognitive-behavioral therapy and psychotherapy integration. In K.S. Dobson (Ed.), *Handbook of cognitive-behavioral therapies* (2nd ed.) (pp. 138–170). New York: Guilford Press.

Blumenthal, D., Gokhale, M., Campbell, E.G., and Weissman, J.S. (2001). Preparing for clinical practice: Reports of graduating residents at academic health centers. *Journal of the American Medical Association, 286*, 1027–1034.

Blunt, C., and Schmiedel, A. (2004). Some cases of severe post-mastectomy pain syndrome may be caused by an axillary haematoma. *Pain, 108*(3), 294–296.

Bombardier, C.H., D'Amico, C., and Jordan, J.S. (1990). The relationship of appraisal and coping to chronic illness adjustment. *Behavior Research and Therapy, 28*(4), 297–304.

BreastCancer.org. (2004). Narbeth, PA (July 12, 2004); Retrieved November 2, 2004, from *http://www.breastcancer.org/treatment.html*

Breslin, E., van der Schans, C., Breukink, S., Meek, P., Mercer, K., Volz, W., and Louie, S. (1998). Perception of fatigue and quality of life in patients with COPD. *The Cardiopulmonary and Critical Care Journal, 114*(4), 958–964.

Bruce, I., Mak, V., Hallett, D., Gladman, D., and Urowitz, M. (1999). Factors associated with fatigue in patients with systemic lupus erythematosus. *Annals of the Rheumatic Diseases, 58*(6), 379–381.

Brunink, S.A. and Schroeder, S.E. (1979). Verbal therapeutic behavior of expert psycho-analytically oriented, gestalt, and behavior therapists. *Journal of Consulting and Clinical Psychology, 47,* 567–574.

Bryant, F.B., and Verhoff, J. (1982). The structure of psychological well-being: A socio-historical analysis. *Journal of Personality and Social Psychology, 43,* 653–673.

Bryant, F.B., and Verhoff, J. (1984). Dimensions of subjective mental health in American men and women. *Journal of Health & Social Behavior, 25,* 116–135.

Burns, D.D. (1980). *Feeling good: The new mood therapy.* New York: Signet.

Buchwald, D.S., Rea, T., Katon, W., Russo, J., and Ashley, R.L. (2000). Acute infectious mononucleosis: Characteristics of patients who report failure to recover. *American Journal of Medicine, 109,* 531–537.

Burns, D.D., and Auerbach, A. (1996). Therapeutic empathy in cognitive-behavioral therapy: Does it really make a difference? In P.M. Salkovskis (Ed.), *Frontiers of Cognitive Therapy* (pp. 135–164). New York: Guilford Press.

Burns, D.D., and Nolen-Hoeksema, S. (1992). Therapeutic empathy and recovery from depression in cognitive-behavioral therapy: A structural equation model. *Journal of Consulting and Clinical Psychology, 60,* 441–449.

Bushby, K.M., Pollitt, C., Johnson, M.A., Rogers, M.T., and Chinnery, P.F. (1998). Muscle pain as a prominent feature of facioscapulohumeral muscular dystrophy (FSHD): Four illustrative case reports. *Neuromuscular Disorders, 8*(8), 574–579.

Caro, I. (1998). Integration of cognitive psychotherapies: Vive la difference!, Right now. *Journal of Cognitive Psychotherapy, 12*(1), 67–76.

Carr, D., Goudas, L., Lawrence, D., Pirl, W., Lau, J., and DeVine, D. (2002). Rockville, MD (July 2002); *Management of cancer symptoms: Pain, depression, and fatigue. Evidence report/technology assessment no. 61* (Prepared by the New England Medical Center Evidence-based Practice Center under contract no. 290-97-0019). Agency for Healthcare Research and Quality Pub. No.02-E032. Retrieved September 22, 2004, from *http://www.ahrq.gov/downloads/pub/evidence/pdf/cansymp/etbls.pdf*

Carver, C.S., and Antoni, M.H. (2004). Finding benefit in breast cancer during the year after diagnosis predicts better adjustment 5 to 8 years after diagnosis. *Health Psychology, 23*(6), 595–598.

Carver, C.S., Scheier, M.F., and Weintraub, J. (1989). Assessing coping strategies: A theoretically based approach. *Journal of Personality and Social Psychology, 56,* 267–283.

Castillo, J., Munoz, P., Guitera, V., and Pascual, J. (1999). Epidemiology of chronic daily headache in the general population. *Headache, 39,* 190–196.

Centers for Disease Control and Prevention (CDC). (2002). (October 24, 2002); *Prevalence of Self-Reported Arthritis or Chronic Joint Symptoms Among Adults—United States,*

2001. Retrieved July 16, 2004, from *http://www.cdc.gov/mmwr/preview/mmwrhtml/ mm514a2.htm*

Centers for Disease Control and Prevention (CDC). (2004a). *Chronic Disease Prevention.* Retrieved July 14, 2004, from *http://www.cdc.gov/nccdphp/*

Centers for Disease Control and Prevention (CDC). (2004b). Atlanta, GA (June 2, 2004); *First joint survey of health in Canada and the United States shows both countries report high level of health.* Retrieved October 27, 2004, from *http://www.cdc.gov/od/oc/media/ pressrel/r040602.htm*

Centers for Disease Control and Prevention (CDC), Division of Viral Hepatitis. (2004c). Washington, DC (August 1, 2004); *Viral hepatitis B fact sheet.* Retrieved October 4, 2004, from *http://www.cdc.gov/ncidod/diseases/hepatitis/b/fact.htm*

Centers for Disease Control and Prevention (CDC), National Center for Health Statistics (NCHS). (2003). Hyattsville, MD (January 28, 2003); *Asthma prevalence, health care use and mortality, 2000–2001.* Retrieved September 22, 2004, from *http://www.cdc.gov/nchs/ products/pubs/pubd/hestats/asthma/asthma.htm*

Chang, V.T., Hwang, S.S., Feuerman, M., and Kasimis, B.S. (2000). Symptom and quality of life survey of medical oncology patients at a veterans affairs medical center: A role for symptom assessment. *Cancer, 88*(5), 1175–1183.

Charlton, J. (1998). *Nothing about us without us.* Berkeley, CA: University of California Press.

Chowdury, R.S., Forsmarch, C.E., Davis, R.H., Toskes, P.P., and Verne, G.N. (2003). Prevalence of gastroparesis in patients with small duct chronic pancreatitis. *Pancreas, 26*(3), 235–238.

Clark, D.A., Beck, A.T., and Alford, B. (1999). *Scientific foundations of cognitive theory and therapy of depression.* New York: John Wiley & Sons.

Cleveland Clinic Health System (CCHS). (2003). Cleveland, OH (November 1, 2003); *A vicious cycle: Chronic illness and depression.* Retrieved October 28, 2004, from *http://www.cchs.net/health/health-info/docs/2200/2282.asp?index=9288&dpath=http: //www.cchs.net/health/health-info/docs/2200/2282.asp?index=9288*

Cohen, A.J. (1998). Caring for the chronically ill: A vital subject for medical education. *Academic Medicine, 73*, 1261–1266.

Coleman, R.M., Roffwarg, H.P., Kennedy, S.J., Guilleminault, C., Cinque, J., Cohn, M, et. al. (1982) Sleep-wake disorders based on polysomnographic diagnosis: A national cooperative study. Journal of the American Medical Association, 247, 997–1003.

Collin, P., Kaukinen, K., Valimaki, M. and Salmi, J. (2002). Endocrinological disorders and celiac disease. *Endrocrine Reviews, 23*(4), 464–483.

Comella, C. (2002). Restless legs syndrome: Treatment with dopaminergic agents. *Neurology, 58*(4), S87–S92.

Contrada, R.J., and Krantz, D.S. (1988). Stress, reactivity, and type A behavior: Current status and future directions. *Annals of Behavioral Medicine, 10*, 64–70.

Costa, P.T., Jr. and VandenBos, G.R. (eds.). (1990). *Psychological aspects of serious illness: Chronic conditions, fatal diseases, and clinical care.* Washington, DC: American Psychological Association.

Craig Hospital. (2004). Englewood, CO. *Fatigue.* Retrieved September 22, 2004, from *http://www.craighospital.org/SCI/METS/fatigue.asp*

Craig Hospital. (n.d.) Englewood, CO (No revision date available); *Colostomies: A Radical Approach to Bowel Mangement.* Retrieved November 1, 2004, from *http://www. craighospital.org/SCI/METS/colostomies.asp*

Curt, G.A., Breitbart, W., Cella, D., Groopman, J.E., Horning, S.J., Itri, L.M., et al. (2000). Impact of cancer-related fatigue on the lives of patients: New findings from the Fatigue Coalition. *Oncologist, 5*(5), 353–360.

Csikszentmihalyi, M. (2000). The contribution of flow to positive psychology. In J.E. Gillham (Ed.). *The science of optimism and hope: Research essays in honor of Martin E.P. Seligman. Laws of life symposia series.* (pp. 387–395). Philadelphia, PA: Templeton Foundation Press.

Dahl, R.C. (2000). Wheat Ridge, CO (July 30, 2004); Retrieved October 13, 2004, from *http://www.csaceliacs.org/GreatMimic.php*

Darko, D., McCutchan, A., Kripke, D., Gillin, J., and Golshan, S. (1992). Fatigue, sleep disturbance, disability, and indices of progression of HIV infection. *American Journal of Psychiatry, 149*(4), 514–520.

Davis, B. (2004). Assessing adults with mental disorders in primary care. *The Nurse Practitioner, 29*(5), 19–27.

Davis, B.E., Nelson, D.B., Sahler, O.J., McCurdy, F.A., Goldberg, R., and Greenberg, L. W. (2001). Do clerkship experiences affect medical students' attitudes toward chronically ill patients? *Academic Medicine, 76*, 815–820.

Davis, C.G., Nolen-Hoeksema, S., and Larson, J. (1998). Making sense of loss and benefiting from the experience: Two construals of meaning. *Journal of Personality and Social Psychology, 75*, 561–574.

Davis, M., Eshelman, E.R., and McKay, M. (1988). *The relaxation and stress reduction workbook.* Oakland, CA: New Harbinger.

Davis, T.H., Jason, L.A., and Banghart, M.A. (1998). The effect of housing on individuals with multiple chemical sensitivities. *Journal of Primary Prevention, 19*, 31–42.

Davison, S.N. (2003). Pain in hemodialysis patients: Prevalence, cause, severity, and management. *American Journal of Kidney Diseases, 42*(6), 1239–1247.

DeCharms, R. (1972). Personal causation training in the schools. *Journal of Applied Social Psychology, 2*(2), 95–113.

DeCharms, R. (1976). *Enhancing motivation: Change in the classroom.* New York: Irvington Publishers.

DeCharms, R. (1992). Personal causation and the origin concept. In C.P. Smith, J.W. Atkinson, D.C. McClelland, and J. Veroff (Eds.), *Motivation and personality: Handbook of thematic content analysis* (pp. 325–333). New York: Cambridge University Press.

DeCharms, R., and Muir, M.S. (1978). Motivation: Social approaches. *Annual Review of Psychology, 29*, 91–113.

DeFronzo, R.A. (1999). Pharmacologic therapy for type 2 diabetes mellitus. *Annals of Internal Medicine, 131*(4), 281–303.

Dellon, A.L., Swier, P., Maloney, C.T., Jr., Livengood, M.S., Werter, S. (2004). Chemotherapy-induced neuropathy: Treatment by decompression of peripheral nerves. *Plastic and Reconstructive Surgery, 114*(2), 478–483.

Devins, G.M., Armstrong, S.J., Mandin, H., Paul, L.C., Hons, R.B., Burgess, E.D., et al. (1990). Recurrent pain, illness intrusiveness, and quality of life in end-stage renal disease. *Pain, 42*(3), 279–285.

Devinsky, O. (2004). No location available (No revision date available); *Fatigue*. Retrieved September 19, 2004, from *http://www.epilepsy.com/epilepsy/interprob_fatigue.html*

DeVivo, M.J., Fine, P.R., Maetz, H.M., and Stover, S.L. (1980). Prevalence of spinal cord injury: A reestimation employing life table techniques. *Archives of Neurology, 37*(11), 707–708.

Diamond, G., Godley, S.H., Liddle, H.A., Sampl, S., Webb, C., Tims, F.M., et al. (2002). Five outpatient treatment models for adolescent marijuana use: A description of the Cannabis Youth Treatment Interventions. *Addiction, 97*(Suppl. 1), 70–83.

Diel, I., Solomayer, E., and Bastert, G. (2000). Treatment of metastatic bone disease in breast cancer: bisphosphonates. *Clinical Breast Cancer, 1*, 43–51.

Dimeo, F., Stieglitz, R., Novelli-Fischer, U., Fetscher, S., and Keul, J. (1999). Effects of physical activity on the fatigue and psychologic status of cancer patients during chemotherapy. *Cancer, 85*(10), 2273–2277.

Dinges, D.F. (1995) An overview of sleepiness and accidents. *Journal of Sleep Research, 4*, 4–14

Dobson, K.S. (2001). *Handbook of cognitive-behavioral therapies* (2nd ed.). New York: Guilford Press.

Dobson, K.S., and Dozois, D.J.A. (2001). Historical and philosophical bases of the cognitive-behavioral therapies. In K.S. Dobson (ed.), *Handbook of cognitive-behavioral therapies* (2nd ed.) (pp. 3–39). New York: Guilford Press.

DoctorOnline.nhs.uk. (2004). No location available (October 14, 2004); *Pain following a stroke*. Retrieved October 14, 2004, from *http://www.doctoronline.nhs.uk/masterwebsite1Asp/targetpages/specialts/pain/stroke*

Donnay, A. (1998, October). *Questionnaire for screening CFS, FMS, and MCS, in adults.* Testimony presented to the U. S. CFS Coordinating Committee, Washington, D.C.

Drossman, D.A., Li, Z., Andruzzi, E., Temple, R.D., Talley, N.J., Thompson, W.G., et al. (1993). U.S. householder survey of functional gastrointestinal disorders: Prevalence, sociodemography, and health impact. *Digestive Diseases and Sciences, 38*(9), 1569–1580.

Drossman, D.A., Sandler, R.S., McKee, D.C., and Lovitz, A.J. (1982). Bowel patterns among subjects not seeking health care. Use of a questionnaire to identify a population with bowel dysfunction. *Gastroenterology, 83*(3), 529–534.

Drossman, D.A., Richter, J.E., Talley, N.J., Thompson, W.G., Corazziari, E., and Whitehead, W.E. (1994). *Functional gastrointestinal disorders: Diagnosis, pathophysiology, and treatment.* Boston: Little Brown.

D'Zurilla, T.J., and Goldfried, M.R. (1971). Problem-solving therapies and behavior modification. *Journal of Abnormal Psychology, 78*, 107–126.

D'Zurilla, T.J., and Nezu, A.M. (2001). Problem-solving therapies. In K.S. Dobson (ed.), *Handbook of cognitive-behavioral therapies* (2nd ed.) (pp. 211–245). New York: Guilford Press.

Ebright, P.R., and Lyon, B. (2002). Understanding hope and factors that enhance hope in women with breast cancer. *Oncology Nursing Forum, 29*(3), 561–568.

Edgar, L., Rosberger, Z., and Nowlis, D. (1992). Coping with cancer during the first year after diagnosis: Assessment and intervention. *Cancer, 69*, 817–828.

Education Development Center, Inc. (EDC). (2000). Newton, MA (April 18, 2000); *Facts about pain in America*. Retrieved October 19, 2004, from *http://www.edc.org/PainLink/plfctr.html*

Ehlert, U., Wagner, D., and Lupke, U. (1999). Consultation-liaison service in the general hospital: Effects of cognitive-behavioral therapy in patients with physical nonspecific symptoms. *Journal of Psychosomatic Research, 47*(5), 411–117.

Eisenberg, N., Shea, C.L., Carlo, G., and Knight, G.P. (1991). Empathy-related responding and cognition: A "chicken and the egg" dilemma. In W.M. Kurtines and J.L. Gewirtz (eds.), *Handbook of moral behavior and development, Vol. 2: Research* (pp. 63–88). New York: Erlbaum.

Elkin, I., Shea, M.T., Watkins, J.T., Imber, S.D., et al. (1989). National Institute of Mental Health treatment of depression collaborative research program: General effectiveness of treatments. *Archives of General Psychiatry, 46*, 971–982.

Ellis, A. (1962). *Reason and Emotion in Psychotherapy*. Oxford, England: Lyle Stewart.

Emedicine Consumer Health. (2004). No location available (August 16, 2004); *Hepatitis C*. Retrieved December 2, 2004, from *http://www.emedicinehealth.com/Articles/11365-1.asp*

Engel, G.L. (1977). The need for a new medical model: A challenge to biomedicine. *Science, 196*, 129–136.

Erdal, K.J., and Zautra, A.J. (1995). Psychological impact of illness downturns: A comparison of new and chronic conditions. *Psychology and Aging, 10*(4), 570–577.

Feldman, N. (2003). Narcolepsy. *Southern Medical Journal, 96*(3), 277–282.

Felton, B.J., Revenson, T.A., and Hinrichsen, G.A. (1984). Stress and coping in the explanation of psychological adjustment among chronically ill adults. *Social Science and Medicine, 18*(10), 889–898.

Fennell, M.J. and Teasdale, J.D. (1987). Cognitive therapy for depression: Individual differences and the process of change. *Cognitive Therapy and Research, 11*, 253–271.

Fennell, P.A. (1993). A systematic, four-stage progressive model for mapping CFIDS experience. *The CFIDS Chronicle, Summer*, 40–46.

Fennell, P.A. (2003). A four-phase approach to understanding chronic fatigue syndrome. In L.A. Jason, P.A. Fennell, and R.R. Taylor (eds.), *Handbook of Chronic Fatigue Syndrome* (pp. 155–175). Hoboken, NJ: John Wiley and Sons.

First, M.B., Spitzer, R.L., Gibbon, M., and Williams, J.B. W. (1995). *Structured Clinical Interview for DSM-IV Axis I Disorders—Patient edition*. New York: Biometrics Research Department.

Follick, M.J., Smith, T.W., and Ahern, D.K. (1985). The Sickness Profile: A global measure of disability in chronic low back pain. *Pain, 21*, 67–76.

Ford, D.E., and Kamerow, D.B. (1989) Epidemiologic study of sleep disturbances and psychiatric disorders: An opportunity for prevention? *Journal of the American Medical Association, 262*, 1479–1484

Fordyce, W. (1976). *Behavioral methods for chronic pain and illness*. St Louis: C.V. Mosby

Fossa, S., Dahl, A., and Loge, J. (2003). Fatigue, anxiety, and depression in long-term survivors of testicular cancer. *Journal of Clinical Oncology, 21*(7), 1249–1254.

Frankenhaeuser, M. (1986). A psychobiological framework for research on human stress and coping. In M.H. Appley and R. Trumbull (Eds.) *Dynamics of stress: Physiological, psychological, and social perspectives* (pp. 101–116) New York: Plenum.

Free, N.K., Green, B.L., Grace, M.C., Chernus, L.A., and Whitman, R.M. (1985). Empathy and outcome in brief focal dynamic therapy. *American Journal of Psychiatry, 142*, 917–921.

Freeman, A., and Greenwood, V. (eds.). (1987). *Cognitive therapy: Applications in medical and psychiatric settings*. New York: Human Sciences Press.

Freidenberg, B.M., Blanchard, E.B., Wulfert, E., and Malta, L.S. (2002). Changes in physiological arousal to gambling cues among participants in motivationally enhanced cognitive-behavior therapy for pathological gambling: A preliminary study. *Applied Psychophysiology and Biofeedback, 27*(4), 251–260.

Friedland, G.H., Pollard, R., Griffith, B., Hughes, M., Morse, G., Bassett, R., Freimuth, W., Demeter, L., Connick, E., Nevin, T., Hirsch, M. and Fischl, M. (1999). Efficacy and safety of delavirdine mesylate with zidovine and didanosine compared with two-drug combinations of these agents in persons with HIV disease with CD4 counts of 100 to 500 cells/mm (ACTG 261). *Journal of Acquired Immune Deficiency Syndrome, 21*(4), 281–292.

Friedman, M., Landsberg, R., Pryor, S., Syed, Z., Ibrahim, H., and Caldarelli, D. (2001). The occurrence of sleep-disordered breathing among patients with head and neck cancer. *Laryngoscope, 111*(11), 1917–1919.

Friedman, R., Sobel, D., Myers, P., Caudill, M., and Benson, H. (1995). Behavioral medicine, health psychology and cost offset. *Health Psychology, 14*, 509–518.

Fromm, K., Andrykowski, M.A., and Hunt, J. (1996). Positive and negative psychosocial sequelae of bone marrow transplantation: Implications for quality of life assessment. *Journal of Behavioral Medicine, 19*, 221–240.

Fukuda, K., Straus, S.E., Hickie, I., Sharpe, M.C., Dobbins, J.G., and Komaroff, A. (1994). The chronic fatigue syndrome: A comprehensive approach to its definition and study. *Annals of Internal Medicine, 121*, 953–959.

Fung, H.B., and Guo, Y. (2004). Enfuvirtide: A fusion inhibitor for the treatment of HIV infection. *Clinical Therapeutics, 26*(3), 352–378.

Furst, G., Gerber, L., Smith, C., Fisher, S., and Shulman, B. (1987). A program for improving energy conservation behaviors in adults with rheumatoid arthritis. *American Journal of Occupational Therapy, 41*(2), 102–111.

Gallagher, K., Burgess, P., Keller, R.B., and Ritchie, R. (2003). Boise, ID (November 19, 2003); *Healthwise topic: Low back pain*. Retrieved October 20, 2004, from *http://www.pamf.org/health/healthinfo/index.cfm?page=articleandsgml_id=hw56429*

Gamble, G.E., Barberan, E., Bowsher, D., Tyrrell, P.J., and Jones, A.K. (2000). Post stroke shoulder pain: More common than previously realized. *European Journal of Pain: Ejp, 4*(3), 313–315.

Gardner, J.R. (1991). The application of self psychology to brief psychotherapy. *Psychoanalytic Psychology, 8*(4), 477–500.

Gaskin, M., Greene, A., Robinson, M., and Geisser, M. (1992). Negative affect and the experience of chronic pain. *Journal of Psychosomatic Research*, 36, 707–713.

Gatchel, R.J., and Blanchard, E.B. (1993). *Psychophysiological disorders: Research and clinical applications*. Washington, DC: American Psychological Association.

Ger, L.P., Ho, S.T., Wang, J.J., and Cherng, C.H. (1998). The prevalence and severity of cancer pain: A study of newly-diagnosed cancer patients in Taiwan. *Journal of Pain and Symptom Management, 15*(5), 285–293.

Gerber, L., and Furst, G. (1992). Scoring methods and application of the Activity Record (ACTRE) for patients with musculoskeletal disorders. *Arthritis Care and Research, 5*, 151–156.

Gibbs, V. (2002). Group treatment for women substance abusers. In D.W. Brook and H.I. Spitz (eds.), *The group therapy of substance abuse* (pp. 243–256). New York: Haworth Press, Inc.

Gidron, Y., Armon, T., Gilutz, H., and Huleihel, M. (2003). Psychological factors correlate meaningfully with percent-monocytes among acute coronary syndrome patients. *Brain, Behavior, and Immunity, 17*, 310–315.

Giles, I., and Isenberg, D. (2000). Fatigue in primary Sjogren's syndrome: Is there a link with the fibromyalgia syndrome? *Annals of the Rheumatic Diseases, 59*(11), 875–878.

Gill, C.J. (1997). Four types of integration in disability identity development. *Journal of Vocational Rehabilitation, 9*, 39–46.

Gillespie, T. (2003). Anemia in cancer: Therapeutic implications and interventions. *Cancer Nursing, 26*(2), 119–128.

Gillin, J.C., Spinweber, C.L., and Johnson, L.C. (1989) Rebound insomnia: A critical review. *Journal of Clinical Psychopharmacology, 9*, 161–172.

Gislason, T. and Almqvist, M (1987) Somatic diseases and sleep complaints. An epidemiological study of 3201 Swedish men. *Acta Medica Scandinavica, 221*, 475–481.

Gitlin, M.J. and Gerner, R.H. (1986). The dexamethasone suppression test and response to somatic treatment: A review. *Journal of Clinical Psychiatry, 47*, 16–21.

Glader, E., Stegmayr, B., and Asplund, K. (2001). A 2-year follow-up study of stroke patients in Sweden. *Stroke, 33*, 1327–1333.

Glaser, R., and Kiecolt-Glaser, J.K. (1994). *Handbook of human stress and immunity.* San Diego: Academic Press.

Glaser, R., Thorn, B.E., Tarr, K.L., Kiecolt-Glaser, J.K., and D'Ambrosio, S.M. (1985). Effects of stress on methyltransferase synthesis: An important DNA repair enzyme. *Health Psychology, 4*, 403–412.

Godshall, S. and Kirchner, J.T. (2000). Infectious mononucleosis: Complexities of a common syndrome. *Postgraduate Medicine, 107*(7), 175–176.

Goff, B., Mandel, L. Melancon, C., and Muntz, H. (2004). Frequency of symptoms of ovarian cancer in women presenting to primary care clinics. *The Journal of the American Medical Association, 291*(22), 2705–2712.

Goksan, B., Karaali-Savrun, F., Ertan, S., and Savrun, M. (2004). Haemodialysis-related headache. *Cephalalgia, 24*(4), 284–287.

Goldfried, M.R., and Davidson, G.C. (1976). *Clinical behavior therapy.* New York: Holt, Rineholt and Winston.

Grayson, C.E. (2000). Elmwood Park, NJ (June, 2004); Retrieved October 13, 2004, from *http://my.webmd.com/content/article/10/1660_51069?z=1660_00000_0000_rl_05*

Greenberg, L.S. and Safran, J.D. (1987). *Emotion in Psychotherapy.* New York: Guilford.

Greenberger, D. and Padesky, C. (1995). *Mind over mood: A cognitive therapy treatment manual for clients.* New York: Guildford Press.

Griffith, C.H., III, and Wilson, J.F. (2001). The loss of student idealism in the 3rd-year clinical clerkships. *Evaluation and the Health Professions, 24*, 61–71.

Grumbach, K., and Bodenheimer, T. (2002). A primary care home for Americans: Putting the house in order. *Journal of the American Medical Association, 288*, 889–893.

Gudbjornsson, B., Broman, J., Hetta, J., and Hallgren, R. (1993). Sleep disturbances in patients with primary Sjogren's syndrome. *British Journal of Rheumatology, 32*(12), 1072–1076.

Guthrie, E. (1996). Emotional disorder in chronic illness. *British Journal of Psychiatry, 168*, 265–273.

Haddock, G., Barrowclough, C., Tarrier, N., Moring, J., O'Brien, R., Schofield, N., et al. (2003). Cognitive-behavioural therapy and motivational intervention for schizophrenia and substance misuse: 18-month outcomes of a randomised controlled trial. *British Journal of Psychiatry, 183*(5), 418–426.

Haboubi, N., Long, J., Koshy, M., and Ward, A. (2001). Short-term sequelae of minor head injury (6 years experience of minor head injury clinic). *Disability and Rehabilitation, 23*(14), 635–638.

Hadjistavropoulos, T. and Craig, K.D (2004) An Introduction to Pain: Psychological Perspectives. In T. Hadjistavropoulos, and K.D. Craig (eds.), *Pain: Psychological Perspectives* (pp. 1–12). Mahwah, New Jersey: Lawrence Erlbaum Associates.

Halmi, K.A., Agras, W.S., Mitchell, J., Wilson, G.T., Crow, S., Bryson S.W., et al. (2002). Relapse predictors of patients with bulimia nervosa who achieved abstinence through cognitive behavioral therapy. *Archives of General Psychiatry, 59*(12), 1105–1109.

Halsted, C.H. (1996). The many faces of celiac disease. *The New England Journal of Medicine, 334*(18), 1190–1191.

Happe, S. (2003). Excessive daytime sleepiness and sleep disturbances in patients with neurological diseases. *Drugs, 63*(24), 2725–2737.

Harris, M.D. (2003). Psychosocial aspects of diabetes with an emphasis on depression. *Current Diabetes Reports, 3*, 49–55.

Harvey, C.K., Cadena, R., and Dunlap, L. (1993). Fibromyalgia. Part I. Review of the literature. *Journal of the American Podiatric Medical Association, 83*, 412–415.

Harvey, C., Rothschild, B.B., Asmann, A.J., and Stripling, T. (1990). New estimates of traumatic SCI prevalence: A survey-based approach. *Paraplegia, 28*(9), 537–544.

Hassoun, Z., Willems, B., Deslauriers, J., Nguyen, B., and Huet, P. (2002). Assessment of fatigue in patients with chronic hepatitis C using the fatigue impact scale. *Digestive Diseases and Sciences, 47*(12), 2674–2681.

Hauri, P.J. (1982). *The sleep disorders.* Kalamazoo, MI: Upjohn.

Healthcommunities.com, Inc. (2004). Northampton, MA (March 9, 2004); *Neurology channel: Multiple sclerosis overview.* Retrieved December 6, 2004, from *http://www.neurologychannel.com/multiplesclerosis/*

Healthwise, Incorporated: Quest Diagnostics Patient Health Library (2004). Boise, ID (February 11, 2003); Retrieved October 21, 2004, from *http://www.questdiagnostics.com/kbase/list/meds/default.htm*

Heijmans, M. and deRidder, D. (1998). Assessing illness representations of chronic illness: Explorations of their disease-specific nature. *Journal of Behavioral Medicine, 21*, 485–503.

Hickie, I., and Davenport, T. (1999). The case of Julio: A behavioral approach based on reconstructing the sleep-wake cycle. *Cognitive and behavioral practice, 6*, 442–450.

Higgins, E.T., and Sorrentino, R.M. (eds.). (1990). *Handbook of motivation and cognition: Foundations of social behavior, Vol. 2.* New York: Guilford Press.

Higuero, T., Merle, C., Thiefin, G., Coussinet, S., Jolly, D., Diebold, M.D., et al. (2004). Jejunoileal Crohn's disease: A case-control study. *Gastroentérologie Clinique et Biologique, 28*(2), 160–166.

Hill, D., Beutler, L.E., and Daldrup, R. (1989). The relationship of process to outcome in brief experiential psychotherapy for chronic pain. *Journal of Clinical Psychology, 45*(6), 951–957.

Hoangmai, P.H., Simonson, L., Elnicki, M., Fried, L.P., Goroll, A.H., and Bass, E.B. (2004). Training U.S. medical students to care for the chronically ill. *Academic Medicine, 79*, 32–41.

Hobfoll, S.E. (1998). *Stress, culture, and community. The psychology and philosophy of stress.* New York: Plenum Press.

Hoffman, C., Rice, D., and Sung, H. (1996). Persons with chronic conditions: Their prevalence and costs. *Journal of the American Medical Association, 276*, 1473–1479.

Holland, J.C., Passik, S., Kash, K.M., Russak, S.M., Gronert, M.K., Sison, A., et al. (1999). The role of religious and spiritual beliefs in coping with malignant melanoma. *Psychooncology, 8*(1), 14–26.

Honda, K., and Goodwin, R. (2004). Cancer and mental disorders in a national community sample: Findings from the National Comorbidity Survey. *Psychotherapy and Psychosomatics, 73*, 235–242.

Howard, J. (1998). Intravenous immunoglobulin for the treatment of acquired myasthenia gravis. *American Academy of Neurology, 51*(6), S30–S36.

Huyser, B., Parker, J., Thoreson, R., Smarr, K., Johnson, J., and Hoffman, R. (1998). Predictors of subjective fatigue among individuals with rheumatoid arthritis. *Arthritis and Rheumatism, 41*(12), 2230–2237.

Indaco, A., Iachetta, C., Nappi, C., Socci, L., and Carrieri, P.B. (1994). Chronic and acute pain syndromes in patients with multiple sclerosis. *ACTA Neurologica (Napoli), 16*(3), 97–102.

Ingram, R.E., Miranda, J, and Segal, Z.V. (1998). *Cognitive vulnerability to depression.* New York: Guilford Press.

Institute for Health and Aging. (1996). Downloaded via the World Wide Web on December 1, 2004 from *nurseweb.ucsf.edu/iha/index.shtml.*

InteliHealth. (2004); *Anemia and Fatigue.* Retrieved September 20, 2004, from *http://www.intelihealth.com/IH/ihtIH/WSIHW000/14294/24016/238187.html?d=dmt content*

I.S.L. Consulting Company, Yahoo!Health. (2003). San Francisco (May 9, 2003); *Bone pain and cancer.* Retrieved September 22, 2004, from *http://health.yahoo.com/health/ centers/bone_health/307.html*

Iverson, G., and McCracken, L. (1997). 'Postconcussive' symptoms in persons with chronic pain. *Brain Injury, 11*(11), 783–790.

iVillage. (2001). No location available (No revision date available); *Fibromyalgia (FM) fact sheet.* Retrieved September 21, 2004, from *http://www.ivillage.com/conditions/auto immune/articles /0,,166085_251196-2,00.html*

Jacobsen, P., Hann, D., Azzarello, L., Horton, J., Balducci, L., and Lyman, G. (1999). Fatigue in women receiving adjuvant chemotherapy for breast cancer: Characteristics, course, and correlates. *Journal of Pain and Symptom Management, 18*(4), 233–242.

Jason, L.A., Fennell, P.A., Klein, S., Fricano, G., Halpert, J.A., and Taylor, R.R. (1999). An investigation of the different phases of the CFS illness. *Journal of Chronic Fatigue Syndrome, 5*, 53–54.

Jason, L.A., Fennell, P.A., Taylor, R.R., Fricano, G., and Halpert, J.A. (2000). An empirical verification of the Fennell phases of the CFS illness. *Journal of Chronic Fatigue Syndrome, 6*, 47–56.

Jason, L.A., Richman, J.A., Rademaker, A.W., Jordan, K.M., Plioplys, A.V., Taylor, R.R., et al. (1999). A community-based study of chronic fatigue syndrome. *Archives of Internal Medicine, 159*, 2129–2137.

Javaheri, S., Parker, T., Liming, J., Corbett, W., Nishiyama, H., Wexler, L., and Roselle, G. Sleep apnea in 81 ambulatory male patients with stable heart failure: Types and their prevalences, consequences, and presentations. *Circulation, 97*(21), 2154–2159.

Jobson Publishing. (2003). Bloomfield, NJ (March 1, 2003); *Power-pak C.E.: Cancer pain.* Retrieved September 23, 2004, from *http://www.powerpak.com/index.asp?show= lesson&lsn_id=2708&page=courses/2708/lesson.htm*

Johnson, C., and Webster, D. (2002). *Recrafting a life: Solutions for chronic pain and illness.* New York: Brunner-Routledge.

Joseph, S., Williams, R., and Yule, W. (1993). Changes in outlook following disaster: The preliminary development of a measure to assess positive and negative responses. *Journal of Traumatic Stress, 6*, 271–279.

Jung, W., and Irwin, M. (1999). Reduction of natural killer cytotoxic activity in major depression: Interaction between depression and cigarette smoking. *Psychosomatic Medicine, 61*, 263–270.

Kabat-Zinn, J. (1990). *Full catastrophe living: Using the wisdom of your body and mind to face stress, pain, and illness*. New York: Dell.

Kabat-Zinn, J. (2005). *Coming to our senses: Healing ourselves and the world through mindfulness*. New York: Hyperion.

Kales, J.D., Kales, A. Bixler, E.O., Soldatos, C.R., Cadieux, R.J., Karshurba, G.J., and Vela-Bueno, A. (1984). Biopsychobehavioral correlates of insomnia: V. Clinical charachteristics and behavioral correlates. American Journal of Psychiatry, 141, 1371–1376.

Kales, A., and Kales, J.D. (1984). Evaluation and treatment of insomnia, New York: Oxford University Press.

Kanner, A., Soto, A., and Gross-Kanner, H. (2004). Prevalence and clinical characteristics of postictal psychiatric symptoms in partial epilepsy. *Neurology, 62*(5), 708–713.

Kassan, S., and Moutsopoulos, H. (2004). Clinical manifestations and early diagnosis of Sjogren Syndrome. *Archives of Internal Medicine, 164*, 1275–1284.

Katz, R.C., Flasher, L., Cacciapaglia, H., and Nelson, S. (2001). The psychosocial impact of cancer and lupus: A cross-validation study that extends the generality of "benefit-finding" in patients with chronic disease. *Journal of Behavioral Medicine, 24*, 561–571.

Keijsers, G., Schaap, C., and Hoogduin, C. (2000). The impact of interpersonal patient and therapist behaviour on outcome in cognitive-behavior therapy: A review of empirical studies. *Behaviour Modification, 24*, 264–297.

Keller, S.E., Shiflett, S.C., Schleifer, S.J., and Bartlett, J.A. (1994). Stress, immunity, and health. In R. Glaser and J.K. Kiecolt-Glaser (eds.), *Handbook of human stress and immunity* (pp. 217–244). San Diego: Academic Press.

Kemp, J.P., Korenblat, P.E., Scherger, J.E., and Minkwitz, M. (1999). Zafirlikast in clinical practice: Results of the accolate clinical experience and pharmacoepidemiology trial (ACCEPT) in patients with asthma. *The Journal of Family Practice, 48*(6), 425–432.

Kiecolt-Glaser, J.K and Glaser, R. (1999). Chronic stress and mortality among older adults. *Journal of the American Medical Association*, Dec 15: 282 (23): 2259–60.

Kiecolt-Glaser, J.K., McGuire, L., Robles, T.F., and Glaser, R. (2002). Psychoneuro-immunology: Psychological influences on immune function and health. *Journal of Consulting and Clinical Psychology, 70*, 537–547.

Kiecolt-Glaser, J.K., Stephens, R.E., Lipetz, P.D., Speicher, C.E., and Glaser, R. (1985). Distress and DNA repair in human lymphocytes. *Journal of Behavioral Medicine, 8*, 311–320.

Kielhofner, G. (1980a). A model of human occupation, part two. Ontogenesis from the perspective of temporal adaptation. *American Journal of Occupational Therapy, 34*, 657–663.

Kielhofner, G. (1980b). A model of human occupation, part three. Benign and vicious cycles. *American Journal of Occupational Therapy, 34*, 731–737.

Kielhofner, G. (2002). A model of human occupation: Theory and application (3rd ed.). Philadelphia: Lippincott, Williams and Wilkins.

Kielhofner, G. (2004). *Conceptual foundations of occupational therapy* (3rd ed.). Philadelphia: F.A. Davis.

Kielhofner, G., and Burke, J. (1980). A model of human occupation, part one: Conceptual framework and content. *American Journal of Occupational Therapy, 34*, 572–581.

Kielhofner, G., Burke, J., and Heard Igi, C. (1980). A model of human occupation, part four. Assessment and intervention. *American Journal of Occupational Therapy, 34*, 777–788.

Kielhofner, G., and Barrett, L. (1998). Meaning and misunderstanding in occupational forms: A study of therapeutic goal-setting. *American Journal of Occupational Therapy*, 52, (5), 345–354.

Kielhofner, G., Mallinson, T., Crawford, C., Nowak, M., Rigby, M., Henry, A., et al. (1998). *A user's manual for the Occupational Performance History Interview (Version 2.0) (OPHI-II)*. Chicago, IL: Model of Human Occupation Clearinghouse, Department of Occupational Therapy, College of Applied Health Sciences, University of Illinois at Chicago.

Kielhofner, G., and Neville, A. (1983). *The modified interest checklist*. Unpublished manuscript, University of Illinois at Chicago.

Koenigs, S.S., Fiedler, M.L., and DeCharms, R. (1977). Teacher beliefs, classroom interaction, and personal causation. *Journal of Applied Social Psychology, 7*(2), 95–114.

Kohut, H. (1966). Forms and transformations of narcissism. *Journal of the American Psychoanalytic Association, 14*, 243–272.

Kohut, H. (1971). *The analysis of the self*. New York: International Universities Press.

Kohut, H. (1977). *The restoration of the self*. New York: International Universities Press.

Kohut, H. (1984). *How does analysis cure?* Chicago: University of Chicago Press.

Kohut, H., and Wolf, E.S. (1978). Disorders of the self and their treatment. *International Journal of Psychoanalysis, 59*, 413–425.

Komaroff, A.L., Fagioli, L.R., Geiger, A.M., Doolittle, T.H., Lee, J., Kornish, R.J., et al. (1996). An examination of the working case definition of chronic fatigue syndrome. *American Journal of Medicine, 100*(1), 56–63.

Kooijman, C.M., Dijkstra, P.U., Geertzen, J.H., Elzinga, A., and van der Schans, C.P. (2000). Phantom pain and phantom sensations in upper limb amputees: An epidemiological study. *Pain, 87*(1), 33–41.

Krishnan, K., Ranga, R., Delong, M., Kraemer, H., Carney, R., Spiegel, D., et al. (2002). Comorbidity of depression with other medical diseases in the elderly. *Biological Psychiatry, 52*, 559–588.

Kutner, N.G. (1978). Medical students' orientation toward the chronically ill. *Journal of Medical Education, 53*(2), 111–118.

Kutty, K. (2004). Sleep and chronic obstructive pulmonary disease. *Current Opinion in Pulmonary Medicine, 10*(2), 104–112.

Lacroix, J.M., Martin, B., Avendano, M., and Goldstein, R. (1991). Symptom schemata in chronic respiratory patients. *Health Psychology, 10*, 268–273.

Lane, C., and Hobfoll, S.E. (1992). How loss affects anger and alienates potential supporters. *Journal of Consulting and Clinical Psychology, 60*(6), 935–942.

Larue, F., Fontaine, A., and Colleau, S.M. (1997). Underestimation and undertreatment of pain in HIV disease: Multicentre study. *British Medical Journal, 314*(7073), 23–28.

Lasfargues, J.E., Custis, D., Morrone, F., Carswell, J., and Nguyen, T. (1995). A model for estimating spinal cord injury prevalence in the United States. *Paraplegia, 33*(2), 62–68.

Lawrence, J.M., Moore, T.L., Madson, K.L., Rejent, A.J., Osborn, T.G., et al. (1993). Arthropathies of cystic fibrosis: Case reports and a review of the literature. *Journal of Rheumatology, 20*(Suppl 38), S12–S15.

Lazarus, R.S., and Folkman, S. (1984). *Stress, Appraisal, and Coping*. New York: Springer.

Lehman, D., Davis, C., DeLongis, A., Wortman, C., Bluck, S., Mandel, D., and Ellard, J. (1993). Positive and negative life changes following bereavement and their relations to adjustment. *Journal of Social and Clinical Psychology, 12*, 90–112.

LeReshe, L (1999). Gender consideration in the epidemiology of chronic pain. In I.K. Crombie, P.R. Croft, S.J. Linton, L. LeResche, and M. von Korff (eds.), *Epidemiology of pain* (2nd ed., pp. 43–52) Seattle, WA: Internaitonal Asosciation for the Study of Pain Press.

Leventhal, H., Meyer, D., and Nerenz, D. (1980). The common-sense representation of illness danger. In S. Rachman (ed.), *Contributions to medical psychology* (Vol. 2) (pp. 7–30). New York: Pergamon.

Leventhal, H., and Nerenz, D. (1985). The assessment of illness cognition. In P. Karoly (ed.), *Measurement strategies in health psychology* (pp. 517–554). New York: Wiley.

Leventhal, H., Nerenz, D.R., and Steele, D.J. (1984). Illness representations and coping with health threats. In A. Baum, S.E. Taylor, and J.E. Singer (eds.), *A Handbook of Psychology and Health, Volume IV: Social Psychological Aspects of Health* (pp. 219–252). Hillsdale, N.J.: Erlbaum.

Levine, S., and Levine, O. (1982). *Who dies? An investigation of conscious living and conscious dying*. New York: Anchor Books.

Levis, D.J. (1980). Implementing the technique of implosive therapy. In A. Goldstein and E.B. Foa (eds.), *Handbook of behavioral interventions: A clinical guide* (pp. 92–151). New York: Wiley.

Lewis, D. (2001). Sleep in patients with asthma and chronic obstructive pulmonary disease. *Current Opinion in Pulmonary Medicine, 7*(2), 105–112.

Lichtenstein, B. (1995). Psychoneuroimmunology and HIV, *STEP Perspect*, Summer, *7*(2), 6–9.

Lindsey, L., and Lewey, S. (1999). *Spinal cord injury info sheet*. Birmingham: Medical RRTC on Secondary Conditions of SCI.

Lindvall, B., Bengtsson, A., Ernerudh, J., and Eriksson, P. (2002). Subclinical myositis is common in primary Sjogren's syndrome and is not related to muscle pain. *Journal of Rheumatology, 29*(4), 717–725.

Linehan, M. (1993a). Cognitive-behavioral treatment of borderline personality disorder. New York: Guilford Press.

Linehan, M. (1993b). *Skills training manual for treating borderline personality disorder*. New York: Guilford Press.

Linton, S. (1998). *Claiming disability: Knowledge and identity*. New York: New York University Press.

Lipton, J.A., and Marbach, J.J. (1984). Ethnicity and the pain experience. *Social Science and Medicine 19*, 1279–1298.

Llewelyn, S.P. and Hume, W.I. (1979). The patient's view of therapy. *British Journal of Medical Psychiatry, 52*, 29–35.

Lock, G.R., Talley, N.H., Fett, S.L, Zinsmeister, A.R., and Melton, L.J. (1997). Prevalence and clinical spectrum of gastroesophageal reflux: a population-based study in Olmstead county. *Gastroenterology, 112*(5), 1448–1456.

Loftus, B. (2004). Houston, TX (2004); *Peripheral polyneuropathy and diabetes*. Retrieved September 29, 2004, from *http://www.loftusmd.com/Articles/Pain/Neuropathy.html*

Lopez, S.J., Floyd, R.K., Ulven, J.C., and Snyder, C.R. (2000). Hope therapy: Helping clients build a house of hope. In C.R. Snyder (ed.), *Handbook of hope: Theory, measures, and applications* (pp. 123–150). San Diego, CA: Academic Press.

Lorig, K., Mazonson, P.D., and Holman, H.R. (1993). Evidence suggesting that health education for self-management in patients with chronic arthritis has sustained health benefits while reducing health care costs. *Arthritis and Rheumatism, 36*, 439–446.

Lorig, K., Seleznick, M., Lubeck, D., Ung, E., Chastain, R.L., and Holman, H.R. (1989). The beneficial outcomes of the arthritis self-management course are not adequately explained by behavior change. *Arthritis and Rheumatism, 32*, 91–95.

Louden, J. (1992). *The woman's comfort book: A self-nurturing guide for restoring balance in your life*. San Francisco: Harper San Francisco.

Luborsky, L., Crits-Christoph, P., Mintz, J., and Auerbach, A. (1988). *Who will benefit from psychotherapy? Predicting therapeutic outcomes*. New York: Basic Books.

Lynn, J., Ely, E.W., Zhong, Z., McNiff, K.L., Dawson, N.V., Connors, A., et al. (2000). Living and dying with chronic obstructive pulmonary disease. *Journal of the American Geriatrics Society, 48*(5 Suppl.), S91-S100.

Manu, P., Lane, T.J., Matthews, D.A., Castriotta, R.J., Watson, R.K., and Abeles, M. (1994). Alpha-delta sleep in patients with a chief complaint of chronic fatigue. *Southern Medical Journal, 87*, 465–470.

March, L.M., and Bagga, H. (2004). Epidemiology of osteoarthritis in Australia. *Medical Journal of Australia, 180*(5 Suppl.), S6–10.

Marcus, B.H., Forsyth, L.H., Stone, E.J., Dubbert, P.M., McKenzie, T.L., Dunn, A., and Blair, S.N. (2000). Physical activity behavior change: Issues in adoption and maintenance. *Health Psychology, 19*(Suppl.), 32–41.

Marks, J.W. (ed.) and Kam, L. (2002). No location available (February 10, 2002); *MedicineNet.com, Crohn's disease.* Retrieved September 23, 2004, from *http://www.medicinenet.com/crohns_disease/article.htm*

Marple, R.I., Pangaro, L., and Kroenke, K. (1994). Third-year medical student attitudes toward internal medicine. *Archives of Internal Medicine, 154*(21), 2459–2464.

Martire, L.M., Lustig, A.P., Schulz, R., Miller, G.E., and Helgeson, V.S. (2004). Is it beneficial to involve a family member? A meta-analysis of psychosocial interventions for chronic illness. *Health Psychology, 23*(6), 599–611.

Matteson, S., Roscoe, J., Hickok, J., and Morrow, G. (2002). The role of behavioral conditioning in the development of nausea. *American Journal of Obstetrics and Gynecology, 186*(Suppl. 2) 239–243.

Maunsell, E., Brisson, J., and Deschenes, L. (1993). Arm problems and psychological distress after surgery for breast cancer. *Canadian Journal of Surgery, 36*(4), 315–320.

McCann, K., and Boore, J. (2000). Fatigue in persons with renal failure who require maintenance haemodialysis. *Journal of Advanced Nursing, 32*(5), 1132–1142.

McClelland, D.C. (1967). *The achieving society.* New York: Free Press.

McClelland, D.C. (1985). How motives, skills, and values determine what people do. *American Psychologist, 40*, 812–825.

McConnell, E.A. (2002). About Addison's disease. *Nursing, 32*(8), 79.

McGrath, N., Anderson, N., Croxson, M., and Powell, K. (1997). Herpes simplex encephalitis treated with acyclovir: Diagnosis and long term outcome. *Journal of Neurology, Neurosurgery and Psychiatry, 63*(3), 321–326.

McLaney, M.A., Tennen, H., Affleck, G., and Fitzgerald, T. (1995). Reactions to impaired fertility: The vicissitudes of primary and secondary control appraisals. *Women's Health: Research on Gender, Behavior, and Policy, 1*, 143–160.

McMillen, J.C., Zuravin, S., and Rideout, G.B. (1995). Perceived benefit from child sexual abuse. *Journal of Consulting and Clinical Psychology, 63*, 1037–1042.

McMillen, J.C., Smith, E.M., and Fisher, R.H. (1997). Perceived benefit and mental health after three types of disaster. *Journal of Consulting and Clinical Psychology, 65*, 733–739.

McNeilly, R.B. (2000). *Healing the whole person: A solution-focused approach to using empowering language, emotions, and actions in therapy.* New York: Wiley.

Medifocus.com, Inc. (2004). Silver Spring, MD (September 2, 2004); *Sjogren's syndrome.* Retrieved December 6, 2004, from *http://www.medifocus.com/guide_detail.php?gid=RH011*

Medinfo/Arboris Ltd. (2002). *Low back pain.* Retrieved July 27, 2004, from *http://www.medinfo.co.uk/conditions/lowbackpain.html*

362   References

Meijer, S.A., Sinnema, G., Bijstra, J.O., Mellenbergh, G.J., and Wolters, W.H. (2002). Coping styles and locus of control as predictors for psychological adjustment of adolescents with a chronic illness. *Social Science and Medicine, 54*(9), 1453–1461.

Mellinger, G.D., Balter, M.B. and Uhlenhuth, E.H. (1985). Insomnia and its treatment: Prevalance and correlates. *Archives of General Psychiatry, 42*, 225–232.

Melzack, R. and Casey, K.L. (1968). Sensory motivational and central conrolled determinants of pain: A new conceptual model. In K. Shalod (ed.), *The skin senses* (pp. 423–443). Springfield, Il.: Charles Thomas.

Melzack, R. (1999). From the gate to the neuromatrix. *Pain, Suppl 6*, S121–S126.

Melzack, R. (1987). The short form of the McGill pain questionnaire, *Pain, 30*, 191–197.

Melzack, R. and Katz, J. (2004). The gate control theory: Reaching for the brain. In T. Hadjistavropoulos and K.D. Craig, (eds.) *Pain: Psychological Perspectives.* (pp. 13–34). Mahwah, New Jersey: Lawrence Erlbaum Associates.

Melzack, R. and Wall, P.D. (1965). Pain mechanisms. *Science* 150, 971–979.

Merck and Co., Inc. (1999). Whitehouse Station, NJ (June, 1999); *Merck Manual of Diagnosis and Therapy, 17ᵗʰ Ed.* Retrieved October 6, 2004, from *http://www.merck.com/mrkshared/mmanual/home.jsp*

Michenbaum, D. (1977). *Cognitive-behavior modification: An integrative approach.* New York: Plenum Press.

Miller, L. (1993). Psychotherapeutic approaches to chronic pain. *Psychotherapy, 30*(1), 115–124.

Miller, S.M., and O'Leary, A. (1993). Cognition, stress, and health. In K.S. Dobson and P. C. Kendall (eds.), *Psychopathology and cognition. Personality, psychopathology, and psychotherapy series* (pp. 159–189). San Diego, CA: Academic Press, Inc.

Minderhoud, I.M., Oldenburg, B., van Dam, P.S., and van Berge Henegouwen, G.P. (2003). High prevalence of fatigue in quiescent inflammatory bowel disease is not related to adrenocortical insufficiency. *American Journal of Gastroenterology, 98*(5), 1088–1093.

Mock, V., Pickett, M., Ropka, M., Lin, E., Stewart, K., Rhodes, V., et al. (2001). Fatigue and quality of life outcomes of exercise during cancer treatment. *Cancer Practice, 9*(3), 119–127.

Mohr, D.C., Dick, L.P., Russo, D., Pinn, J., Boudewyn, A.C., Likosky, W., and Goodkin, D.E. (1999). The psychosocial impact of multiple sclerosis: Exploring the patient's perspective. *Health Psychology, 18*, 376–382.

Moldofsky, H. (1993). Fibromyalgia, sleep disorder, and chronic fatigue syndrome. *Ciba Foundation Symposium, 173*, 262–279.

Moldofsky, H. (2002). Management of sleep disorders in fibromyalgia. *Rheumatic Diseases Clinics of North America, 28*, 353–365.

Monk, T.H., Leng, V.C., Folkard, S., and Weitzman, E.D. (1983). Circadian rhythms in subjective alertness and core body temperature. *Chronobiologia, 10*, 49–55.

Montplaisir, J., and Godbout, R. (1989). Restless legs syndrome and periodic movements during sleep. In M. Kryger, T. Roth, and W.C. Dement, (eds.), *Principles and practice of sleep medicine* (pp. 402–409). Philadelphia: Saunders.

Moorey, S. (1996). When bad things happen to rational people: Cognitive therapy in adverse life circumstances. In P. Salkovskis (ed.), *Frontiers of Cognitive Therapy* (pp. 450–469). New York: Guilford Press.

Moorey, S., and Greer, S. (2002). *Cognitive behavior therapy for people with cancer.* Oxford, England: Oxford University Press.

Morgan, K., Dallosso. H., Ebrahim, S., Arie, T., and Fentem, P.H. (1988). Prevalence, frequency, and duration of hypnotic drug use among elderly living at home. *British Medical Journal, 296*, 601–602

Morin, C.M., *Insomnia: Psychological Assessment and Management.* New York: Guilford Press.

Morin, C.M. and Espie, C.A. (2003) Insomnia: A clinical guide to assessment and treatment. New York: Kluwer.

Morin, C.M., Rogrigue, S., and Ivers, H. (2003). The role of stress, arousal, and coping skills in primary insomnia. *Psychosomatic Medicine, 65*, 259–267.

Morris, R.J., and Magrath, K.H. (1983). The therapeutic relationship in behavior therapy. In M.J. Lambert (ed.), *Psychotherapy and patient relationships* (pp. 145–189). Homewood, IL: Dorsey Press.

Moss, D.P. (1992). Cognitive therapy, phenomenology, and the struggle for meaning. *Journal of Phenomenological Psychology, 23*(1), 87–102.

Moynihan, C., Bliss, J.M., Davidson, J., et al. (1998). Evaluation of adjuvant psychological therapy in patients with testicular cancer: A randomized trial. *British Medical Journal, 316*, 429–435.

Mucsi, I., Molnar, M., Rethelyi, J., Vamos, E., Csepanyi, G., Tompa, G., Barotfi, S., Marton, A., and Novak, M. (2004). Sleep disorders and illness intrusiveness in patients on chronic dialysis. *Nephrol Dial Transplantation, 19*, 1815–1822.

Myasthenia Gravis Foundation of America (2001). St. Paul, MN (October 5, 2004); Retrieved October 27, 2004, from *http://www.myasthenia.org/information/*

Nadler, J.P., Gathe, J.C., Pollard, R.B., Richmond, Q.L., Griffith, S., Lancaster, C.T., et al. (2003). Twice-daily amprenavir 1200mg versus amrenavir 600mg/ritonavir 100mg, in combination with at least 2 other antiretroviral drugs, in HIV-I-infected patients. *BMC Infectious Diseases, 3*(1), 10.

National Diabetes Information Clearinghouse (NDIC). (2004). *National Diabetes Statistics: NIH Publication No. 04-3892.* Retrieved July 16, 2004, from *http://diabetes.niddk.nih.gov/dm/ pubs/statistics/index.htm*

National Institute of Allergy and Infectious Diseases (NIAID), National Institutes of Health. (2004a). Bethesda, MD (July 13, 2004); *Facts and figures: HIV/AIDS statistics.* Retrieved December 6, 2004 from *http://www.niaid.nih.gov/factsheets/aidsstat.htm*

National Institute of Allergy and Infectious Diseases (NIAID), National Institutes of Health. (2004b). Bethesda, MD (November 18, 2004); *Research on: HIV infection in women.* Retrieved December 6, 2004 from *http://www.niaid.nih.gov/factsheets/womenhiv.htm*

National Institute of Arthritis and Musculoskeletal and Skin Diseases (NIAMS). (1998). Bethesda, MD (May 2004); *Handout on Health: Rhematoid Arthritis: NIH Publication No. 04-4179.* Retrieved July 16, 2004, from *http://www.niams.nih.gov/hi/topics/arthritis/rahandout.htm*

National Institute of Arthritis and Musculoskeletal and Skin Diseases (NIAMS), National Institutes of Health. (1999). Bethesda, MD (June, 2004); *NIH Publication NO. 04 5326: Questions and Answers About Fibromyalgia.* Retrieved October 5, 2004, from *http://www.niams.nih.gov/hi/topics/fibromyalgia/fibrofs.htm*

National Institute of Diabetes and Digestive and Kidney Diseases (NIDDK), National Institutes of Health. (1992). Bethesda, MD (June, 2001); *National Digestive Diseases Information Clearinghouse: NIH Publication No. 95-3421: Harmful effects of medicines on the adult digestive system.* Retrieved October 5, 2004, from *http://www.intelihealth.com/IH/ihtIH/WSIHW000/8270/28972/188585 .html?d=dmt Content#Readings*

National Institute of Diabetes and Digestive and Kidney Diseases (NIDDK). (2000). Bethesda, MD (No revision date available); *Office of Health Research Reports: NIH Publication No. 903054: Addison's Disease*. Retrieved October 12, 2004, from *http://www.addisons.org.au/core.htm*

National Institute of Diabetes and Digestive and Kidney Diseases (NIDDK), National Institutes of Health. (2003). Bethesda, MD (January 2003); *National Digestive Diseases Information Clearinghouse: NIH Publication No. 03-3410: Crohn's Disease*. Retrieved July 27, 2004, from *http://digestive.niddk.nih.gov/ddiseases/pubs/crohns/*

National Institute of Diabetes and Digestive and Kidney Diseases (NIDDK), National Institutes of Health. (2004a). Bethesda, MD (June 2004); *National Digestive Diseases Information Clearinghouse: NIH Publication No. 04-3054: Addison's Disease: Adrenal Insufficiency*. Retrieved September 20, 2004, from *http://www.niddk.nih.gov/health/endo/pubs/addison/addison.htm*

National Institute of Diabetes and Digestive and Kidney Diseases (NIDDK), National Institutes of Health. (2004b). Bethesda, MD (April 2004); *National Digestive Diseases Information Clearinghouse: NIH Publication No. 04-3873: National Diabetes Statistics*. Retrieved December 2, 2004, from *http://diabetes.niddk.nih.gov/dm/pubs/statistics/index.htm#7*

National Institute of Mental Health (NIMH). (2004). Bethesda, MD (October 6, 2004); *Publications*. Retrieved September 14, 2004, from *http://www.nimh.nih.gov/publicat/index.cfm*

National Institute of Neurological Disorders and Stroke (NINDS), National Institutes of Health. (2003). Bethesda, MD (July 26, 2003); *Low Back Pain Fact Sheet*. Retrieved July 27, 2004, from *http://www.ninds.nih.gov/health_and_medical/pubs/back_pain.htm*

National Institute of Neurological Disorders and Stroke (NINDS), National Institutes of Health. (2003). Bethesda, MD (December 1, 2003); *Central pain information page*. Retrieved October 21, 2004, from *http://www.ninds.nih.gov/health_and_medical/disorders/centpain_doc.htm*

National Institute of Neurological Disorders and Stroke (NINDS), National Institutes of Health. (2003). Bethesda, MD (August 21, 2003); *Spinal cord injury: Hope through research*. Retrieved October 12, 2003, from *http://www.ninds.nih.gov/health_and_medical/pubs/sci.htm*

National Institute of Neurological Disorders and Stroke (NINDS), National Institutes of Health. (2004). Bethesda, MD (July 29, 2004); *NINDS Muscular Dystrophy (MD) Information Page*. Retrieved October 11, 2004, from *http://www.ninds.nih.gov/health_and_medical/disorders/md.htm*

National Mental Health Association (NMHA). (2004). Alexandria, VA (2004); *Co-occurrence of depression with medical, psychiatric, and substance use disorders*. Retrieved October 28, 2004, from *http://www.nmha.org/infoctr/factsheets/28.cfm*

National Multiple Sclerosis Society. (2004). New York (January 2004); *Library & literature: Pain*. Retrieved October 7, 2004, from *http://www.nationalmssociety.org/Sourcebook-Pain.asp*

National Multiple Sclerosis Society. (2004). New York (October 8, 2004); Retrieved October 27, 2004, from *http://www.nationalmssociety.org/Meds-Mitoxantrone.asp*

National Women's Health Information Center (NWHIC). (2002). Fairfax, VA (November, 2002); Heart and cardiovascular disease. Retrieved December 2, 2004 from *http://www.4woman.gov/faq/heartdis.htm*

New York Thyroid Center. (n. d.). New York (n. d.); *Thyroid disorders: An overiview*. Retrieved December 6, 2004, from *http://www.cumc.columbia.edu/dept/thyroid/disorders.html*

Nicassio, P.M., and Smith, T.W. (eds.). (1995). *Managing chronic illness: A biopsychosocial perspective*. Washington, DC: American Psychological Association.

Nicassio, P., and Wallston, K. (1992). Longitudinal relationships among pain, sleep problems, and depression in rheumatoid arthritis. *Journal of Abnormal Psychology, 101*(3), 514–520.

Niemeyer, R.A. and Feixas, G. (1990). The role of homework and skill acquisition in the outcome of group cognitive therapy for depression. *Behavior Therapy, 21*, 281–292.

Ogle, K.S., Mavis, B., and Rohrer, J. (1997). Graduating medical students' competencies and educational experiences in palliative care. *Journal of Pain and Symptom Management, 14*(5), 280–285.

Oliver, M. (1990). *The politics of disablement*. London: Macmillan.

Oncology Channel, Healthcommunities.com, Inc. (2004). Northampton, MA (March 9, 2004); *Pain*. Retrieved September 22, 2004, from *http://www.oncologychannel.com/pain/*

O'Neill, W.M., and Sherrard, J.S. (1993). Pain in human immunodeficiency virus disease: A review. *Pain. 54*(1), 3–14.

Orlinsky, D.E. (1994). Research-based knowledge as the emergent foundation for clinical practice in psychotherapy. In P.F. Talley, H.H. Strupp, et al. (eds.) *Psychotherapy Research and Practice: Bridging the Gap*. pp. 99-123. New York: Basic Books.

Otto, M.W., Reilly-Harrington, N.A., Kogan, J.N., and Winett, C.A. (2003). Treatment contracting in cognitive-behavior therapy. *Cognitive and Behavioral Practice, 10*(3), 199–203.

Ozdil, S., Demir, K., Boztas, G., Danalioglu, A., Karaca, C., Akyuz, F., et al. (2003). Crohn's disease: Analysis of 105 patients. *Hepatogastroenterology, 50*(Suppl. 2), 287–291.

Pain Relief Foundation. (2003a). Liverpool, UK (2003); *Dealing with pain series 2003: Central post stroke pain*. Retrieved October 23, 2004, from *http://www.painrelieffoundation.org.uk/docs/painseries% 20– %20cpsp.pdf*

Pain Relief Foundation. (2003b). Liverpool, UK (2003); *Dealing with pain series 2003: Painful diabetic neuropathy*. Retrieved Septmeber 27, 2004, from *http://www.painrelieffoundation.org.uk/docs/painseries % 20 -% 20diabneuro.pdf*

Palm, O., Moum, B., Ongre, A., and Gran, J.T. (2002). Prevalence of ankylosing spondylitis and other spondyloarthropathies among patients with inflammatory bowel disease: A population study (the IBSEN study). *Journal of Rheumatology, 29*(3), 511–515.

Papageorgious, C., and Wells, A. (1998). Effects of attention training on hypochondriasis: A brief case series. *Psychological medicine, 28*, 193–200.

Parasa, R.B., and Maffulli, N. (1999). Musculoskeletal involvement in cystic fibrosis. *Bulletin (Hospital for Joint Diseases (New York, NY)), 58*(1), 37–44.

Parish, J., and Somers, V. (2004). Obstructive sleep apnea and cardiovascular disease. *Mayo Clinic Proceedings, 79*(8), 1036–1046.

Park, C.L., Cohen, L., and Murch, R. (1996). Assessment and prediction of stress-related growth. *Journal of Personality, 64*, 71–105.

Parloff, M.B., Waskow, I.E., and Wolfe, B.E. (1978). Research on therapist variables in relation to process and outcome. In S.L. Garfield and A.E. Bergin (eds.), *Handbook of psychotherapy and behavior change* (2nd ed.). New York: Wiley.

Patten, S.B., Beck, C.A., Williams, J.V., Barbui, C., and Metz, L.M. (2003). Major depression in multiple sclerosis: A population-based perspective. *Neurology, 61*(11), 1524–1527.

Paul, R. and Elder, L. (2002). *Critical thinking: Tools for taking charge of your professional and personal life*. Upper Saddle River, NJ: Financial Times Prentice Hall.

Paul, R., Cohen, R., Goldstein, J., and Gilchrist, J. (2000). Fatigue and its impact on patients with myasthenia gravis. *Muscle and Nerve, 23*(9), 1402–1406.

Pawlikowska, T., Chalder, T., Wessely, S., Wright, D., Hirsch, S., and Wallace, P. (1994). A population based study of fatigue and psychological distress. *British Medical Journal, 308*, 763–766.

Persons, J.B. and Burns, D.D. (1985). Mechanisms of action of cognitive therapy: The relative contributions of technical and interpersonal interventions. *Cognitive Therapy and Research, 9*, 539–551.

Persons, J.B., Burns, D.D., and Perloff, J.M. (1988). Predictors of dropout and outcome in cognitive therapy for depression in a private practice setting. *Cognitive Therapy and Research, 12*, 557–575.

Pesek, J.R., Jason, L.A., and Taylor, R.R. (2000). An empirical investigation of the envelope theory. *Journal of Human Behavior in the Social Environment, 3*, 59–77.

Pham, H.H., Simonson, L., Elnicki, D.M., Fried, L.P., Goroll, A.H., and Bass, E.B. (2004). Training U.S. medical students to care for the chronically ill. *Academic Medicine, 79*, 32–40.

Pimentel, M., Wallace, D., Hallegua, D., Chow, E., Kong, K., Park, S. et al. (2004). A link between irritable bowel syndrome and fibromyalgia may be related to findings on lactose breathing testing. *Annals of Rheumatic Diseases, 63*(4), 450–452.

Plach, S.K., Heidrich, S.M., and Waite, R.M. (2003). Relationship of social role quality to psychological well-being in women with rheumatoid arthritis. *Research in Nursing and Health, 26*(3), 190–202.

Pollard, R.B., Robinson, P., and Dransfield, K. (1998). Safety profile of nevirapine, a nonnucleoside reverse transcriptase inhibitor for the treatment of human immunodeficiency virus infection. *Clinical Therapeutics, 20*(6), 1071–1092.

Prochaska, J.O., and DiClemente, C.C. (1986). Toward a comprehensive model of change. In W.R. Miller and N. Heather (eds.), *Treating addictive behaviors: Process of change* (pp. 3–27). New York: Plenum.

Prolo, P., Chiapelli, F., Fiorucci, A., Dovio, A., Sartori, M.L. and Angeli, A. (2002). Psychoneuroimmunology: New Avenues of Research for the twenty-first century. *Annals of the New York Academy of Sciences. 996*, 400–408.

Quismorio, F.P., Jr., Lupus Foundation of America, Inc. (2001). Washington, DC (2001); *Joint and muscle pain in systemic lupus erythematosus (SLE)*. Retrieved October 6, 2004, from *http://www.lupus.org/education/brochures/jointpain.html#1*

Ramsay, J.R. (1998). Postmodern cognitive therapy: Cognitions, narratives, and personal meaning-making. *Journal of Cognitive Psychotherapy, 12*(1), 39–55.

Raue, P.J., Castonguay, L.G., and Goldfried, M.R. (1993). The working alliance: A comparison of two therapies. *Psychotherapy Research, 3*, 197–207.

Ravilly, S., Robinson, W., Suresh, S., Wohl, M.E., and Berde, C.B. (1996). Chronic pain in cystic fibrosis. *Pediatrics, 98*(4 Pt 1), 741–747.

Rea, T., Russo, J., Katon, W., Ashley, R., and Buchwald, D. (2001). Prospective study of the natural history of infectious mononucleosis caused by Epstein-Barr virus. *The Journal of the American Board of Family Practice, 14*(4), 234–242.

Rees, P.M. (2003). Contemporary issues in mild traumatic brain injury. *Archives of Physical Medicine and Rehabilitation, 84*(12), 1885–1894.

Rehm, L.P., Kaslow, N.J., and Rabin, A.S. (1987). Cognitive and behavioral targets in a self-control therapy program for depression. *Journal of Consulting and Clinical Psychology, 55*, 60–67.

Revenson, T.A., Wollman, C.A., and Felton, B.J. (1983). Social supports as stress buffers for adult cancer patients. *Psychosomatic Medicine, 45*, 321–331.

Riley, T.R., and Koch, K. (2003). Characteristics of upper abdominal pain in those with chronic liver disease. *Digestive Diseases and Sciences, 48*(10), 1914–1918.

Rinat Neuroscience. (2004). Palo Alto, CA (2004); *Peripheral neuropathy.* Retrieved September 23, 2004, from *http://www.rinatneuro.com/products/neuropathy.html*

Rodin, J., McAvay, G., Timko, C. (1998). A longitudinal study of depressed mood and sleep disturbances in elderly adults. *Journal of Gerontology, 43*, P45–P53.

Rogers, C. (1951). *Client-centered therapy.* Boston: Houghton-Mifflin.

Rogers, W. (1984). Changing health-related attitudes and behavior: The role of preventive health psychology. In J.H. Harvey, J.E. Maddux, R.P. McGlynn, and C.D. Stoltenberg (eds.), *Social perception on clinical and counseling psychology* (Vol. 2, pp. 91–112). Lubbock, TX: Texas Tech University Press.

Rollman, G.B. (2004). Ethnocultural variations in the experience of pain. In T. Hadjistavropoulos & K.D. Craig (eds.). *Pain: Psychological Perspectives.* Mahwah, NJ: Lawrence Erlbaum.

Rose, L., Pugh, L., Lears, K., and Gordon, D. (1997). The fatigue experience: Persons with HIV infection. *Journal of Advanced Nursing, 28*(2), 295–304.

Rosen, R.C., and Kostis, J.B., (1985) Biobehavioral sequellae associated with adrenergic-inhibiting antihypertensive agents. A critical Review. *Health Psychology, 4*, 579–604

Rosenstock, I.M. (1974). Historical origins of the health belief model. *Health Education Monographs, 2*, 354–95.

Ryan, V.L. and Gizynski, M.N. (1971). Behavior therapy in retrospect: Patients' feelings about their behavior therapists. *Journal of Consulting and Clinical Psychology, 37*, 1–9.

Rubinstein, M., and Selwyn, P. (1998). High prevalence of insomnia in an outpatient population with HIV infection. *Journal of Acquired Immune Deficiency Syndromes and Human Retrovirol, 19*(3), 260–265.

Safran, J.D., and McMain, S. (1992). A cognitive interpersonal approach to the treatment of personality disorders. *Journal of Cognitive Psychotherapy, 6*(1), 59–68.

Safran, J. and Segal, Z. (1996). *Interpersonal Process in Cognitive Therapy.* Northvale, N.J. Jason Aronson, Inc.

Salkovskis, P.M. (1996). *Frontiers of cognitive therapy.* New York: Guilford Press.

Salkovskis, P.M., and Freeston, M.H. (2001). Obsessions, compulsions, motivation, and responsibility for harm. *Australian Journal of Psychology, 53*(1), 1–6.

Salovey, P., Rothman, A.J., Detweiler, J.B., and Steward, W.T. (2000). Emotional states and physical health. *American Psychologist, 55*(1), 110–121.

Salvio, M.A., Beutler, L.E., Wood, J.M., Engle, D. (1992). The strength of the therapeutic alliance in three treatments for depression. *Psychotherapy Research, 2*, 31–36.

Sandler, R.S. (1990). Epidemiology of irritable bowel syndrome in the United States. *Gastroenterology, 99*(2), 409–415.

Sandroni, P., Benrud-Larson, L.M., McClelland, R.L., and Low, P.A. (2003). Complex regional pain syndrome type I: Incidence and prevalence in Olmsted county, a population-based study. *Pain, 103*(1–2), 199–207.

Sankar, A., and Becker, S.L. (1985). The home as a site for teaching gerontology and chronic illness. *Journal of Medical Education, 60*(4), 308–313.

Savard, J., and Morin, C. Insomnia in the context of cancer: A review of a neglected problem. *Journal of Clinical Oncology, 19*(3), 895–908.

Savard, J., Laroch, L., Simard, S., Ivers, H., and Morin, C.M. (2003) Chronic insomnia and immune functioning. *Psychosomatic Medicine. 65*, 211–221.

Scharloo, M., Kaptein, A.A., Weinman, J., Hazes, J.M., Willems, L.N., Bergman, W., et al. (1998). Illness perceptions, coping and functioning in patients with rheumatoid arthritis, chronic obstructive pulmonary disease and psoriasis. *Journal of Psychosomatic Research, 44*(5), 573–585.

Scher, A.I., Stewart, W.F., Liberman, J., and Lipton, R.B. (1998). Prevalence of frequent headache in a population-based study of the prevalence of different CDH types. *Headache, 38,* 497–506.

Schmader, K.E. (2002). Epidemiology and impact on quality of life of postherpetic neuralgia and painful diabetic neuropathy. *Clinical Journal of Pain, 18*(6), 350–354.

Schwartz, A. (1999). Fatigue mediates the effects of exercise on quality of life. *Quality of Life Research, 8,* 529–538.

Schwartz, A. (2000). Daily fatigue patterns and effect of exercise in women with breast cancer. *Cancer Practice, 8*(1), 16–24.

Schwartz, A., Mori, M., Gao, R., Nail, L., and King, M. (2001). Exercise reduces daily fatigue in women with breast cancer receiving chemotherapy. *Medicine and Science in Sports & Exercise, 33*(5), 718–723.

Schwartzman, R.J., Grothusen, J., Kiefer, T.R., and Rohr, P. (2001). Neuropathic central pain: Epidemiology, etiology, and treatment options. *Archives of Neurology, 58*(10), 1547–1550.

Scott, F.T., Leedham-Green, M.E., Barrett-Muir, W.Y., Hawrami, K., Gallagher, W.J., Johnson, R., et al. (2003). A study of shingles and the development of postherpetic neuralgia in East London. *Journal of Medical Virology, 70*(Suppl 1), S24–30.

Sears, S.R., Stanton, A.L., and Danoff-Burg, S. (2003). The yellow brick road and the emerald city: Benefit finding, positive reappraisal coping, and posttraumatic growth in women with early-stage breast cancer. *Health Psychology, 22,* 487–497.

Seligman, M.E.P. (1998). *Learned optimism.* New York: Pocket Books.

Seligman, M.E.P. (2002). *Authentic happiness: Using the new positive psychology to realize your potential for lasting fulfillment.* New York: Free Press.

Seligman, M.E.P., and Csikszentmihalyi, M. (2000). Positive psychology: An introduction. *American Psychologist, 55*(1), 5–14.

SeniorJournal.com. (2004). *Arthritis sufferers still hurt, despite advances in treatment: New study.* Retrieved October 13, 2004, from *http://www.seniorjournal.com/NEWS/ Health/4-10-05ArthritisHurts.htm*

Shaker, R., Castell, D., Schoenfeld, P., and Spechler, S. (2003). Nighttime heartburn is an under-appreciated clinical problem that impacts sleep and daytime function: the results of a Gallup survey conducted on behalf of the American Gastroenterological Association. *American Journal of Gastroenterology, 98*(7), 1487–93.

Sin, D., Fitzgerald, F., Parker, J., Newton, G., Floras, J., and Bradley, T. (1999). Risk factors for central and obstructive sleep apnea in 450 men and women with congestive heart failure. *American Journal of Respiratory and Critical Care Medicine, 160,* 1101–1106.

Small, S., and Lamb, M. (1999). Fatigue in chronic illness: The experience of individuals with chronic obstructive pulmonary disease and with asthma. *Journal of Advanced Nursing, 30*(2), 469–478.

Smith, C.P., Atkinson, J.W., McClelland, D.C., and Veroff, J. (1992). *Motivation and personality: Handbook of thematic content analysis.* New York: Cambridge University Press.

Smith, M.B. (1966). Explorations in competence: A study of Peace Corps teachers in Ghana. *American Psychologist, 21,* 555–566.

Smith, M.B. (1974). Competence and adaptation. *American Journal of Occupational Therapy, 28,* 11–15.

Smith, N., Kiehofner, G., and Watts, J. (1986). The relationship between volition, activity pattern and life satisfaction in the elderly. *American Journal of Occupational Therapy, 40,* 278-283.

Smith, T.W., and Nicassio, P.W. (1995). Psychological practice: Clinical application of the biopsychosocial model. In P.M. Nicassio and T.W. Smith (eds.), *Managing chronic illness: A biopsychosocial perspective* (pp. 1-31). Washington, DC: American Psychological Association.

Snyder, C.R. (1989). Reality negotiation: From excuses to hope and beyond. *Journal of Social and Clinical Psychology, 8,* 130-157.

Snyder, C.R., Rand, K.L., and Sigmon, D.R. (2002). Hope theory: A member of the positive psychology family. In C.R. Snyder and S.J. Lopez (Eds.), *Handbook of positive psychology* (pp. 257-276). London: Oxford University Press.

Snyder, C.R., Sympson, S.C., Ybasco, F.C., Borders, T.F., Babyak, M.A., and Higgins, R. L. (1996). Development and validation of the State Hope Scale. *Journal of Personality and Social Psychology, 70*(2), 321-335.

Solaro, C., Brichetto, G., Amato, M.P., Cocco, E., Colombo, B., D'Aleo, G., et al. (2004). The prevalence of pain in multiple sclerosis: A multicenter cross-sectional study. *Neurology, 63*(5), 919-921.

Sperry, L. (1999). *Cognitive behavior therapy of DSM-IV personality disorders: Highly effective interventions for the most common personality disorders.* New York: Brunner-Routledge.

Stanton, A.L., Danoff-Burg, S., Cameron, C.L., et al. (2000a). Emotionally expressive coping predicts psychological and physical adjustment to breast cancer. *Journal of Consulting and Clinical Psychology, 68,* 875-882.

Stanton, A.L., Kirk, S.B., Cameron, C.L., et al. (2000b). Coping through emotional approach: Scale construction and validation. *Health Psychology, 12,* 16-23.

Steel, R.K., Musliner, M.C., and Boling, P.A. (1995). Home care in the urban setting–a challenge to medical education. *Bulletin of the New York Academy of Medicine, 72*(1), 87-94.

Steer, S., Jones, H., Hibbert, J., Kondeatis, E., Vaughan, R., Sanderson, J., et al. (2003). Low back pain, sacroiliitis, and the relationship with HLA-B27 in Crohn's disease. *Journal of Rheumatology, 30*(3), 518-522.

Stone, P., Richardson, A., Ream, E., Smith, A.G., Kerr, D.J., and Kearney, N. (2000). Cancer-related fatigue: Inevitable, unimportant and untreatable? Results of a multicentre patient survey. Cancer Fatigue Forum. *Annals of Oncology, 11*(8), 971-975.

Strowig, S.M., Aviles-Santa, M.L., and Raskin, P. (2002). Comparison of insulin monotherapy and combination therapy with insulin and metform or insulin and troglitazone in type 2 diabetes. *Diabetes Care, 25*(10), 1691-1698.

Stucky, C., Gold, M., and Zhang, X. (2001). Mechanisms of pain. Proceedings of a National Academy of Sciences of the United States of America, 98, 11845-11846

Sullivan, P., and Dowrkin, M. (2003). Prevalence and correlates of fatigue among persons with HIV infection. *Journal of Pain and Symptoms Management, 25*(4), 329-333.

Surveillance, Epidemiology, and End Results (SEER): Program of the National Cancer Institute. (2001). Bethesda, MD (January 1, 2001); Retrieved July 16, 2004, from *http://seer.cancer.gov/faststats/html/pre_all.html*

Sweetwood, H. Grant, I., Kripke, D.F., Gerst, M.S., and Yager, J. (1980). Sleep disorder over time: Psychiatric correlates among males. *British Journal of Psychiatry, 136,* 456-462.

Taft, C.T., Murphy, C.M., Musser, P.H., and Remington, N.A. (2004). Personality, interpersonal, and motivational predictors of the working alliance in group cognitive-behavioral therapy for partner violent men. *Journal of Consulting and Clinical Psychology, 72*(2), 349-354.

Taibi, D., Bourguignon, C., and Taylor, A. (2004). Valerian use for sleep disturbances related to rheumatoid arthritis. *Holistic Nursing Practice, 18*(3), 120-126.

Tan, T.L., Kales, J.D., Kales, A., Soldator, C.R., and Bixler, E.O. (1984) biopsychobehavioral correlates of insomnia: IV. Diagnosis based on DSM-III *American Journal of Psychiatry*, 141, 357-362.

Taylor, J.D., Feldman, D.B., Saunders, R.S., and Ilardi, S.S. (2000a). Hope theory and cognitive behavioral therapies. In C.R. Snyder (ed.), *Handbook of hope: Theory, measures, and applications* (pp. 109-122). San Diego, CA: Academic Press.

Taylor, R.R., Friedberg, F., and Jason, L.A. (2001). *A clinician's guide to controversial illnesses: Chronic fatigue syndrome, fibromyalgia, and multiple chemical sensitivities.* Sarasota, FL: Professional Resource Press.

Taylor, S.E. (1983). Adjustment to threatening events: A theory of cognitive adaptation. *American Psychologist, 38*, 1161-1173.

Taylor, S.E., and Aspinwall, L.G. (1990). Psychosocial aspects of chronic illness. In P.T. Costa and G.R. Vanden Bos (eds.), (1996), *Psychological aspects of serious illness: Chronic conditions, fatal diseases, and clinical care. Master lectures in psychology* (pp. 3-60). Washington, DC: American Psychological Association.

Taylor, S.E., Kemeny, M.E., Reed, G.M., Bower, J.E., and Gruenewald, T, L. (2000b). Psychological resources, positive illusions, and health. *American Psychologist, 55*(1), 99-109.

Taylor, S.E., Lichtman, R., and Wood, J. (1984). Attributions, beliefs about control, and adjustment to breast cancer. *Journal of Personality and Social Psychology, 46*, 489-471.

Tengrup, I., Tennvall-Nittby, L., Christiansson, I., and Laurin, M. (2000). Arm morbidity after breast-conserving therapy for breast cancer. *Acta Oncologica, 39*(3), 393-397.

Tennen, H., Affleck, G., Urrows, S., Higgins, P., and Mendola, R. (1992). Perceiving control, construing benefits, and daily processes in rheumatoid arthritis. *Canadian Journal of Behavioral Science, 24*, 186-203.

The Cleveland Clinic. (2003). Cleveland, OH (November, 2003); Retrieved October 19, 2004, from *http://my.webmd.com/content/article/59/66840?printing=true*

Theander, K., and Unosson, M. (2004). Fatigue in patients with chronic obstructive pulmonary disease. *Journal of Advanced Nursing, 45*(2), 172-177.

Thompson, S.C. (1985). Finding positive meaning in a stressful event and coping. *Basic and Applied Social Psychology, 6*, 279-295.

Thomson Healthcare. (2004). No location available (No revision date available); PDRhealth. Retrieved December 2, 2004, from www.pdrhealth.com

Tollison, C. (1993) The magnitude of the pain problem: The problem in perspective. In R. Weiner (ed.), *Innovations in pain management: A practical guide for clinicians* (vol. 1) (pp. 3-9). Orlando, FL: Paul M. Deutsch Press.

Tomich, P.L., and Helgeson, V.S. (2002). Five years later: A cross-sectional comparison of breast cancer survivors with healthy women. *Psycho-Oncology, 11*, 154-169.

Tomich, P.L., and Helgeson, V.S. (2004). Is finding something good in the bad always good? Benefit finding among women with breast cancer. *Health Psychology, 23*, 16-23.

Thyroid Foundation of America. (2004). Boston (August 8, 2004). *Thyroid disorders and treatments: Thyroid related disorders.* Retrieved October 14, 2004, from *http://www.tsh.org/disorders/related/arthritis.html*

Tjemsland, L., Soreide, J.A., Matre, R., and Malt, U.F. (1997). Properative psychological variables predict immunological status in patients with operable breast cancer. *Psycho-Oncology, 6*, 311-320.

Trivalle, C., Doucet, J., Chassagne, P., Landrin, I., Kadri, N., Menard, J., et al. (1996). Differences in the signs and symptoms of hyperthyroidism in older and younger patients. *Journal of the American Geriatrics Society, 44*(1), 50-53.

Tsay, S. (2003). Acupressure and fatigue in patients with end-stage renal disease: a randomized controlled trial. *International Journal of Nursing Studies, 41*, 99-106.

Turk, D.C. (2002) A diathesis-stress model of chronic pain and disability following traumatic injury. *Pain Research and Management, 7*, 9-10.

Turk, D.C. and Flor, H. (1999) The biobehavioral perspective of pain. In R.J. Gatchel and D.C. Turk (eds.) *Psychosocial factors in pain: Clinical perspectives* (pp. 18-34). New York: Guilford Press.

Turk, D.C., and Salovey, P. (1995). Cognitive-behavioral treatment of illness behavior. In P.M. Nicassio and T.W. Smith (eds.), *Managing chronic illness: A biopsychosocial perspective* (pp. 245-284). Washington, DC: American Psychological Association.

Turk, D.C., Meichenbaum, D., and Genest, M. (1983). Pain and behavioral medicine: A cognitive behavioral perspective. New York: Guilford Press.

Turkat, I.D., and Brantley, P.J. (1981). On the therapeutic relationship in behavior therapy. *The Behavior Therapist, 47*, 16-17.

Turvey, C.L., Schultz, K., Arndt, S., Wallace, R.B., and Herzog, R. (2002). Prevalence and correlates of depressive symptoms in a community sample of people suffering from heart failure. *Journal of the American Geriatrics Society, 50*, 2003-2008.

University of Alabama at Birmingham (UAB). (2004). No location available (No revision date available); UAB health system. Retrieved December 2, 2004, from www.health.uab.edu

University of Chicago. (n.d.) Chicago; *Crohn's disease*. Retrieved September 23, 2004, from *http://gi.bsd.uchicago.edu/diseases/inflambowel/crohns.html*

Updegraff, J.A., Taylor, S.E., Kemeny, M.E., and Wyatt, G.E. (2002). Positive and negative effects of HIV infection in women with low socioeconomic resources. *Personality and Social Psychology Bulletin, 28*, 382-394.

U.S. Department of Health and Human Services (USDHHS). (1996). *Physical activity and health: A report of the surgeon general*. Atlanta, GA: Centers for Disease Control and Prevention, National Center for Chronic Disease Prevention and Health Promotion.

U.S. Department of Health and Human Services, AIDS info. (2004). Rockville, MD (October 29, 2004); *Guidelines for the Use of Antiretroviral Agents in HIV Infected Adults and Adolescents*. Retrieved October 21, 2004, from *http://www.aidsinfo.nih.gov/guidelines/default_db2.asp?id=50*

U.S. National Library of Medicine, National Institutes of Health. (1999). Bethesda, MD (October, 2004); *Drug Information*. Retrieved October 25, 2004, from *http://www.nlm.nih.gov/medlineplus/druginfo/uspdi/202194.html#SXX19*

U.S. National Library of Medicine (NLM), National Institutes of Health. (2003). Bethesda, MD (June 12, 2003); MedlinePlus medical encylcopedia: Diabetes. Retrieved December 2, 2004, from *http://www.nlm.nih.gov/medlineplus/ency/article/001214.htm*

U.S. National Library of Medicine, National Institutes of Health. (2000). Bethesda, MD (September, 2004); *American Accreditation HealthCare Commission (A.D.A.M.), Medical Encyclopedia: Cholelithiasis*. Retrieved October 7, 2004, from *http://www.nlm.nih.gov/medlineplus/ency/imagepages/17039.htm*

U.S. National Library of Medicine (NLM), National Institutes of Health. (2004). Bethesda, MD (September 28, 2004); MedlinePlus medical encylcopedia: Mononucleosis. Retrieved October 6, 2004, from *http://www.nlm.nih.gov/medlineplus/ency/article/ 000591.htm#Alternative%20Names*

van der Naalt, J., van Zomeren, A., Sluiter, W., and Minderhoud, J. (1999). One year outcome in mild to moderate head injury: The predictive value of acute injury characteristics related to complaints and return to work. *Journal of Neurology, Neurosurgery, and Psychiatry, 66*(2), 207-213.

Vlaeyen, J.W.S., and Linton, S.J. (2000). Fear-avoidance and its consequences in chronic musculoskeletal pain: A state of the art. *Pain, 85,* 317-332.

Vignola, A., Lamoreaux, C., Bastien, C.H., and Morin, C.M., (2000) Effects of chronic insomnia and use of benzodiazepines on daytime performance in older adults. *Journal of Gerontology, 55,* P54-P63.

Volicer, L., Harper, D., Manning, B., Goldstein, R., and Satlin, A. (2001). Sundowning and circadian rhythms in Alzheimer's Disease. *The American Journal of Psychiatry, 158*(5), 704-711.

Waddell, G. (1987). A new clinical model for the treatment of low back pain. *Spine, 12,* 632-644.

Waddell, G. (1991). Low back disability. A syndrome of Western civilization. *Neurosurgery Clinics of North America, 2,* 719-738.

Waddell, G. (1992) Biopsychosocial analysis of low back pain. *Clinical Rheumatology, 6,* 523-557.

Wanklyn, P., Forster, A., and Young, J. (1996). Hemiplegic shoulder pain (HSP): Natural history and investigation of associated features. *Disability and Rehabilitation, 18*(10), 497-501.

Ward, N., and Winters, S. (2003). Results of a fatigue management programme in multiple sclerosis. *British Journal of Nursing, 12*(18), 1075-1080.

Weijman, I., Ros, W., Rutten, G., Schaufeli, W., Schabracq, M., and Winnubst, J. (2003). Fatigue in employees with diabetes: Its relation with work characteristics and diabetes related burden. *Occupational and Environmental Medicine, 60*(1), i93-i98.

Weinberger, J., and McClelland, D.C. (1990). Cognitive versus traditional motivational models: Irreconcilable or complementary? In E.T. Higgins and R.M. Sorrentino (eds.), *Handbook of motivation and cognition: Foundations of social behavior* (pp. 562-597). New York: Guilford Press.

Weisberg, J., and Keefe, F. (1999). Personality, individual differences, and psychopathology in chronic pain. In R. Gatchel and D. Turk (eds.), *Psychosocial factors in pain. Critical perspectives.* (pp. 56-73). New York: Guilford Press.

Weishaar, M.E. (1996). Cognitive risk factors in suicide. In P.M. Salkovskis (ed.), *Frontiers of cognitive therapy* (pp. 226-249). New York: Guilford Press.

Weissman, A.N., and Beck, A.T. (1978). *Development and validation of the Dysfunctional Attitude Scale: A preliminary investigation.* Paper presented at the annual meeting of the American Educational Research Association, Toronto.

Wells, A. (2000). *Emotional disorders and metacognition. Innovative cognitive therapy.* Chichester: John Wiley and Sons.

Wells, N. (2000). Pain intensity and pain interference in hospitalized patients with cancer. *Oncology Nursing Forum, 27*(6), 985-991.

Wendell, S. (1996). *The rejected body: Feminist philosophical reflections on disability.* NY and London: Routledge.

Wheeler, A.H., Stubbart, J.R., and Hicks, B. (2004). Charlotte, NC (October 14, 2004); *Pathophysiology of chronic back pain.* Retrieved October 19, 2004, from *http://www.emedicine.com/neuro/topic516.htm*

White, C.A. (2001). *Cognitive behavior therapy for chronic medical problems: A guide to assessment and treatment in practice.* Chichester, England: John Wiley and Sons.

White, P.D., Thomas, J.M., Kangro, H.O., Bruce-Jones, W.D., Amess, J., Crawford, D.H., et al. (2001). Predictions and associations of fatigue syndromes and mood disorders that occur after infectious mononucleosis. *Lancet, 358,* 1946-1954.

White, R.W. (1959). Motivation reconsidered: The concept of competence. *Psychological Review, 66,* 297-333.

Wider, M., Ahlstrom, G., and Ek, A.C. (2004). Health-related quality of life in persons with long-term pain after a stroke. *Journal of Clinical Nursing, 13*(4), 497-505.

Winterowd, C., Beck, A.T. and Gruener, D. (2003). *Cognitive Therapy with Chronic Pain Patients.* New York: Springer.

Wiesel, P.H., Norton, C., Glickman, S., and Kamm, M.A. (2001). Pathophysiology and management of bowel dysfunction in multiple sclerosis. *European Journal of Gastroenterology and Hepatology, 13,* 441-448.

Williams, H. (2002). North Yorkshire, United Kingdom. *Encephalitis and fatigue.* Retrieved September 20, 2004, from *http://www.encephalitis.info/the_illness/Possible%20Outcomes/Fat.htm*

Williams, R.L., (1988) Sleep disturbances in vartious medical and surgical conditions. In R.L. Williams, I. Karacan and C.A. Moore (eds.), *Sleep disorders: Diagnosis and treatment* (pp. 265-291). New York: Wiley.

Wilson, G.T. (1987). Clinical issues and strategies in the practice of behavior therapy. In G.T. Wilson, C.M. Franks, P.C. Kendall, and J.P. Foreyt (eds.), *Review of behavior therapy: Theory and practice* (Vol. 11, pp. 288-317). New York: Guilford Press.

Witt, J., and Murray-Edwards, D. (2002). Living with fatigue: Managing cancer-related fatigue at home and in the workplace. *American Journal of Nursing,* 28-31.

Witte, K., Desilva, R., Chattopadhyay, S., Ghosh, J., Cleland, J., and Clark, A. (2004). Are hemantinic deficiencies the cause of anemia in chronic heart failure? *American Heart Journal, 147*(5), 924-930.

Wolf, E.S. (1988). *Treating the Self.* New York: Guilford.

Wolfe, F., Hawley, D.J., and Wilson, K. (1996). The prevalence and meaning of fatigue in rheumatic disease. *Journal of Rheumatology, 23*(8), 1407-1417.

Wolfe, F., Ross, K., Anderson, J., Russell, I.J., and Hebert, L. (1995). The prevalence and characteristics of fibromyalgia in the general population. *Arthritis and Rheumatism, 38*(1), 19-28.

Wolfe, G. (1999). Fatigue: Fatigue in patients with HIV /AIDS. *The Journal of Care Management, 3*(1), 8-11.

Wooten, V. (1989). Medical causes of insomnia. In M.H. Kryger, T. Roth, and W.C. Dement (eds.), *Principles and practice of sleep medicine,* (pp. 465-475) Philadelphia: Saunders

Wrongdiagnosis.com. (2003). *Complications of hepatitis.* Retrieved October 4, 2004, from *http://www.wrongdiagnosis.com/h/hepatitis/complic.htm*

Yalom, I.D. (1980). *Existential psychotherapy.* New York: Basic Books.

Zeiss, A.M., Lewinsohn, P.M., Munos, R.F. (1979). Nonspecific improvement effects in depression using interpersonal skills training, pleasant activity schedules, or cognitive training. *Journal of Consulting and Clinical Psychology, 47,* 427-439.

Zonderman, J. and Vender, R.S. (2000). *Understanding Crohn disease and ulcerative colitis.* Jackson: University Press of Mississippi.

Index